Nutraceuticals

Nutraceuticals

A guide for healthcare professionals

Second edition

Brian Lockwood

BPharm, PhD, MRPharmS

Senior Lecturer in Pharmacy,
School of Pharmacy and Pharmaceutical Sciences,
University of Manchester,
Manchester, UK

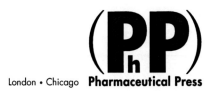

London • Chicago   **Pharmaceutical Press**

Published by Pharmaceutical Press

1 Lambeth High Street, London SE1 7JN, UK
1559 St. Paul Avenue, Gurnee, IL 60031, USA

© Pharmaceutical Press 2007

(PP) is a trade mark of Pharmaceutical Press
Pharmaceutical Press is the publishing division of the Royal
Pharmaceutical Society of Great Britain

First edition published 2002
Second edition published 2007

Typeset by Type Study, Scarborough, North Yorkshire

ISBN 978 0 85369 659 9

A catalogue record for this book is available from the British Library

To my father Thomas George Lockwood MRPharmS (deceased) who retired from the register after 60 years, and died just before completion of the book. He had a great interest in scientific and literary knowledge, and worked prodigiously on both pharmaceutical and non-pharmaceutical matters for the good of others.

Contents

Preface

This book was written in response to the obvious need for a scientifically based text on the evidence for the use of nutraceuticals for the prevention and treatment of important disease states. The use of nutraceuticals is by now an established complementary therapy, with a few being used as if they were conventional pharmaceuticals, and a number of others being purchased and used by the general public as self-medication. Although nutraceuticals are constantly discussed in the media and freely available, comprehensive knowledge concerning their activities, mode of action and safety is not yet widely available. The main aim of this book was, therefore, to explore, discuss and possibly substantiate claims that a number of nutraceuticals can actually treat or prevent the underlying causes of disease.

Consumers clearly hope that they will benefit from intake of these products either through long-term use or via a conscious decision to change lifestyle. That is why I have decided here, unlike a number of other books on the subject, to organise the information according to disease states. In addition, any evidence quoted should be of understandable quality. The inclusion of directly attributable information sources was considered vital for this, producing a usable text for both patient, consumer and healthcare practitioners wanting to find further details by checking the original publications. Wherever possible, I have tried to focus on clinical and human research, although results from animal studies are included, particularly for the chapter on animal health, but also when there are major findings or there are insufficient human data.

Previous books have either focused on the individual chemical entities and their applications, or consist of information in therapeutic areas which is not directly attributed to published data, hence not allowing easy access to original material. In contrast, this text aims to cover a wide range of nutraceuticals, specifically focusing on their use in specific therapeutic categories. Although the book was designed as a text to inform readers as to the claimed benefits of specific nutraceuticals in various therapeutic contexts, it was still thought necessary to include monographs on individual compounds. This gives us the opportunity to describe their properties and to define the characteristics that are often important in a number of disease states, either due to a particular activity that results in applications in more than one therapeutic area, or because they possess a number of attributes with wide-ranging applications. The monographs include information on biological sources, which are important for those wishing to supplement their diets with specific foods containing nutraceuticals, manufacturing and analytical details, metabolism, bioavailability and pharmacokinetics. Much of this information has been compiled into tables to allow easy comparison between the entities discussed.

The major change in this text with respect to the previous book is the inclusion of soy and tea. Over the last 10–20 years a body of scientific and medical literature has been published concerning the proposed health benefits of soy and tea products. This weight of evidence, still increasing annually, has determined that any text on the subject of nutraceuticals takes into account commercially available products from these two sources. At the time of writing (2006) it can be said that roughly 20–30% of all studies and reviews on nutraceuticals are derived from these two supplements.

In addition to the growth in evidence for these two supplements, there is now also more evidence concerning, for example, flax lignans and resveratrol, which justifiably warrants their inclusion in any relevant text. Looking to the future, we can also see more evidence being published on minor or new nutraceuticals, such as theanine and NADH, which have been the subject of clinical trials.

Since 2002 there has been rapid expansion of publications in the overall area of nutraceuticals, and this book attempts to reflect this new material, particularly in reporting more detailed pharmacological profiling of the nutraceuticals. Chapters on a number of pertinent aspects of nutraceutical use have been included, apart from their applications in specific therapeutic categories, namely combination therapy and synergy, safety, adverse effects and quality issues, along with a section on minor nutraceuticals.

Increasing evidence that health is related to diet have resulted in a range of government initiatives designed to encourage healthy eating, and positive steps are being taken by an increasing number of individuals. However, for many people living in an increasingly sophisticated world, supplementation with formulated nutraceuticals is a more realistic solution than making major modifications to the diet.

It is hoped that this work will be useful to pharmacists, medical practitioners and nursing staff, as well as respective students. A chapter on veterinary nutraceuticals specifies particular applications for domesticated animals, but many of the included human nutraceuticals are now also being used for animals.

Most information is summarised to allow readers to refer to data on the large number of nutraceuticals currently available; some are the subject of vast numbers of clinical trials and scientific publications, while others have only been described in limited published data. Some of the information has been published recently in peer-reviewed articles (for example in *Nutrition* or the *Pharmaceutical Journal* and business-related science journals) along with chapters in books, and a chapter in the *Encyclopedia of Pharmaceutical Technology*. These publications were often in association with co-authors, and are referenced in relevant sections. Over the last 3–4 years numerous publications have appeared on the subject of nutraceuticals, and it has been an ongoing task to keep updating sections in this book, with references up to mid-2006 being incorporated. Inevitably a number of articles will have been superseded by more up-to-date studies during the publication process.

Brian Lockwood
January 2007

Acknowledgements

I wish to thank the John Rylands University Library of Manchester for exceptional staff, answering all my enquiries, no matter how many, always correctly, and supplying all required documents with a smile!

I also thank all the co-authors of previously published relevant material, and my (ex)postgraduate students Kenza and Proramate, technicians Ann and Karen for continual help with computing problems, and many of the staff of the School of Pharmacy and Pharmaceutical Sciences, University of Manchester for useful discussions, and for helping in numerous other ways.

Some of the material in this text has been modified from articles published in the *Pharmaceutical Journal*, however, the majority has either not been previously published, or is completely rewritten from articles or book chapters published elsewhere, which are referred to in the text.

About the author

Brian Lockwood is a practising academic pharmacist, who has lectured widely on plant and complementary medicines, both nationally and internationally. He is author and co-author of a number of books, book and encyclopoedia chapters, and articles in scientific and professional journals on the subject of nutraceuticals. He has taught in Manchester for 26 years, and also spent a number of months and years in a further eight Schools of Pharmacy, dealing with most aspects of plant medicines.

Abbreviations

ACE	angiotensin-converting enzyme
ADAS-Cog	Alzheimer Disease Assessment Scale, Cognitive Section
ADP	adenosine diphosphate
AHR	airway hyperresponsiveness
ALA	α-linolenic acid
AMD	age-related macular degeneration
AO	antioxidant
AOAC	Association of Official Analytical Chemists
ARM	age-related maculopathy
ATP	adenosine triphosphate
AUC	area under the curve (blood concentration-time profile)
AUC_∞	maximum AUC at ∞
BMC	bone mineral content
BMD	bone mineral density
BMU	bone multicellular units
BSE	bovine spongiform encephalitis
CAM	complementary and alternative medicine
CE	capillary electrophoresis
CFA	cetylated fatty acid
CFS	chronic fatigue syndrome
CGI	Clinical Global Impression
CHD	coronary heart disease
CHF	congestive heart failure
CLA	conjugated linoleic acid
C_{max}	maximum concentration (blood concentration-time profile)
CDS	cognitive dysfunction syndrome
CMO	cetyl myristoleate
CoA	coenzyme A
COMT	catechol-O-methyl transferase
COPD	chronic obstructive pulmonary disease
Co Q10	coenzyme Q10
COX	cyclooxygenase

CSM	Committee on Safety of Medicines
CVD	cardiovascular disease
CVI	chronic venous insufficiency
CVS	cardiovascular system
CYP	cytochrome P
Defra	Department for Environment, Food and Rural Affairs
DGLA	dihomo γ-linolenic acid
DHA	docosahexaenoic acid
DHEA	dehydroepiandrosterone
DHEAS	dehydroepiandrosterone sulfate
DHLA	dihydrolipoic acid
DHT	5α-dihydrotestosterone
DMS	dimethyl sulfide
DMSO	dimethyl sulfoxide
$DMSO_2$	dimethyl sulfone
DNA	deoxyribonucleic acid
DSHEA	Dietary Supplement Health and Education Act
DVT	deep vein thrombosis
EC_{50}	50% effective dose
ECG	epicatechin gallate
EGC	epigallocatechin
EGCG	epigallocatechin gallate
EGF	epidermal growth factor
EIA	exercise-induced asthma
EPA	eicosapentaenoic acid
ER	oestrogen receptor
ERE	oestrogen response element
$ES_{all\ scales}$	integrated summary of clinical tests
FAO	Food and Agriculture Organization of the UN
FDA	Food and Drug Administration
FEV_1	forced expiratory volume per second
FIM	Foundation for Innovation in Medicine
FMD	flow-mediated dilation
FOSHU	Foods for Specified Health Use
FSA	Food Standards Agency (UK)
FVC	forced vital capacity
GAG	glycosaminoglycan
GAIT	glucosamine/chondroitin arthritis intervention trial
GCG	gallocatechin gallate
GH	growth hormone
GI	glycaemic index

GLA	γ-linolenic acid
GRAS	Generally Recognized as Safe
GSPE	grape seed proanthocyanidin extract
GT-ase	glucosyltransferase
HDL-C	high-density lipoprotein–cholesterol
5-HETE	5-hydroxyeicosatetraenoic acid
HMG-CoA	hydroxymethyl glutaryl CoA
HPLC	high-performance liquid chromatography
HRT	hormone replacement therapy
IgA	immunoglobulin A
IGF	insulin-like growth factor
IL	interleukin
IMT	intima media thickness
JHCI	Joint Health Claims Initiative
LA	linoleic acid
LD_{50}	lethal dose for 50%
LDL	Low-density lipoprotein
LDL-C	Low-density lipoprotein–cholesterol
LH	luteinising hormone
LI	Lequesne Index
LMWCS	low molecular weight chondroitin sulfate
LOX	lipoxygenase
LT	leukotriene
LTB4	leukotriene B4
LTB5	leukotriene B5
MAO	monoamine oxidase
MHRA	Medical and Healthcare Products Agency
MI	mycocardial infarction
MMSE	Mini-Mental State Examination
MRP	multi-drug resistance protein
MS	mass spectrometry
MSM	methylsulfonylmethane
NADH	reduced form of nicotinamide adenine dinucleotide
NF-κB	nuclear factor-κB
NGF	nerve growth factor
NHS	National Health Service (UK)
NIDDM	non-insulin-dependent diabetes mellitus
NIH	National Institutes of Health (US)
NNK	4-(methylnitrosamine)-1-(3-pyridyl)-1-butanone
NO	nitric oxide
NREA	Nutraceutical Research and Education Act

NSAID	non-steroidal anti-inflammatory drug
OA	osteoarthritis
8-OHdG	8-hydroxyguanosine
8OHdG/dG	8-hydroxydeoxyguanosine/deoxyguanosine
6-OHMS	6-hydroxymelatonin sulfate
OKG	ornithine ketoglutarate
OPG	osteoprotegerin
ORAC	oxygen radical absorbance capacity
OVX	ovariectomised
PCB	polychlorinated biphenyls
PEF	peak expiratory flow
PG	prostaglandin
PGE1	prostaglandin E1
PGE2	prostaglandin E2
PGE3	prostaglandin E3
PGH2	prostaglandin H2
PS	phosphatidylserine
PKC	protein kinase C
PMN	polymorphonuclear neutrophils
POM	prescription-only medicine (UK)
PPAR α	peroxisome proliferator-activated receptor α
PS	phosphatidylserine
PTH	parathyroid hormone
PTK	protein tyrosine kinase
PUFA	polysaturated fatty acid
RA	rheumatoid arthritis
RANK	receptor activator of nuclear factor-kappa
RNA	ribonucleic acid
ROS	reactive oxygen species
SAD	seasonal affective disorder
SAMe	S-adenosyl methionine
SAR	seasonal allergic rhinitis
SDG	secoisolariciresinol-diglycoside
SHBG	sex hormone-binding globulin
6-SMT	6-sulfatoxymelatonin
SOD	superoxide dismutase
SPE	solid phase extraction
$t_{\frac{1}{2}}$	half-life
t_{max}	time of C_{max}
TNFα	tumour necrosis factor alpha
UV	ultraviolet

VCAM-1	vascular cell adhesion molecule-1
VLDL	very low-density lipoprotein
VLDL-C	very low-density lipoprotein–cholesterol
VO$_2$ max	maximal oxygen uptake
WHO	World Health Organization
WOMAC	Western Ontario and McMaster Universities OA Index

1

Introduction

Over the last 20 years the number of nutraceuticals available for self-medication in pharmacies or for sale in supermarkets and healthfood shops has grown enormously, fostered by wide media coverage of their benefits.[1] There has been a boom in their sales as patients rush to self-medicate, either in the hope that these products will be effective in treating diseases unsatisfactorily treated with pharmaceuticals, or that the adverse effects of some pharmaceuticals may be avoided. With an ageing population throughout the Western world, a number of diseases are becoming increasingly prevalent, and current and predicted patient numbers are often vast. For example, it has been predicted that arthritis will affect most of the population at some time during their lifetime. And it is in disease states such as arthritis that nutraceuticals are increasingly used.

This text will outline the major nutraceuticals with therapeutic applications in a number of important therapeutic areas. The pharmaceutically important issues, adverse reactions and drug interactions, and the quality of available nutraceuticals are now being addressed, as evidence is now becoming available.

Foods or medicines? The relationship between nutraceuticals, foods and medicines

'Nutraceutical' is the term used to describe a medicinal or nutritional component that includes a food, plant or naturally occurring material, which may have been purified or concentrated, and that is used for the improvement of health, by preventing or treating a disease. It is often thought that nutraceuticals have to occupy a narrow strip of legislative ground between pharmaceuticals and food, but in reality their position is much more complex.

Figure 1.1 shows the inter-relationship between nutraceuticals and other health products. This relationship is confused due to the overlap between the various entities, in terms of legal status, origins, marketing

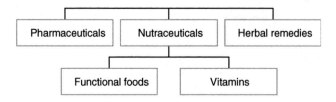

Figure 1.1 The relationship between nutraceuticals and other health products.

and public perception. Pharmaceuticals are usually classed as medicines by law, but some are freely available without legal constraints and some are legally classed as medicines. For example, in certain countries melatonin is classed as a medicine and is not freely available. Most nutraceuticals, however, are openly on sale and available via the Internet.

Herbal remedies may be classed as medicines because of their perceived risks with self-medication. For example, plants containing potent pharmacological entities such as digitalis are classed as medicines. Functional foods are closely related to nutraceuticals as they often contain nutraceuticals in a food-based formulation, such as carotenoids, but others are novel biotechnological entities derived from foods, for instance, pre- and probiotics. A new term for these has recently been coined – 'Phoods' – which presumably aims to blur the distinction between pharmaceuticals and foods in the minds of consumers.[2] Further new terms to attract consumers include cosmeceuticals and aquaceuticals, which aim to convey pharmaceutical activity and quality in the areas of cosmetics and soft drinks, respectively. Vitamins can also be classed as medicines, but may be freely available. The distinction between certain vitamins and nutraceuticals is blurred (e.g. β-carotene, which is a vitamin A precursor). Many nutraceuticals are derived from plants or foods and marketing usually follows legal status, medicines and non-medicines being clearly separate. Public perception may involve little distinction between any of these entities, except when legal status affects availability. Most people are guided by the marketing: nutraceuticals usually appear to be packaged and labelled as if they were medicines.

Many terms and definitions are used in different countries and this can become quite confusing. Dr Stephen De Felice, the founder and chairman of the Foundation for Innovation in Medicine (Cranford, NJ, USA), an educational organisation set up in 1976 to encourage medical health research, coined the term 'nutraceutical'.[3] De Felice defined a 'nutraceutical' as a 'food, or parts of a food, that provide medical or health benefits, including the prevention and treatment of disease'.

Another definition from the USA is 'diet supplement that delivers a concentrated form of a presumed bioactive agent from a food, presented in a non-food matrix, and used to enhance health in dosages that exceed those that could be obtained from normal food'.[4]

A 'functional food' is a natural or formulated food that has enhanced physiological performance or prevents or treats a particular disease. This term was first used in Japan, and by 1998 it was the only country to legally define 'Foods for specified health use' (FOSHU). Functional foods consist of food- and drink-based formulations, as opposed to tablets and capsules, etc. Often these products contain established nutraceuticals and are recommended for the same range of therapeutic categories as the nutraceuticals contained therein.

In Canada, a functional food has been defined as 'similar in appearance to conventional foods, . . . consumed as part of a usual diet', whereas a nutraceutical is 'a product produced from foods but sold in pills, powders, (potions) and other medicinal forms not generally associated with food'.[5]

In the UK the Department for Environment, Food and Rural Affairs (Defra) defines a functional food as a 'food that has a component incorporated into it to give it a specific medical or physiological benefit, other than purely nutritional benefit'.[6]

Thus both in Canada and in Britain a functional food is essentially a food, and a nutraceutical is an isolated or concentrated form. In the USA, however, 'medical foods' and 'dietary supplements' are regulatory terms (see below), and 'nutraceuticals', 'functional foods', and other such terms are determined by consultants and marketers, based on consumer trends.[7]

In many countries food labelling regulations do not allow food labels to carry health claims. In the UK, the Joint Health Claims Initiative (JHCI) provides guidance on claims that are allowed for functional foods, such as fortified breakfast cereals and 'bio'-yoghurts. In some cases although *medical* claims such as 'helps prevent heart disease' are not allowed, *health promoting* claims, such as 'helps lower cholesterol' can be made, if scientific evidence exists. Inevitably many inaccurate claims are made for supplements and the consumer research provider Mintel found that most British consumers were sceptical about health claims and found them misleading.[8]

Companies marketing nutraceuticals cannot advertise specific medical claims for their products without a medicine licence. When launching a new product they have the option of either not doing any research at all or researching it thoroughly and possibly obtaining a patent. Unfortunately many companies tend towards the former route because of the expense, the problems of obtaining a patent on a natural product and the fact that even if they do the research they cannot put their claims on the label without a product licence. To bring a medicine to market can take about ten years and cost US$0.8–1.7 billion,[9] but to market an unlicensed nutraceutical can take a fraction of this time and money. Look at, for example, the case of Cholestin, a cholesterol-lowering supplement marketed by Pharmanex in 1996. This product was made from red yeast rice, a food that has been used for centuries in China. The red yeast rice is made by a natural fermentation process, which generates multiple statins and provides the cholesterol-lowering benefit. When the pharmaceutical company Merck tested this supplement, they found that the active ingredient was lovastatin, a known cholesterol-lowering agent available on prescription, which is made from the isolation of one of these statins and included in their product Mevacor. In 1998, the US Food and Drug Administration (FDA) banned Pharmanex from importing red yeast rice for the manufacture of Cholestin on the grounds that one of the many beneficial constituents in red yeast rice is chemically identical to lovastatin. However, in February 1999, a district court ruled that Cholestin was indeed a dietary supplement, based on the US Dietary Supplement Health and Education Act of 1994[10] and Cholestin remains available. As can be seen from this example the difference between pharmaceuticals and nutraceuticals is sometimes difficult to define, depending only on regulatory issues.

Depending on issues such as claims, presentation and dosage, a particular substance could be a food or a medicine. There are also a vast number of products in a borderline area.[11] These substances probably include many nutraceuticals and need to be classified as medicines, foods or in some other category. In the UK, unlicensed supplements are marketed without medical claims and as such are legally regarded as food supplements and are controlled by Defra. However, they can still be packaged to look like medicines, with a recommended dose, which can confuse the public. In the past, as long as the products did not claim to have medicinal uses, the Medicines and Healthcare Products Regulatory Agency (MHRA) – the body responsible for regulating medicinal products – has not required that such products should satisfy medical legislation.[12] However, more emphasis is now being placed on the *function* of the marketed products as the UK moves in line with the rest of Europe. Control of herbal products has now moved to the European Commission and it is likely that supplements will follow.

Article 1 of Directive 65/65 EEC[13] defines a medicinal product as 'any substance or combination of substances presented for treating, or preventing disease in human beings or animals' and 'any substance or combination of substances which may be administered to human beings or animal with a view to making diagnosis or to restoring, correcting or modifying physiological functions in human beings or animals is likewise considered a medicinal product'. The second definition describes a product which has a medical function irrespective of whether these claims have been stated or not, which would include many supplements being taken for medical purposes.

In Britain, medicines licensed for human use are regulated according to The Medicines Act 1968[14] and the Medicines for Human Use (Marketing Authorisations Etc.) Regulations 1994 SI3144 (The Regulations).[15] In 1995 these regulations came in to effect implementing all the controls as listed in Directive 65/65 EEC. According to these regulations there are controls over variation and renewal of UK licences as well as labelling and package inserts.

In the USA, a new product may be eligible for regulatory status as a food, a dietary supplement or as a medical food.[16] The US Congress passed the Dietary Supplement Health and Education Act (DSHEA) in 1994. This set up a new regulatory body for dietary supplements under the US FDA. Unlike foods, dietary supplements are allowed to use 'nutritional support statements'. These may offer nutritional support in nutrient-deficiency disease, or state a description of the intended role, mechanism of action or effect on general health as a result of taking the product. For those dietary supplements for which such a statement is used the label must also state: 'This statement has not been evaluated by the Food and Drug Administration. This product is not intended to diagnose, treat, cure or prevent any disease.'

In effect, because legally they are in a class by themselves, dietary supplements in the USA can be marketed without the FDA being satisfied that they are safe. This makes it relatively easy for a manufacturer to market a product without investing the time and money required for its safety.

The Foundation for the Innovation in Medicine (FIM) introduced the Nutraceutical Research & Education Act in Congress on 1 October 1999.[17] This Act promotes clinical research and development of dietary supplements, and foods with health benefits (nutraceuticals) to establish a new legal classification, and give exclusive rights to the company doing the research for a set time period.

Of all three categories (food, dietary supplement or medical food) medical foods have the fewest formal regulatory controls. US Congress

1990 defines a medical food as: 'a food which is formulated to be consumed or administered enterally under the supervision of a physician and which is intended for the specific dietary management of a disease or condition for which distinctive nutritional requirements, based on recognised scientific principles, are established by medical evaluation'.[16] These products are usually promoted through healthcare professionals including pharmacists, and in the UK this would make them 'prescription only' or 'pharmacy medicines'.

If the present restrictions on health claims were lifted, the market would probably be flooded with products that have no evidence for their claims. It is very unlikely that this will happen, but it has been suggested that a move from nutraceutical supplements being sold in healthfood shops and most pharmacies to the production of nutraceuticals aimed at the prescription market could occur. This would not necessarily be in the manufacturers' best interests, as it would limit the size of the market. In either case, whether prescribed by a doctor or self-selected, the logical place for the supply of these nutraceutical supplements is the pharmacy where pharmacists are able to offer professional advice.

The use of nutraceutical supplements – demographic trends

In a survey carried out by Mintel Market Research in November 1998,[18] 57% of 979 adults agreed that they would like to use supplements more often, but were unsure of what to buy. This indicated a need for more information to be available. The following year a market trend survey carried out by Mintel Market Research in March 1999[19] found that the prime target users of supplements were middle-aged females with an above average income and above average education. There were also occasional users who used supplements at a time of illness or stress, rather like a medicine. These users were more varied in age and income and were less likely to take supplements on a long-term basis.

In 2003, the Mintel Survey of Complementary Medicines in the UK found that 51% of consumers consulted their GP concerning complementary medicines, and 40% consulted their pharmacists. This trend was repeated in other European countries: 37% consulted with their pharmacists in Germany, 30% in France, and 15% in Spain. Consumers over 64 years old consulted with their GPs, but 25–44 year olds, particularly women with children, preferred to consult with their pharmacist. Interestingly, there was a greater proportion of people earning over €52 500 taking them 'once a day or more', than all lower income groups.[20] The Mintel Survey on Vitamins and Mineral Supplements – UK, which includes some nutraceuticals, found that 25% of all adults were 'convinced they were beneficial', and 86% of 55 year olds and over and 65% of 20–24 year olds took them 'once a day or more'. According to this survey the consumption of these products was greater among lower income groups than among higher income groups, but the biggest users were those with no children, not working, and the sole occupant of the household.[21]

Consumers use nutraceutical supplements for many varied reasons. These include supplementation of a poor diet, to improve overall health, to delay the onset of age-related diseases, after illness, for stress, recommended by a health professional, in pregnancy and slimming, to improve sports performance and to treat symptoms (colds, coughs, arthritis, etc.).

In the USA and in Europe the use of alternative or complementary medicines, including supplements and nutraceuticals, is increasing. Many theories have been put forward as to why consumers choose alternative over conventional remedies.[22] It is thought that many patients are not satisfied with the treatment they are given by their doctors due to adverse effects or because it has been ineffective. Another reason for choosing alternative over conventional remedies is that patients may feel that conventional medicine is impersonal or technologically orientated. Some patients prefer to have personal control over their healthcare and therefore are happier to self-select than be told what to take by their doctor.

A number of surveys have been published concerning the use of nutraceuticals by various sections of populations. One survey from 1988 to 1990, of a cohort of 2152 middle to older age adults living in Wisconsin found that the use of nutraceutical supplements was more prevalent among women, people with more than 12 years of education, those with relatively low body mass index, people with active lifestyles, and people who had never smoked rather than current smokers.[23] A similar study carried out in Japan on 45–74 year olds from 1995 to 1998 found that nutraceutical supplement users were likely to have never smoked or to have formerly smoked. Female users were likely to have been moderate consumers of alcohol. The prevalence of users was found to be higher among the elderly, the self-employed, those with lower body mass index, those carrying out greater physical activity, those with a lower frequency of eating ready-prepared food, those with a higher frequency of eating out, and those of both sexes with higher stress levels.[24]

Another US study carried out between 1993 and 1996 found that the use of nutraceutical supplementation was high amongst all ethnic groups, but use tended to increase with age, education, physical activity, fruit and dietary fibre intake, and to decrease with obesity, smoking and dietary fat intake. Overall, participants with healthy lifestyles were more likely to use these supplements.[25] Use of these supplements by young male (18–47 years) US Army Special Operations candidates was reported in 1999. Eighty-five per cent of them reported using a supplement, 64% reported current use and 35% reported daily use. Of these participants it was found that users were significantly less likely to smoke and were more likely to exercise daily.[26]

Another survey specifically targeting the elderly (65 years or older) in Piedmont County, North Carolina in 1996, found that users were more likely to be white women, were high school educated, were under-weight, took prescription medicines, had five or more health visits in the previous year, and had supplemental health insurance.[27]

Surveys have also been carried out concerning the use of specific nutraceuticals, notably creatine, cod liver oil and evening primrose oil. Creatine use amongst members of health clubs was found to be more likely in men using resistance training, and was associated with the consumption of dehydroepiandrosterone (DHEA) and other supplements used to increase strength. The primary source of information guiding their use was found to be popular magazines, as opposed to qualified medical advice.[28] In a Norwegian study, women using cod liver oil were found to be non-smokers of higher educational experience, of high physical activity levels and normal body mass index, with concomitant consumption of healthy food.[29]

Demographic surveys of many alternative or complementary medicines have been conducted in a range of locations, but there is usually a problem in clearly defining and categorising individual types of product. Nevertheless, the usual outcome of these surveys is that the typical patient is middle aged, middle income and female.

A recent survey carried out in Washington State, USA, on patients aged 50–76 years with a variety of medical conditions established the incidence of use of a number of nutraceuticals by both men ($n = 29\ 435$) and women ($n = 32\ 152$).[30] It can be seen from Table 1.1, which summarises their results, that many common disease states are being treated in this population by self-medication with nutraceuticals. For example, two widespread conditions – joint pain and insomnia – are often treated in this way. Glucosamine, chondroitin and methylsulfonylmethane (MSM) are used for joint pain, particularly that caused

Table 1.1 Use of nutraceuticals for treating specific diseases

Medical condition	Incidence of use (%)	Nutraceuticals used
Prostate cancer	5.3	Lycopene, dehydroepiandrosterone
Enlarged prostate	16.9	Lycopene
Osteoarthritis	29.7	Glucosamine, chondroitin, methylsulfonylmethane
Neck, back, or joint pain	25.3	Glucosamine, chondroitin, methylsulfonylmethane
Degenerative eye conditions	9.9	Lutein
Perimenopause	4.6	Soy products
Memory loss	8.9	Fish oil, coenzyme Q10
Insomnia	20.0	Melatonin

Data extracted from Gunther S, Patterson R E, Kristal A R, Stratton K L, White E. Demographic and health-related correlates of herbal and specialty supplement use, *Journal of the American Dietetic Association* 2004; 104: 27–34, with permission from the American Dietetic Association.

by rheumatoid or osteoarthritis, and melatonin is used for insomnia. There is also a substantial incidence of degenerative eye conditions in this population, which is often treated with lutein. It was also noted that there is increased incidence of use of complementary medicines by female patients; this was also shown to be the case with nutraceuticals.[30]

An overview of these publications tends to show that users of nutraceutical supplements are better educated, more healthy, and live more healthy lifestyles than their counterparts not taking supplementation, but confusingly a survey in Holland showed that consumption of cholesterol-lowering margarines were more likely to be reported by individuals with poorer subjective health, and smokers![31]

Safety

This text highlights why the safety of these supplements must be ensured. Many consumers are unaware of the difference between licensed and unlicensed products and the differences between food legislation versus medicine legislation. Pharmacists in the UK are being encouraged to use the Yellow Card Scheme to report suspected drug reactions from both unlicensed and licensed supplements as well as conventional medicines. This scheme is run by the MHRA on behalf of the Committee on Safety of Medicines (CSM) and relies on health professionals reporting side-effects they suspect to be related to the medicine a patient is taking. The upsurge of interest in nutraceutical supplements shows that many members of the public are seeking to improve their health either through diet or through 'natural' remedies. It cannot be over-emphasised that while many components of foods may be safe at the normal levels of intake, once these levels are increased to 'pharmacological' levels, other effects may appear. It is therefore imperative that these nutraceuticals are properly researched and that health professionals, as well as the public, are well-informed of the benefits and drawbacks of these medications.

Scientific evidence

Various types of studies have been carried out on nutraceuticals. These include:

- Studies on *in vitro* cell cultures acting as models of target cells, either animal or human derived. The problem with this type of study is that it does not account for important *in vivo* factors which may be important for the action of the compound, for example absorption or metabolism.
- Studies on live animals in the laboratory. In this case such a model cannot be used to predict effects in humans due to physiological differences.
- Epidemiological studies of populations taking a compound in supplements or through their diet. Ideally there should be evidence of a link between very low levels of a particular nutraceutical with an increased incidence/prevalence of a disease.
- Clinical trials comparing a potential compound with a placebo, showing that providing the supplement will reduce the risk of developing osteoporosis, for example. In these cases it is often necessary to use subjects already with the disease or at greater risk of developing it, as it would be impractical to observe onset of the disease in healthy volunteers. There may, however, be physiological differences between the healthy and disease state which preclude the assumption that an intervention will prevent disease.[1]

All the above study designs may have problems in terms of controlling the doses that should be used for testing, as there are often small traces of nutraceuticals found in all foods which may be taken over long periods of time. Many of the methods used to detect levels of these compounds or effects on outcome measures may lack the sensitivity to draw any conclusions.

The use of clinical trials

In order to provide conclusive evidence of the role of a particular nutraceutical either to prevent or treat disease, several factors must be known. There must be an inverse relationship between body levels of the supplement and risk of disease and the levels required must be established. Research teams use many different types of evaluation. Animal studies are often used, which although conclusive may be irrelevant to humans. Another method is the *in vitro* study, using cell and tissue responses, but this may be different to the response of that tissue when exposed *in vivo*, nor does it take into account the absorption of that substance after digestion. Epidemiological studies are another widely used type of study. For example, Japanese women who consume soya in large amounts and suffer very little from sex hormone-related cancers have been compared with Western women who have very few soya products in their diet and a high incidence of such cancers.[32] Although small-scale human studies are popular with researchers, some maintain that only large clinical trials can provide conclusive evidence for the effects of nutraceuticals in the prevention and cure of disease.[33]

When studying a nutraceutical for its disease prevention properties, such as antioxidants used to prevent the development of atherosclerosis or cancer, ideally a healthy population should be studied until sufficient numbers have developed the disease. This is highly impractical and a very large population would be required over a very long time. Therefore researchers resort to the study of subjects who already have the disease or who are at high risk of developing the disease.[33] It is assumed that if high-risk subjects or patients with the disease are cured then healthy subjects would benefit from the supplement in question as a preventative measure. But just because high-risk patients are cured, can it be assumed that healthy patients will also derive benefit? Moreover, if high-risk subjects or people with the disease are not helped does this mean that healthy subjects will not derive benefit either?

There is another important factor to consider when carrying out clinical trials for nutraceuticals. Whereas with medicines it can safely be assumed that the subject is receiving no other source of the test substance, a nutraceutical is often a pharmacological dose of a substance that is present in much smaller amounts in the body, for example, melatonin. In this case it is very difficult to assess the baseline levels of the placebo group, which may vary considerably between subjects, depending on the time of day or the diet.

A combination of several types of double-blind trials is required to evaluate any particular nutracetical:[34]

• Cross-cultural epidemiological studies must show the association between low levels of that nutrient in a sample population, and high levels of disease.
• In the same study group there must be a relationship between low initial levels of the nutrient and subsequent high risk for the disease.
• Supplementation of the nutrient to a sample population must show a reduced incidence of the disease, compared with a group that receives only placebo.

In addition to clinical trials, meta-analyses of clinical trials, often those involving small patient numbers, combine study results in order to draw conclusions about therapeutic efficacy. A number of meta-analyses and systematic reviews have been carried out on the use of nutraceuticals in many disease states, and this effectively increases the number of subjects studied. Additionally, these may help to explain contradictory results reported by individual trials.

Literature retrieval

In addition to using standard literature retrieval protocols, information in the book has been routinely collected from government and institutional publications, frequently available on the internet, and commercial data, manufacturers' data, trade publications and nutraceutical retailers. The data were cross-referenced from many sources, when relevant information was not readily found, for example the results of analysis of a nutraceutical are usually not easily found using a single search strategy, and a variety of synonyms may also be required.

A chapter on meta-analyses and evidence from the Cochrane Library and the Cochrane Database of Systematic Reviews is included (see Chapter 19), in order to supply the most critical data available on the demonstrable effects of nutraceuticals.

Market trends

The markets for nutraceuticals and functional foods are rapidly expanding. Combined, they represented annual global sales of US$95

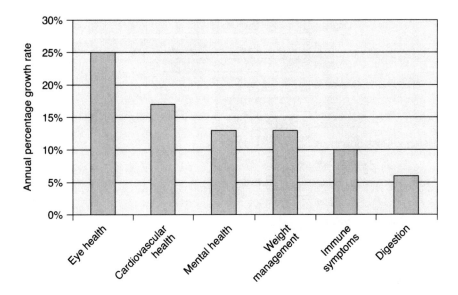

Figure 1.2 Predicted growth rate of nutraceutical usage. Permission to use this data from Dr C Gaertner, Cognis, is gratefully acknowledged.

billion in 2001, and this has been projected to grow to US$127 billion by 2005. The global nutraceutical market reached US$47 billion in 2002, and is expected to reach US$75 billion by 2007. The global market for functional foods was estimated to be US$30 billion in 2003, and Leatherhead Food RA consider that it will eventually reach 5% of all food expenditure in developed countries.[35] The predicted annual growth rates of various nutraceutical categories have been estimated to range from 6% for products treating digestive ailments, up to 25% for eye health products (Figure 1.2).

An alternative view of current and predicted sales claims that the joint health supplements – glucosamine, chondroitin and MSM – appear to be the major product group, followed by the polyunsaturated fatty acids (PUFAs). However, fish oils and MSM have been predicted to show the greatest increase in sales.[36]

The contemporary use of soy, for example, is not simply a matter of geographical habitat or cultural lifestyle. The availability of specific foods and nutraceuticals refined from soy allows all consumers to derive the proposed benefits. This also applies to green tea, fish oils, flax seed and others. However, a more active approach has to be taken with those only normally available in formulated dosages such as glucosamine, chondroitin and MSM, for example.

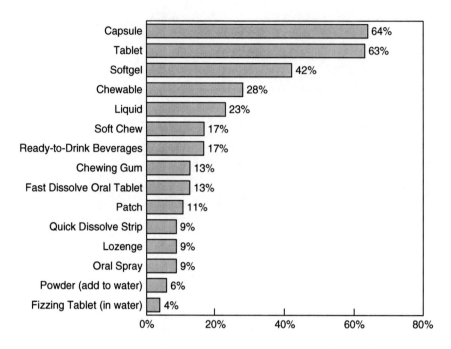

Figure 1.3 Consumer preference for various nutraceutical formulations (USA survey, 2004). Permission to reproduce from Nutraceuticals World, Ramsey, NJ, USA is gratefully acknowledged.

In combination with supplying increasing amount of product information by a variety of strategies and developing products for new therapeutic categories, manufacturers are increasingly marketing novel formulations. Tablets, capsules and softgels are still the most widely available formulations, but new formulations such as soft chews, and fast dissolving tablets and strips are becoming available. As with pharmaceuticals, nutraceutical manufacturers are extolling the virtues of controlled release formulations for release of precise levels of active entities over a particular time period, in order to achieve maximum therapeutic effects. An example of the use of this technology is the Novasoy soya isoflavone range.[37]

Consumers and suppliers are also increasingly willing to choose less conventional formulations (Figure 1.3). An American survey of consumer preferences for different formulations in 2004 revealed that younger consumers in particular are trying new delivery systems such as patches, chewing gums and fizzing tablets, instead of conventional dosage forms such as tablets and capsules.[38]

Major nutraceuticals and their applications

The therapeutic applications, dosage range and available formulations for the major nutraceuticals are discussed in Chapter 2. The major nutraceuticals have a number of origins, being either endogenous human metabolites, dietary constituents, animal or plant constituents normally not present in the diet in therapeutic levels, or synthetic compounds (notably MSM).[39]

For both patients and pharmacists, the choice of nutraceutical is based upon the disease state, and the efficacy and safety data. The information in this book is set out according to disease states, which is a logical arrangement for patients and pharmacists wishing to identify a suitable product for treating a particular ailment. The nutraceuticals discussed will be those popularly available, whether or not there is a large body of clinical or scientific evidence to substantiate their use.

Overview

The following chapters in this book will attempt to answer a number of important questions;

- What are nutraceuticals?
- Do they work?
- Should consumers ask for medical advice?
- Are they safe?
- Are there any adverse effects, or interactions with conventional pharmaceuticals?
- What is the quality of available products?
- Can patients or consumers simply modify their diets to obtain the perceived benefits?

Overall, lifestyle and dietary choices are probably the main determinants of health/bad health, and therefore the main question today is:

- Can nutraceuticals help in the prevention of diseases and in their treatment?

References

1. Rapport L, Lockwood B. *Nutraceuticals*. London: Pharmaceutical Press, 2002.
2. Packaged Facts (2006) www.packagedfacts.com (accessed 12 April 2006).

3.   Mannion M. Nutraceutical revolution continues at Foundation for Innovation in Medicine Conference. *Am J Nat Med* 1998; 5: 30–33.

4.   Zeisel S H. Regulation of 'nutraceuticals'. *Science* 1999; 285: 1853–1855.

5.   Mazza G. *Functional Foods.* Lancaster, Pennsylvania: Technomic Publishing, 1998.

6.   Cockbill C A. Food law and functional foods. *Br Food J* 1994; 96: 3–4.

7.   Aarts T A. How long will the 'Medical Food' window of opportunity remain open? *J Nutr Function Med Foods* 1998; 1: 45–57.

8.   Mintel Market Intelligence. *Functional Foods* March 2000.

9.   Food and Drug Administration (2004). Challenge and opportunity on the critical path to new medical products, 1–37. http://www.fda.gov/oc/initiatives/criticalpath/ (accessed 15 June 2006).

10. Heber D, Yip I, Ashley J M *et al.* Cholesterol-lowering effcts of a proprietary Chinese red-yeast-rice dietary supplement. *Am J Clin Nutr* 1999; 69: 231–236.

11. Mason P. The regulation of herbal products in Europe – from diversity to harmonisation? *Pharm J* 2000; 264: 856–857.

12. Barnes J, Anderson L A, Phillipson J D. *Herbal Medicines: A Guide for Healthcare Professionals*, 2nd edn. London: Pharmaceutical Press, 2002.

13. Council Directive 65/65/EEC. *Off J EC* 1965; 22: 369.

14. The Medicines Act, 1968. London; HMSO.

15. Statutory Instrument (SI) 1994: 3144, *The Medicines for Human Use (Marketing Authorisations etc) Regulations.*

16. Litov R E. Developing claims for new phytochemical products. In: Bidlack W R, Omaye S T, Meskin M S, Jahner D, eds. *Phytochemicals. A New Paradigm.* Lancaster, Pennsylvania: Technomic Publishing, 1998, 173–178.

17. Foundation for Innovation in Medicine (2006) www.fimdefelice.org (accessed 12 April 2006).

18. Mintel Market Intelligence. *Complementary Medicines* March 1999.

19. Mintel Market Intelligence. *Functional Foods* March 1999.

20. Mintel Market Intelligence. *Complementary Medicines* March 2003.

21. Mintel Market Intelligence. *Vitamins and Mineral Supplements* May 2003.

22. Asin JA. Why patients use alternative medicine, results of a national study. *JAMA* 1998; 279: 1548–1553.

23. Lyle B J, Mares-Perlman J A, Klein B E K *et al.* Supplement users differ from nonusers in demographic, lifestyle, dietary and health characteristics. *J Nutr* 1998; 128: 2355–2362.

24. Ishihara J, Sobue T, Yamamoto S *et al.* Demographics, lifestyles, health characteristics, and dietary intake among dietary supplement users in Japan. *Int J Epidemiol* 2003; 32: 546–553.

25. Foote J A, Murphy S P, Wilkens L R *et al.* Factors associated with dietary supplement use among healthy adults of five ethnicities: the Multiethnic Cohort Study. *Am J Epidemiol* 2003; 157: 888–897.

26. Arsenault J, Kennedy J. Dietary supplement use in U.S. Army Special Operations candidates. *Military Med* 1999; 164: 495–501.

27. Gray S L, Hanlon J T, Fillenbaum G G *et al.* Predictors of nutritional supplement use by the elderly. *Pharmacotherapy* 1996; 16: 715–720.

28. Sheppard H L, Raichada S M, Kouri, K M *et al.* Use of creatine and other supplements by members of civilian and military health clubs: A cross-sectional survey. *Int J Sport Nutr Exerc Metab* 2000; 10: 245–259.

29. Brustad M, Braaten T, Lund E. Predictors for cod-liver oil supplement use – the Norwegian Women and Cancer Study. *Eur J Clin Nutr* 2004; 58: 128–136.

30. Gunther S, Patterson R E, Kristal A R, Stratton K L, White E. Demographic and health-related correlates of herbal and specialty supplement use. *J Am Diet Assoc* 2004; 104: 27–34.

31. de Jong N, Ocke M C, Branderhorst H A C *et al.* Demographic and lifestyle characteristics of functional food consumers and dietary supplement users. *Br J Nutr* 2003; 89: 273–281.

32. Mason P. Isoflavones. *Pharm J* 2001; 266: 16–19.

33. Young J. Functional foods and the European consumer. In: Buttriss J, Saltmarsh M, eds. *Functional Foods II, Claims and Evidence.* Cambridge: The Royal Society of Chemistry, 2000, 75–78.

34. Mason P. *Handbook of Dietary Supplements*, 2nd edn. London: Pharmaceutical Press, 2001.

35. Iisakke K. Nutraceuticals and functional foods demand for ingredients. *NutraCos* 2003, Nov/Dec, 2–4.

36. Challener C. Speciality supplements are the bright spot in US dietary supplement market. *Chemical Market Rep* 2003; July 14: 3–8.

37. Jones M. Controlled delivery technology in nutraceutical applications: A users perspective. *NutraCos* 2003; May/June: 7–9.

38. Write T. New age delivery. *Nutraceuticals World* 2005; September: 42, 44.

39. Lockwood G B. Nutraceutical supplements. In: *Encyclopedia of Pharmaceutical Technology.* Boca Raton, FL: Taylor and Francis, 2005: 1–23.

2

Monographs – general and specific properties

This chapter outlines the structure(s) and general properties of the major nutraceuticals. Brief information on metabolism and pharmacokinetics, and therapeutic uses and legal classification are also included in this chapter. More detailed information on the sources, manufacture and analytical techniques is collated in Chapter 3, followed by Chapter 4 listing comparative data for most nutraceuticals on their metabolism, bioavailability and pharmacokinetics.

The available information for the different entities varies widely: data for some are limited or even completely missing, whereas complex supplements such as grape seed proanthocyanidin extract (GSPE) and food-derived nutraceuticals such as soy and tea have been the subject of extensive research into their composition, properties and related epidemiology because of their consumption in wide-ranging populations and over long periods of time.

Glucosamine

Structure and properties

Glucosamine (Figure 2.1) is an amino monosaccharide, consisting of glucose and the amino acid glutamic acid.[1] It is found naturally in the body and is present in almost all human tissue, especially in cartilage, tendons and ligament tissues. It is a precursor of the disaccharide units of articular cartilage glycoaminoglycan (GAG), which forms most of the

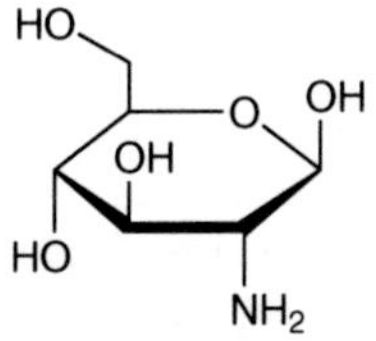

Figure 2.1 The structure of glucosamine.

cartilage tissue.[1,2] The sulfate, hydrochloride and *N*-acetyl forms are usually used for therapeutic purposes.

Glucosamine is not found in significant amounts in the usual diet and must be synthesised by the body. This ability declines with age and predisposes the body to degenerative joint disease or arthritis.

Metabolism and pharmacokinetics

The bioavailability of glucosamine in humans is 44% after oral ingestion, and urinary excretion during the first 24 hours has been shown to be 1.2% of the dosage (7.5 g).[3]

> Therapeutic areas: Joint, skin and animal health
>
> Legal classification: No restriction; may be obtainable on prescription in the UK
>
> Recommended oral dose: 1500 mg/day
>
> Formulations available: Tablet, capsule, patch, gel, effervescent tablet, sustained release tablet

Chondroitin

Structure and properties

Chondroitin sulfate (Figure 2.2) is a GAG made up from alternate sequences of differently sulfated units of uronic acid and *N*-acetyl-galactosamine.[4] It is commercially obtained from bovine or calf cartilage.[4] Chondroitins of different origins have different constitutions, resulting in disaccharide units with different numbers and positioning

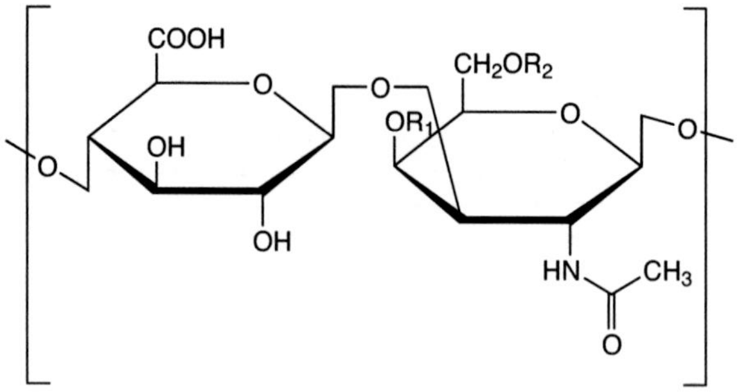

Consists of 15-150 monomer units. R_1 represents either SO_3 or H, R_2 represents either H or SO_3.

Figure 2.2 The structure of chondroitin.

of sulfate groups, and different polymer lengths. Studies have typically used material of molecular weight 14 000,[5] but the size of commercially available material varies widely. This wide range in molecular weights may have a marked effect on a preparation's ability to treat joint ailments.

Metabolism and pharmacokinetics

The bioavailability following oral administration of 3 g showed a half-life of 363 minutes, and bioavailability of 13%.[6]

> Therapeutic areas: Joint and veterinary health
> Legal classification: No restriction
> Recommended oral dose: 1200–1500mg/day
> Formulations available: Tablet, nasal drops

Methylsulfonylmethane

Structure and properties

Methylsulfonylmethane (MSM) is derived from dimethyl sulfoxide (DMSO), and is a by-product of the wood pulp industry that is used as an industrial solvent. Other well-established names for MSM include dimethyl sulfone ($DMSO_2$) or methyl sulfone. MSM was developed after previous experience with DMSO.

The history of DMSO and its clinical applications have been reviewed.[7] Its use in rheumatoid arthritis was questioned after side-effects were reported. The possible side-effects of DMSO, plus the unpleasant garlic odour reported by both users and partners, suggested MSM, the major metabolite of DMSO, as a replacement. Approximately 15% of DMSO that enters the body is converted to MSM (Figure 2.3).[8]

MSM occurs naturally in a number of foods, such as meat, milk and capers for example, and is one of the compounds responsible for the pungent urinary odour after consumption of asparagus.

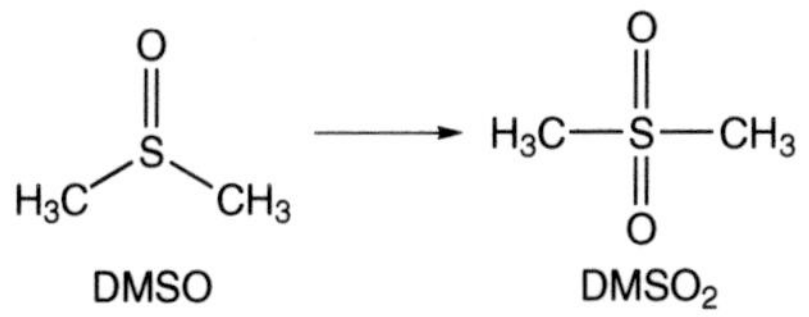

Figure 2.3 Degradation of dimethyl sulfoxide (DMSO).

Metabolism and pharmacokinetics

MSM exists in human plasma at levels of about 4 mg/person, and 4–11 mg are excreted every 24 hours in the urine.[7]

Many studies have looked at the conversion of DMSO to MSM, both in animals and in humans. Reduced serum levels and recovery of DMSO and MSM reported after dermal administration suggest that absorption and bioavailability are lower after dermal application than after oral administration. This may be due to retention in the skin at the site of application (which could be beneficial for dermatological conditions) or possible volatilisation from the skin. Much lower percentage levels are found as the metabolite dimethyl sulfide (DMS), which is responsible for producing the oyster/garlic odour and taste in the mouth that occurs a short time after receiving DMSO.[7] It has been shown that MSM does not produce this unpleasant effect and no part of it is converted into the odorous DMS.[8]

In all species studied MSM persists in tissues far longer than its parent compound DMSO.[9] It has been shown that excretion in the urine of orally administered DMSO was complete after 120 hours, whereas that of the metabolite MSM lasted longer than 480 hours.

> Therapeutic areas: Joint and veterinary health
> Legal classification: No restriction
> Recommended oral dose: Up to 2 g/day
> Formulations available: Tablet, capsule, cream, powder

Coenzyme Q10

Structure and properties

Coenzyme Q10 (Co Q10) (synonyms: ubiquinone, ubidecarone) (Figure 2.4) is an endogenously synthesised lipid soluble antioxidant. It is also present in a number of foods, and this may cause ingestion of 3–5 mg/day. The food types containing Co Q10 are widely diverse,

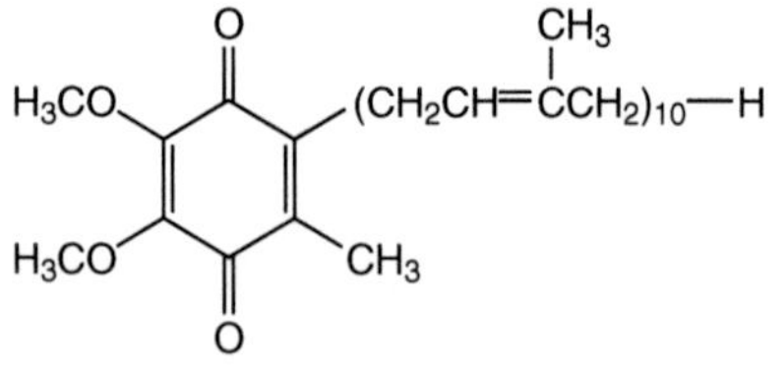

Figure 2.4 The structure of coenzyme Q10.

including fatty fish, cereals, poultry and vegetables, particularly spinach.[10] It is present in human plasma at a level of 1 mg/L.[11]

Metabolism and pharmacokinetics

When ingested as a supplement or present in food, Co Q10 is absorbed and then contributes to plasma concentrations. The metabolism has been studied in a range of animals, and the major metabolites found in bile and urine have been identified as carboxylated derivatives.[12] Coenzyme Q9 has also been identified in rats.[11] After administration of Co Q10 capsules (30 mg), or cooked pork heart (natural source of Co Q10, equivalent to 30 mg) to human subjects, maximum serum concentrations of approximately 1 mg/L were detected at 6 hours, and levels in pork heart-fed subjects was slightly higher.[11]

> Therapeutic areas: Cardiovascular health, cancer prevention, respiratory, skin and animal health (antioxidant)
> Legal classification: No restriction
> Recommended dose: 100–360 mg/day
> Formulations available: Tablet, capsule, chewtab, drops, gel, gum, softgel

Melatonin

Structure and properties

Melatonin (Figure 2.5) is the primary hormone secreted by the pineal gland. It is biosynthesised from the amino acid trytophan, via the intermediate serotonin. This biosynthesis and the subsequent release of melatonin is usually inhibited by exposure to light and stimulated by darkness, via a multisynaptic neural pathway connecting the pineal gland to the retina.[13] However, the 24-hour cycle (or circadian rhythm) of melatonin secretion is observed even when subjects are kept in darkness, so it is thought that light adjusts this rhythm rather than primarily causing it.[14] Melatonin secretion usually starts as soon as darkness falls and usually peaks between 2 and 4 am.

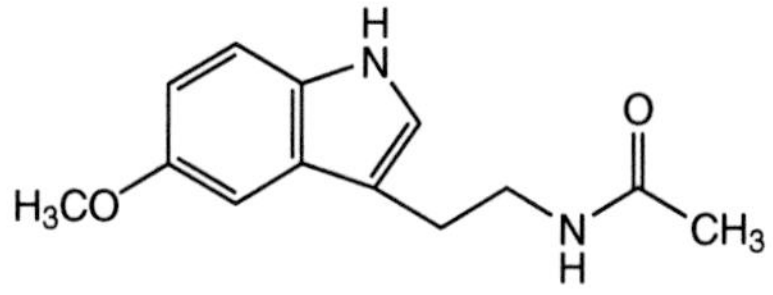

Figure 2.5 The structure of melatonin.

The amount of melatonin produced varies with age. Babies secrete low levels, but from the age of about three months, melatonin concentrations begin to increase, reaching a maximum between one and three years of age. Young adults secrete 5–25 µg of melatonin daily and this decreases markedly with advancing age.[15]

As it is a hormone, melatonin has been called a drug, however it is also a nutrient. The consumption of plant materials containing high levels of melatonin could alter serum concentrations. Melatonin has been identified in bananas, tomatoes, cucumbers and beetroots, but unrealistically large amounts of these foods would have to be eaten to achieve pharmacological doses.[15,16]

Metabolism and pharmacokinetics

Melatonin is rapidly metabolised by the liver, with more than 85% being excreted as 6-sulfatoxymelatonin (6-SMT) in urine. This is used as a research tool to measure plasma melatonin.[17] Low doses of between 0.1 and 0.3 mg result in serum concentrations similar to the usual, physiological, night time peak, but doses of between 1 and 5 mg (pharmacological doses) result in serum concentrations up to 100 times higher than this concentration.[14] Oral doses of melatonin have a short half-life and are quickly cleared, and even very high nightly doses of 50 mg are cleared by the following morning. However, after two weeks of high daily dosing, lipid storage occurs.[15]

> Therapeutic areas: Cardiovascular health, cancer prevention, sport enhancement, sleep improvement, and bone health (antioxidant)
>
> Legal classification: In the UK, the Medicines and Healthcare Products Regulatory Agency (MHRA) has restricted melatonin to prescription, available on a named patient basis only. There are no licensed products in the UK, so it is unlawful to promote melatonin. However, in the USA it may be sold as a food supplement, under the Dietary Supplement Health and Education Act of 1994. British residents can legally bring melatonin purchased in the USA home, for personal use.[18]
>
> Recommended dose: 0.3–25 mg/day
>
> Formulations available: Tablet, patch, liquid

Carnitine

Structure and properties

Carnitine (Figure 2.6) is an essential cellular component, synthesised from lysine and methionine in the liver and kidney, from where it is

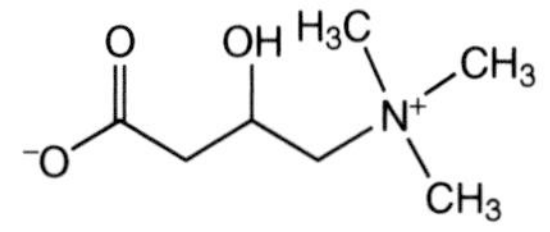

Figure 2.6 The structure of carnitine.

released into the systemic circulation, and is also synthesised in the brain.[19,20]

Carnitine exists in two isomeric forms, the D- and L-forms, which have different biochemical and pharmacological properties. Naturally occurring carnitine is almost always the L-isomer, whereas the D-isomer is usually obtained from chemical synthethesis. The L-isomer is a substrate for carnitine-acetyltransferase and is the only isomer with biological activity, but the D-isomer acts as a competitive inhibitor, interfering with fatty acid oxidation and energy production.[21] Some people do not excrete the D-isomer efficiently and it has also been reported that administration of the D-isomer causes a depletion of L-carnitine in the heart muscle, leading to abnormalities.[22] D-Carnitine and DL-carnitine are therefore toxic and not safe for human consumption. They have been banned in the USA.[21]

Ninety-eight per cent of carnitine is found in the cardiac and skeletal muscle, with a further 1.5% in liver and kidneys and 0.5% in extracellular fluid. Carnitine can also be obtained from the diet, predominantly from food of animal origin, such as meat and dairy produce. In humans, 100–200 μmol carnitine is synthesised daily and an omnivorous diet supplies approximately 300–400 μmol daily.[23]

The main function of carnitine is in fatty acid metabolism. The biochemical reactions of this nutrient are based on the reversible reaction between carnitine and long-chain fatty acyl groups:

Carnitine + Acyl-coA ⇌ Acyl-L-carnitine + Coenzyme A

Carnitine is therefore involved with many coenzyme A-dependent pathways.[24]

The first recognised function of carnitine was its involvement in long-chain fatty acid oxidation, at the mitochondrial level, providing energy. Carnitine acts as a carrier of the acyl and acetyl groups across the mitochondrial membrane. Once inside the mitochondria, β-oxidation can occur to provide energy from the long-chain fatty acids.[25] This is the main energy source in skeletal and cardiac muscle.[20]

Metabolism and pharmacokinetics

A small amount of carnitine is excreted by the kidneys in the urine as free carnitine or as acylcarnitine, but more than 85% is reabsorbed by the proximal renal tubule.[19,26] The bioavailability of dietary carnitine has been shown to be 54–87%, depending on food level, and the bioavailability from supplements (0.5–0.6 g) has been estimated as 14–18% of the dose.[27]

Although the amount ingested determines the absorption rate, oral doses of greater than 2 g have no advantage, since at this dose mucosal absorption appears to be saturated.[20] In vegetarians metabolic needs are usually met by endogenous biosynthesis.[28] Carnitine levels would have to drop by more than 50% to lead to a marked metabolic change, and this does not usually occur even in strict vegetarians.[21] Plasma carnitine levels are higher in men than in women, and older women (above 40 years) have lower levels still.[19,26]

Physical activity causes increased serum levels of acetyl-L-carnitine, C-4/C-8 acetylcarnitines, propionylcarnitine and γ-butyrobetaine, and decreased levels of serum carnitine compared with levels before exercise.[29]

> Therapeutic areas: Sport enhancement, cardiovascular and bone health, weight optimisation, veterinary health
>
> Legal classification: Widely used in carnitine-deficiency conditions, and in many countries in Europe (including the UK) L-carnitine is available as a prescription-only medicine (POM). In the UK doctors can prescribe 'Carnitor' (POM), while health food shops sell unbranded carnitine with no legal restrictions.
>
> Recommended dose: 2–4 g/day
>
> Formulations available: Tablet

Acetyl-L-carnitine

Structure and properties

Acetyl-L-carnitine (Figure 2.7) is the acetyl derivative of L-carnitine (see above) and has some similar functions, but it is not technically an essential nutrient. It occurs naturally in the brain, liver and kidney, and is synthesised in mitochondria.[30]

Primary deficiency of acetyl-L-carnitine is caused by impairment of the membrane transportation of carnitine, and symptoms may include chronic muscle weakness, recurrent episodes of coma and hypoglycaemia, as well as encephalopathy and cardiomyopathy. Inherited

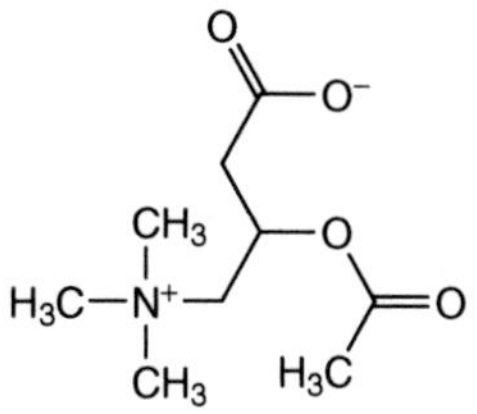

Figure 2.7 The structure of acetyl-L-carnitine.

disorders of metabolism can lead to secondary deficiency of carnitine.[31] Side-effects associated with the ingestion of this compound are relatively uncommon and mild.[32]

Metabolism and pharmacokinetics

Acetyl-L-carnitine is rapidly hydrolysed to carnitine. Pharmacokinetics of acetyl-L-carnitine are similar to those of carnitine.[27]

> Therapeutic areas: Mental health, sport enhancement, weight management
> Legal classification: No restriction
> Recommended dose: 1.5–3 g/day
> Formulations available: Capsule

Octacosanol/policosanol

Structure and properties

Octacosanol (Figure 2.8) is a 28-carbon aliphatic primary alcohol $(CH_3(CH_2)_{26}CH_2OH)$, which is present in the superficial waxy layers of fruit, leaves and epidermis of many plants, as well as whole grains. The main commercial source is a by-product from the sugarcane industry, but it is also found in the leaves of alfalfa and wheat, in wheatgerm and also in various animal sources. It is also a component of paraffin.[33,34] As only very small amounts are available in the diet, to gain any health benefits from octacosanol it must be ingested as a supplement. Most studies assessing these benefits have been carried out using either a wheatgerm oil extract or policosanol, which is a natural mixture of

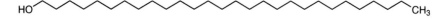

Figure 2.8 The structure of octacosanol.

primary alcohols purified from sugarcane (*Saccharum officinarum* L.) wax, whose main component is octacosanol. Both wheatgerm extract and policosanol are reported to contain 8% hexacosanol, 67% octacosanol, 12% triacosanol and 13% other long-chain alcohols.[35]

Metabolism and pharmacokinetics

There are limited data available in this area. The supposed active metabolite, octacosanoic acid, has been detected in the liver, along with octacosanol, within 24 hours. After oral administration to rodents, absorption of octacosanol has been 'assumed' to range between 10% and 35%, and bioavailability ranges between 5% and 12%.[36]

> Therapeutic areas: Cardiovascular health, sport enhancement
> Legal classification: No restriction
> Recommended dose: 100 mg/day
> Formulations available: Tablet, capsule

S-Adenosyl methionine

Structure and properties

S-Adenosyl methionine (SAMe) (synonym: ademetionine) (Figure 2.9) is synthesised from methionine and adenosine triphosphate (ATP) by *S*-adenosylmethionine synthetase, and it is involved in transmethylation, transsulfuration and aminopropylation reactions. It occurs in every living cell and acts either as a group donor or enzyme inducer.[37]

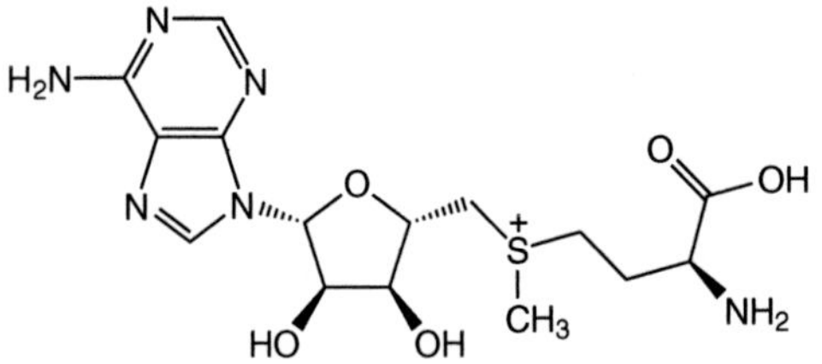

Figure 2.9 The structure of *S*-adenosyl methionine (SAMe).

Metabolism and pharmacokinetics

The major metabolic pathway involves decarboxylation, yielding methylthioadenosine, or putrescine and polyamines.[37] SAMe is very unstable in the body, and has very poor absorption and bioavailability. Maximum plasma concentrations occur 3–6 hours after oral administration of 400 mg, with a half-life of 1.7 hours, and volume of distribution of 0.4 L/kg.[38]

> Therapeutic areas: Joint and mental health
> Legal classification: No restriction
> Recommended dose: 200–1200 mg/day
> Formulations available: Tablet

Polyunsaturated fatty acids

Fatty acids derive from triglycerides (animal fats and plant oils) in the diet, and many can also be synthesised *de novo*. There is, however, a group that can only be obtained from the diet as the body lacks the ability to synthesise them, and these are known as essential fatty acids.

Many of those of interest derive from fish and plant oils and include linoleic acid, eicosapentaenoic acid (EPA), docosahexaenoic acid (DHA), α-linolenic acid (ALA) and γ-linolenic acid (GLA).

All possess multiple unsaturated double bonds and hence are termed polyunsaturated fatty acids (PUFAs). The first of these double bonds in EPA, DHA and ALA is located at the third carbon atom from its terminal, hence they are described as omega-3 or *n*-3 PUFAs. Linoleic acid and GLA have their first double bonds at the sixth carbon, and are termed omega-6 or *n*-6 PUFAs.

Metabolic pathways have been identified which outline how the *n*-3 and *n*-6 PUFAs act as precursors for the formation of prostaglandins:

- The *n*-6 PUFA linoleic acid is converted to GLA, then dihomo γ-linolenic acid (DGLA) and finally arachidonic acid (AA) through the action of a series of enzymes. Cyclooxygenase-2 (COX-2) then converts AA to prostaglandin E_2 (PGE_2). DGLA also forms the precursor of prostaglandin E_1 (PGE_1) through the action of cyclooxygenase-1 (COX-1) enzymes.
- The *n*-3 PUFA ALA is converted to EPA and then DHA which can compete with and inhibit the action of COX-2, and reduce PGE_2 formation.

These prostaglandins are released into the immediate bone tissue environment and have conflicting actions.

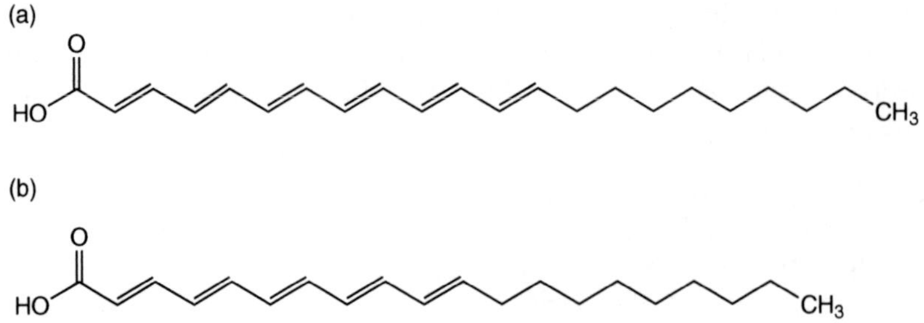

(a)

(b)

Figure 2.10 The structures of (a) docosahexaenoic acid (DHA) and (b) eicosapentaenoic acid (EPA).

n-3 Fatty acids from fish oils

Structure and properties

Docosahexaenoic acid (DHA) (Figure 2.10) is one of the major components of grey matter in the brain, and is important in the retina, testes, and present at high levels in fish oil. The major source is marine algae, consequently the largest commercial source is fish feeding off the algae. Many of the important body functions are thought to require adequate tissue levels of DHA, particularly brain and eye functions, and there is a growing trend to enrich a large number of foods with DHA, the virtues of which are widely extolled in the media. DHA is produced in the body from EPA by desaturation and elongation reactions.[39]

Metabolism and pharmacokinetics

DHA-containing fatty acid triglycerides are hydrolysed by pancreatic lipase in the duodenum to release free DHA. Relative absorption rates for DHA are dependent on the form administered; up to 95% of free DHA is absorbed, and less for triglycerides and ester forms. Maximum plasma concentration occurs 5 hours after ingestion of a single dose of fish oil. EPA is converted to DHA.[39] Administration of 3–12 g fish oil daily for 28 days produced rapid increases of EPA and DHA plasma concentrations at all dosages. EPA accumulation was higher than DHA, and dose-dependent increases were recorded, but DHA showed similar plasma levels at all dosage levels.[40]

Therapeutic areas: Joint, cardiovascular, eye and mental health, cancer prevention, bone, respiratory, skin and veterinary health
Legal classification: No restriction
Recommended dose: 2.5 g/day
Formulations available: Oil, soft capsule

γ-Linolenic acid

Structure and properties

The structure of γ-linolenic acid (GLA) is shown in Figure 2.11.

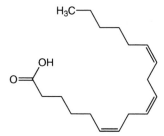

Figure 2.11 The structure of γ-linolenic acid (GLA).

Metabolism and pharmacokinetics

GLA is an essential intermediate between linoleic acid and DGLA, and thence prostaglandins, thromboxanes and leukotrienes. It is often claimed to be beneficial in disease states where it is not biosynthesised from linoleic acid, and consequently supplementation may be beneficial. Atopic eczema and premenstrual syndrome are two of the most popular applications. GLA is not widely found in substantial amounts in nature, but is present in evening primrose seed oil, starflower oil and black-currant seed oil.[10] Supplementation with GLA is usually carried out by use of the complete oil source, with no prior purification of the GLA.

GLA is an important intermediate in the production of prostaglandins and eicosanoids, via the metabolites DGLA and AA,[41] and disruption of its production by the action of delta-6-desaturase on linoleic acid is thought to be responsible for a number of human disease states. This disruption is believed to be circumvented by oral GLA supplementation.

Therapeutic areas: Skin health, joint health
Legal classification: No restriction, Epogam and Efamast lost their licences as
    POM medicines in 2002
Recommended dose: 360–2800 mg/day
Formulations available: Oil, soft capsule

Flaxseed/α-linolenic acid

Structure and properties

Flaxseed, also known as linseed, is produced from the flax plant (*Linum usitatissimum*), and has traditionally been used for a number of medical and non-medical applications.[42] Over recent years flaxseed applications have been 'rediscovered' in the area of health and are often promoted by producers.

Flaxseed oil contains more than 50% ALA (Figure 2.12), which is an essential *n*-3 fatty acid. Other sources of ALA include candlenut, hemp seed, pumpkin seed, canola, walnut and soybean.[42]

Because ALA is an essential fatty acid humans need to make sure there is enough in the diet. Health recommendations to replace saturated fats with unsaturated fats have often resulted in replacement by *n*-6 rather than *n*-3 PUFAs. This has led to the modern, Western diet including far more *n*-6 fatty acids than *n*-3, in a ratio of approximately 20–30:1. Ideally the ratio should be almost equal. Moreover, fish consumption, which was a source of *n*-3 oils, has decreased in recent years. Due to modern food industry and agricultural methods, the *n*-3 content of many foods, including meat, fish, eggs and vegetables is much lower than it used to be. As a result many people are deficient in the *n*-3 essential fatty acid ALA.[43]

Both *n*-6 and *n*-3 fatty acids are precursors of longer chain eicosanoids, such as prostaglandins, thromboxanes and leukotrienes.

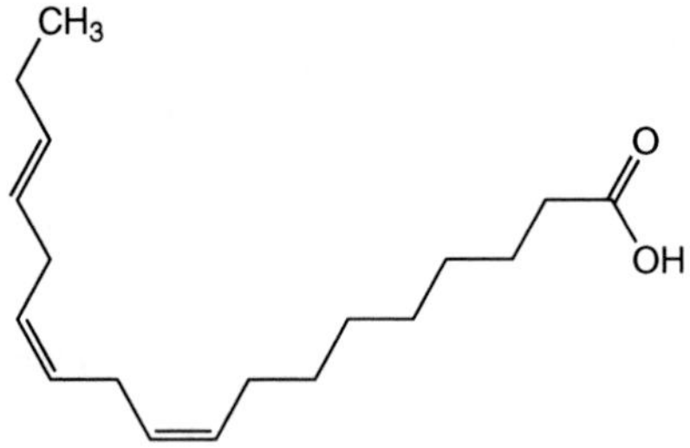

Figure 2.12 The structure of α-linolenic acid (ALA).

Those derived from *n*-6 fatty acids have opposing properties to those derived from *n*-3 and therefore a balance is required. A diet rich in *n*-6 and lacking in *n*-3 tends to lead to thrombi, blood aggregation and cardiovascular disease, as well as allergies, inflammation and diabetes. Fish oils have long been recognised as a source of long-chain *n*-3 PUFAs, and many researchers have studied these oils. However, flaxseed provides the richest plant source precursor, ALA, which is converted to these long-chain fatty acids, and provides a way to correct deficiency and prevent diseases associated with decreased *n*-3 fatty acids.

One advantage of ALA over fish oils is that the problem of reduced plasma vitamin E does not occur when plant sources are used, because ALA does not cause reduction, as is the case with fish oil supplements.[43] Moreover, as well as being a precursor for longer chain *n*-3 fatty acids, ALA has clinically relevant effects in its own right, which offers another benefit over *n*-3-containing fish oils.[44]

Metabolism and pharmacokinetics

After ingestion, ALA is absorbed and partly converted to EPA or DHA. However, after high intake of linoleic acid, desaturase enzyme degrades both ALA and linoleic acid, causing reduction in synthesis of DHA from the ALA.[39]

> Therapeutic areas: Cancer prevention, respiratory health (antioxidant)
> Legal classification: No restriction
> Recommended dose: 1–2 g/day
> Formulations available: Soft capsule

Conjugated linoleic acid

Conjugated linoleic acid (CLA) is a collective term used to describe the mixture of positional and geometric isomers of linoleic acid with conjugated double bonds (Figure 2.13). The two bioactive isomers of CLA are *cis*-9,*trans*-11 and *trans*-10,*cis*-12, and these two isomers usually predominate in commercial mixtures.

The main dietary sources of CLA are the meat and dairy products of grazing animals in whose stomachs bacteria are able to modify dietary linoleic acid. CLA concentrations in dairy products are usually of the order of 3–9 mg/g, and are formed as a result of rumen gut microbial isomerisation of dietary linoleic acid. The levels of CLA in human plasma are directly related to milk fat intake; no isomerisation from linoleic acid occurs in the human gut.[45]

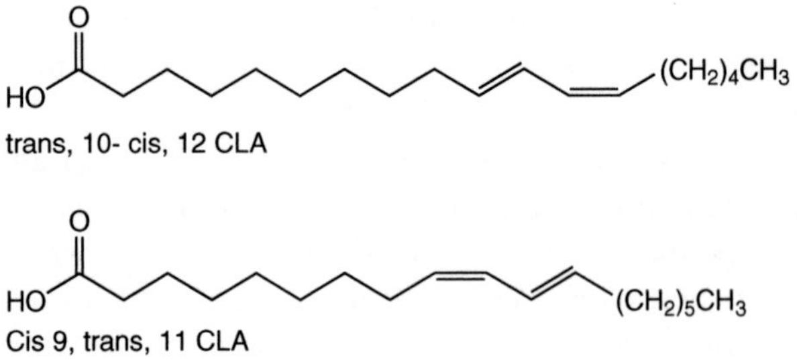

trans, 10- cis, 12 CLA

Cis 9, trans, 11 CLA

Figure 2.13 The structures of *trans*-10,*cis*-12 and *cis*-9,*trans*-11 conjugated linoleic acid (CLA).

Metabolism and pharmacokinetics

Limited data are available.

> Therapeutic areas: Weight management, sport enhancement
> Legal classification: No restriction
> Recommended dose: 1–2 g/day
> Formulations available: Soft capsule

Flax lignans

Structure and properties

The two major lignans are secoisolariciresinol diglucoside (SDG) and matairesinol, and their major metabolites are enterolactone and enterodiol (Figure 2.14). These are often referred to as mammalian lignans, and have not been found in plants. Six other lignans have been identified, and these are also converted to enterolactone and enterodiol to some extent, and also to enterofuran.[46] A number of lignans have been found in a range of commonly consumed cereals and they have been identified as enterolactone precursors.[47]

Metabolism and pharmacokinetics

The metabolites are shown in Figure 2.14. Administration of 10 g flaxseed to humans resulted in large increases in faecal lignan excretion, from 727 to 12 871 nmol/day. Wide variations in individual abilities to metabolise lignans have been reported in populations, and this is possibly caused by variations in the endogenous microflora of different individuals.[46]

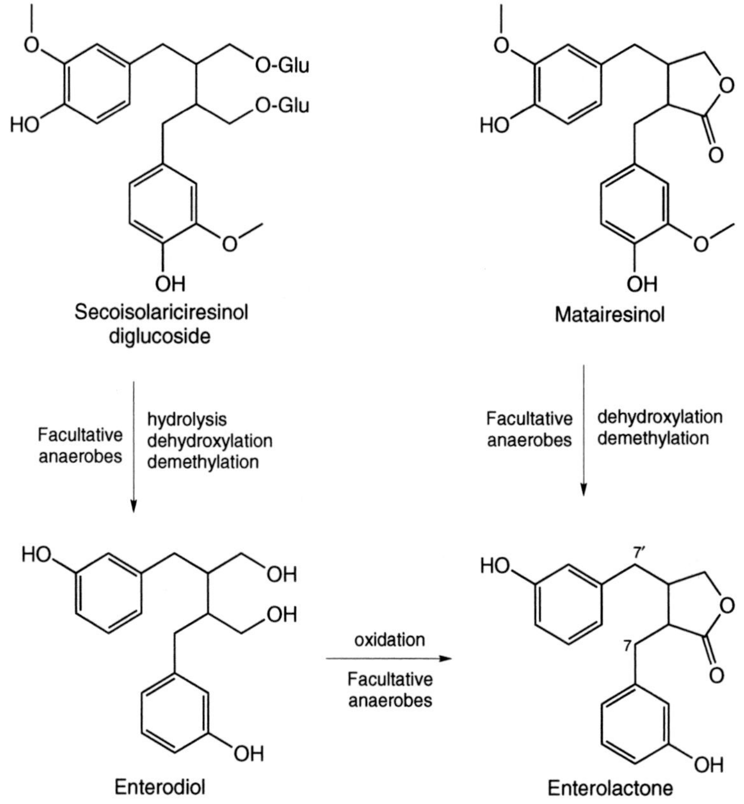

Figure 2.14 The metabolism of flax lignans. Reproduced from Rowland I, Faughnan M, Hoey L et al. Bioavailability of phyto-oestrogens. Br J Nutr 2003; 89: S45–S58. with permission.

Therapeutic areas: Cardiovascular health, cancer prevention, women's health (antioxidant and weakly oestrogenic)
Legal classification: No restriction
Recommended dose: Present at about 1% in flaxseed oil
Formulations available: Soft capsule

Pycnogenol

Structure and properties

Pycnogenol is the trade name of a standardised extract of the bark of the French maritime pine, *Pinus pinaster* Aiton subspecies Atlantica des Villar. The standardised extract is a concentrate of polyphenols, mainly

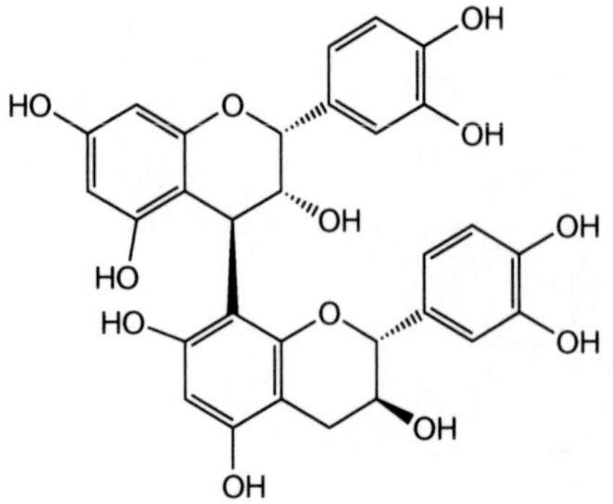

Procyanidin B3

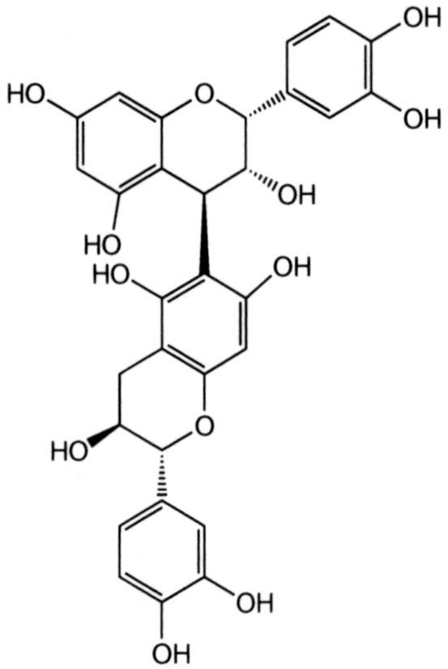

Procyanidin B6

Figure 2.15 The structures of procyanidins B3 and B6.

phenolic acids and procyanidins. The phenolic acids are either derivatives of benzoic acid, such as p-hydroxybenzoic acid, procatechuic acid,
vanillic acid or gallic acid, or cinnamic acid derivatives such as
p-coumaric acid, caffeic acid and ferulic acid. These acids exist in the
free form and as glucosides and glucose esters. The procyanidins are
polymers of catechin or epicatechin monomers, composed of 2–12
monomers. The major dimers include procyanidin B1, consisting of
catechin and epicatechin, followed by B3, consisting of two catechin
monomers linked by a C4–C8 bond, and lower concentrations of the

equivalent dimers C4–C6 linked, namely B6 and B7. Monomeric catechin, free taxifolin and its glucoside, and vanillin have also been found.[48] The structures of two proanthocyanidins found in Pycnogenol are shown in Figure 2.15.

Metabolism and pharmacokinetics

Metabolites of procyanidins (see Table 4.1) were identified after oral intake by humans, and maximum excretion was seen after between 8 and 15 hours, indicating slow absorption and metabolism.[49]

> Therapeutic areas: Cardiovascular, eye, respiratory, and oral health (antioxidant)
> Legal classification: No restriction
> Recommended dose: 25–200 mg/day
> Formulations available: Capsule

Resveratrol

Structure and properties

Resveratrol (Figure 2.16) has been identified in the leaves, skins and petals of *Vitis vinifera*, and also in wines and grape juice, but is also in other foods, such as peanut butter. In grape products, levels are higher after infection of the vine with *Botrytis cinerea*, and in red wines manufactured with extended time in contact with the skins.[50] In addition to resveratrol, a number of closely related stilbene analogues are also present.

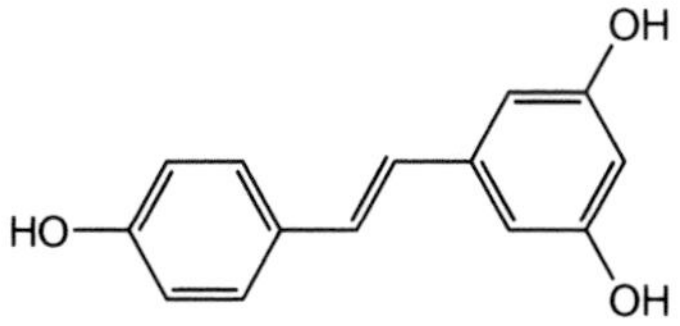

Figure 2.16 The structure of resveratrol.

Metabolism and pharmacokinetics

A number of degradation products have been identified (see Table 4.1). After oral administration of 25 mg resveratrol to humans, the highest plasma concentrations were detected after 30 minutes, which returned to baseline after 2 hours.[50] Most work has been carried out in rats, and it appears to be well absorbed after oral administration; plasma values peaked at about 60 minutes.[51]

> Therapeutic areas: Cardiovascular health, cancer prevention, women's health (antioxidant and weakly oestrogenic)
> Legal classification: No restriction
> Recommended dose: 15–200 mg/day
> Formulations available: Tablet, capsule

Grape seed proanthocyanidin extract

Structure and properties

Proanthocyanidins occur naturally in many fruits, vegetables, nuts, seeds, flowers and bark.[52] It is thought that protection from diseases results from the increase of antioxidants in the body. Grape seed proanthocyanidin extract (GSPE) contains proanthocyanidins based on either catechin or epicatechin (Figure 2.17). The monomers join together to form dimers, trimers and other oligomers, and many different

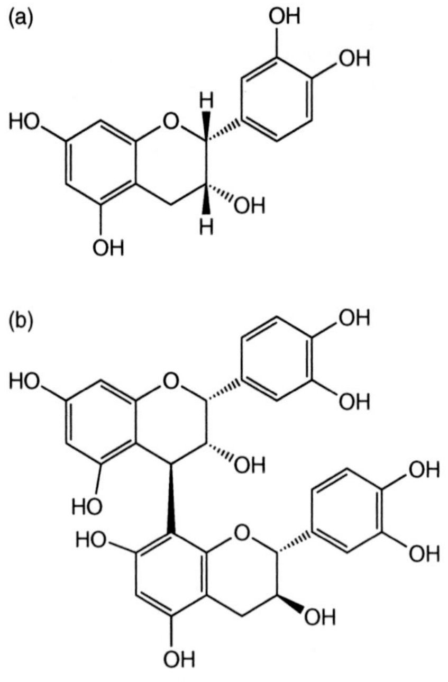

Figure 2.17 The structures of (a) epicatechin and (b) procyanidin B2.

structures are formed due to changes in stereochemistry. Dimeric procyanidins have been classified as procyanidins B1, B2, B3 and B4 depending on the configuration of catechin and epicatechin subunits. A number of these catechin derivatives are present as their gallates in addition to the free form.

Metabolism and pharmacokinetics

The proanthocyanidins are poorly absorbed in the small intestine, and it is thought that ingestion results in metabolism by colonic bacteria. 3-Hydroxyphenylpropionic acid has been identified as the major metabolite.[53]

> Therapeutic areas: Cardiovascular and skin health (antioxidant)
> Legal classification: No restriction
> Recommended oral dose: 1500 mg/day
> Formulations available: Tablet, capsule, patch, gel, effervescent tablet, sustained release tablet

Lycopene

Structure and properties

Lycopene (Figure 2.18) is a natural red pigment synthesised by plants and microorganisms, but not by animals. It is found in red fruits and vegetables, particularly the tomato, and is one of over 600 carotenoids found in nature which function as pigments in photosynthesis and in photoprotection.[54] Of these, about 24 are present in foods. Examples include β-carotene found in carrots, broccoli and other green-leafed vegetables and lutein found in spinach, peas and watercress.[55] Unlike many of the other carotenoids, however, lycopene is not a precursor of vitamin A.

As humans are unable to synthesise carotenoids such as lycopene, they must be obtained from dietary intake. One group has estimated the

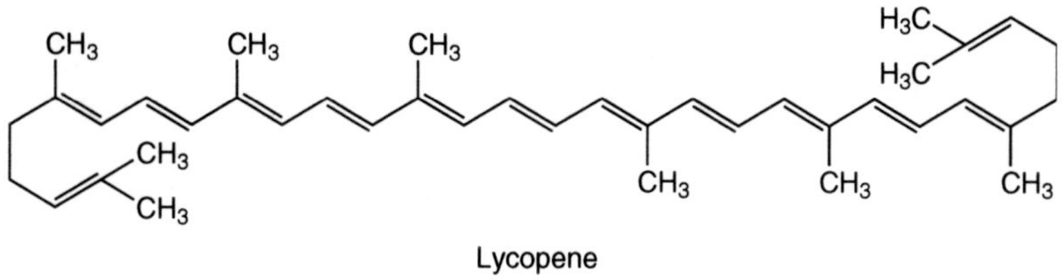

Lycopene

Figure 2.18 The structure of lycopene.

Table 2.1 Lycopene contents of some tomato products

Tomato product	Lycopene content (μg/g)
Fresh tomatoes	8.8–42.0
Tomato sauce	62.0
Tomato paste	54.0–1500.0
Tomato juice	50.0–116.0
Ketchup	99.0–134.4
Pizza sauce	127.1

From ref. 58.

usual dietary intake in Germany to be approximately 5 mg daily[56] but others have estimated the average daily intake in North America to be as high as 25 mg, with processed products accounting for at least 50% of the total intake. Based on these findings the recommended daily intake is about 35 mg, which is rarely met.[57]

Processed tomato products such as tomato ketchup, tomato paste and tomato juice are all good sources of lycopene and, unlike some other nutrients, lycopene is not lost through cooking or food processing. Indeed, the lycopene bioavailability increases with heat processing and therefore tomato-based products are a better source than raw tomatoes (Table 2.1).[58] Studies have shown that heat processing causes isomerisation of the ingested *trans*-lycopene to the *cis*-form, which may be responsible for the increased absorption.[57]

Metabolism and pharmacokinetics

Lycopene is one of the carotenoids present in humans in the greatest amount, and plasma concentrations range from 0.22 to 1.06 μmol/L. After administration of tomato juice containing high levels of lycopene, peak plasma concentrations were reported from 24 to 48 hours, and elimination half-life was estimated to be 48–72 hours.[59]

After ingestion, lycopene is metabolised to a series of epoxides and diols (see Table 4.1).[60]

Although most studies have been carried out using high-dose lycopene (16.5–75 mg/day), in a recent study using low-dose lycopene (5 mg/day) over a period of six weeks, it was found that tomato juice and softgel capsules led to higher rates of absorption than fresh tomatoes.[56]

A lipid-rich diet also increases the bioavailability of lycopene and therefore the addition of oil to sauces and soups is beneficial. The presence of β-carotene and other carotenoids in the diet also enhance the bioavailability of lycopene, and the carotenoids seem to act synergistically.[54] Once ingested, lycopene is found distributed non-uniformly in most human tissues. It concentrates in adrenal glands, testes, liver and prostate.[54]

> Therapeutic areas: Cardiovascular and respiratory health, cancer prevention (antioxidant)
> Legal classification: No restriction
> Recommended dose: 10–40 mg/day
> Formulations available: Tablet, capsule, oral gel

Lutein

Structure and properties

Lutein (Figure 2.19) (and zeaxanthin) are highly concentrated in the eye, specifically the macula, and function as antioxidants. They exist in a number of foods, such as green vegetables, particularly spinach.[61]

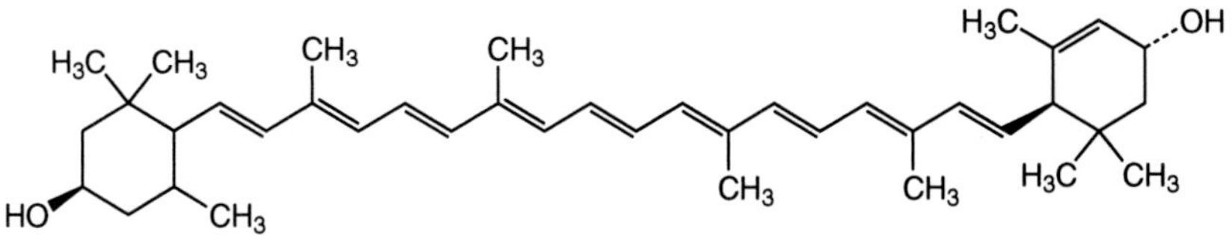

Figure 2.19 The structure of lutein.

Metabolism and pharmacokinetics

Limited data are available. The bioavailability of lutein has been shown to depend upon the chemical and physical nature of the food source, and co-consumed material, particularly the fat content.

> Therapeutic areas: Cardiovascular, eye and skin health (antioxidant)
> Legal classification: No restriction
> Recommended dose: 10–40 mg/day
> Formulations available: Capsule

Zeaxanthin and astaxanthin

Structure and properties

The structures of zeaxanthin and astaxanthin are shown in Figure 2.20.

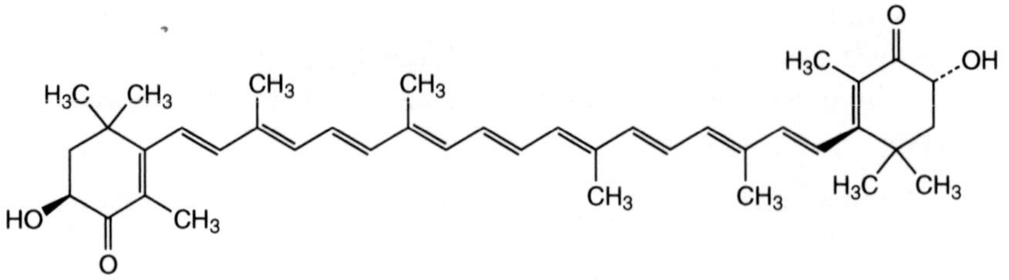

Figure 2.20 The structures of astaxanthin and zeaxanthin.

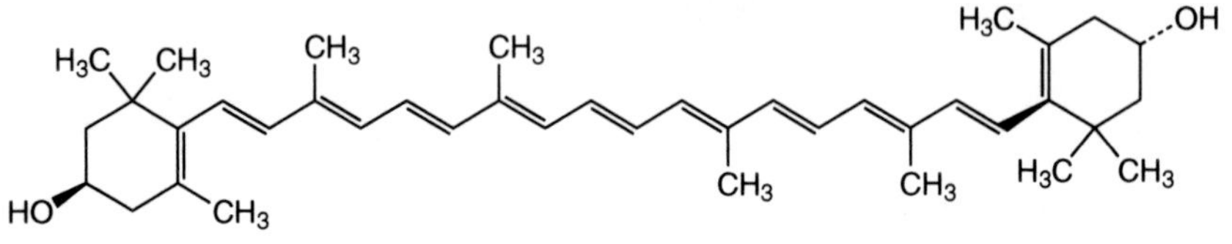

Metabolism and pharmacokinetics

The major metabolites of zeaxanthin have been shown to be lutein and 3′-dehydro-lutein, and the time courses of plasma concentrations were similar for both. Half-life for accumulation was 5 days.[62]

> Therapeutic areas: Eye health (antioxidant)
> Legal classification: No restriction
> Recommended dose: 10–40 mg/day
> Formulations available: Capsule

α-Lipoic acid

Structure and properties

Lipoic acid (synonym: thiotic acid) (Figure 2.21) is present in all kinds of prokaryotic and eukaryotic cells, and is linked to lysine residues on proteins. In humans it is involved in energy production, and acts as a redox couple in combination with its reduced form, dihydrolipoic acid. It is found in high amounts in metabolic organs such as the heart (pig heart contains 1.1–1.6 mg/kg).

α-Lipoic acid is an antioxidant found naturally in meat, liver and yeast,[63] which is readily absorbed from the diet, but also synthesised by animals and humans. In many tissues it is rapidly converted to dihydrolipoic acid, which acts synergistically with other antioxidants.

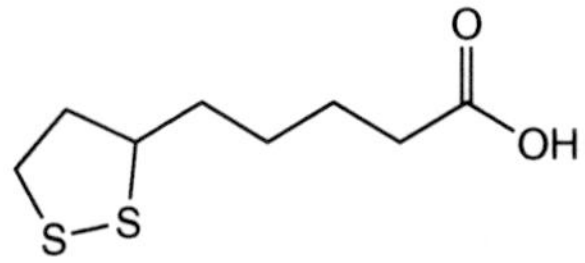

Figure 2.21 The structure of lipoic acid.

Dihydrolipoic acid is a non-essential nutrient created by the human body and so deficiencies are not known to occur.

Metabolism and pharmacokinetics

The primary metabolites found in humans are the result of *S*-methylation and β-oxidation (see Table 4.1). Urinary excretion of lipoic acid and its major metabolites account for only 12.4% of the administered dose.[64] Pharmacokinetic parameters for lipoic acid and its metabolites have been reported in humans after administration of 600 mg doses once daily for 4 days. The parameters were the same on both day 1 and day 4, and there were prolonged half-lives for the major metabolites compared with that of lipoic acid.[64] After oral administration to humans, the absolute bioavailability was calculated as 20–38%, depending on isomer and formulation.[65]

> Therapeutic areas: Eye and veterinary health (antioxidant)
> Legal classification: No restriction
> Recommended dose: 50–100 mg/day
> Formulations available: Tablet, capsule, liquid

Dehydroepiandrosterone

Structure and properties

Dehydroepiandrosterone (DHEA) (synonym: Prasterone) (Figure 2.22) and its metabolite DHEA sulfate (DHEAS) are endogenous hormones

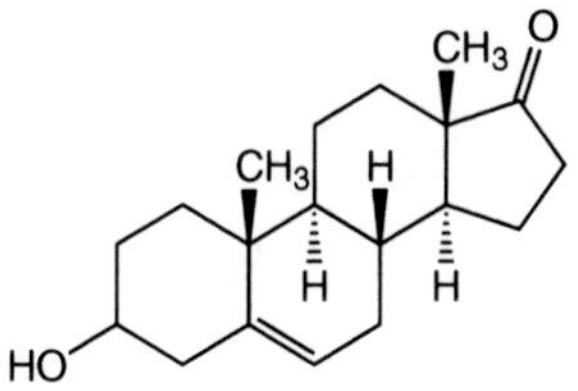

Figure 2.22 The structure of dehydroepiandrosterone (DHEA).

synthesised and excreted mainly in the adrenal gland, in response to adrenocorticotropic hormone.[66]

Metabolism and pharmacokinetics

DHEA is converted to DHEAS, and further to androstenedione, and androstenediol, and testosterone. The elimination half-life of DHEA is 15–38 minutes, and for DHEAS it is 7–22 hours. Oral absorption is excellent.[66]

> Therapeutic areas: Cardiovascular and mental health, veterinary health
> Legal classification: POM in UK
> Recommended dose: 5–25 mg/day
> Formulations available: Tablet

Soy isoflavones

Structure and properties

Although soy is grown in many countries of the world, and the USA is now a major producer, the major consumers are traditionally the inhabitants of East Asia. Soy is available in a wide variety of different food

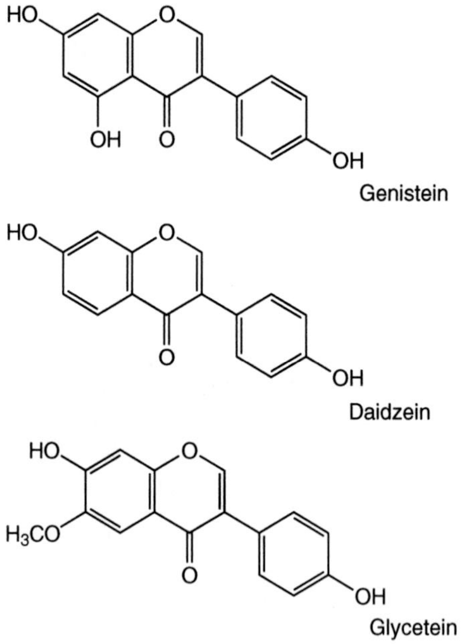

Genistein

Daidzein

Glycetein

Figure 2.23 The structures of genistein, daidzein and glycitein.

forms, for example whole soybeans, soy sauce, tofu (soybean curd), tempeh, soymilk, miso (fermented soybean paste) and natto (fermented soybeans).[67]

The major isoflavones present in soybeans are genistein, daidzein and, to a lesser extent glycitein (Figure 2.23). Genistein is found in the highest proportion. This conjugates to form its β-glycoside genistin in biological fluids. Daidzein and its β-glycoside daidzin are less abundant in soy foods but still present in significant quantity.[68] A third isoflavone, glycitin (and its aglycone glycitein), is found in soy but this has been much less researched as it is only found in relatively small amounts. These isoflavones are available as extracted compounds, in a range of foods, in traditional and modern commercial products, and in soy protein.

The isoflavone content of raw soybean is around 1 mg/g but is highly variable, varying between 0.4 to 2.4 mg/g depending on growing conditions and crop variety. Highly processed products contain much lower isoflavone contents due to manufacturing methods such as alcohol washing of soy concentrates. This process vastly reduces the levels of isoflavone present in the food.

Genistein is found at levels of 1–150 mg/100 g in the mature soybean. Daidzein and its β-glycoside daidzin are less abundant in soy at levels of 0.5–91 mg/100 g.[69] The third isoflavone, glycitin and its aglycone glycitein, are also present in relatively small amounts.

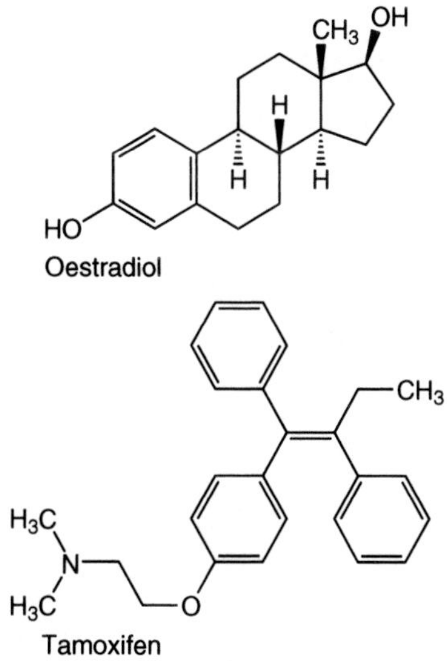

Figure 2.24 The structures of oestradiol and tamoxifen.

The structural similarity between the isoflavones and oestradiol is the basis for the proposition that the isoflavones may be able to replace human oestrogenic activity.

17β-Oestradiol (Figure 2.24) is one of the most potent endogenous oestrogens in humans. The structures of isoflavones are similar to the structure of 17β-oestradiol in two ways: (1) Both have an aromatic ring with a hydroxyl group attached to it; (2) A nearly identical distance exists between the two hydroxyl groups in both.[70]

Comparisons, both structurally and pharmacologically, can be drawn with the oestrogen antagonist tamoxifen, commonly used as a chemopreventative and chemotherapeutic drug for breast cancer (see Figure 2.24).

Metabolism and pharmacokinetics

The bioavailability of the isoflavones can depend on relative uptake rates of the conjugated and free forms of genistein and daidzein, hydrolysis of glycosides by gut bacteria and gut wall enzymes, further metabolism in the liver, and excretion rates.[71]

Genistein and daidzein are efficiently absorbed from the gut and small intestine. In non-fermented soy foods such as soybeans, genistein is conjugated in several different forms but predominantly as the β-glucuronide.[72] Absorption requires prior hydrolysis by β-glucuronidase to the aglycone. This results in a number of metabolic products such as equol (Figure 2.25), which is produced by gastrointestinal flora. This also possesses oestrogenic properties.[73]

In non-fermented soy products the conjugated isoflavones predominate, whereas in fermented products such as soy sauce and miso, the aglycone forms are more abundant. Fermented soy foods therefore already contain the aglycone form of genistein, theoretically allowing this to be absorbed straight into the blood.[74] Cooking also generates this absorbable form by degrading the heat-labile malonyl glucosides of

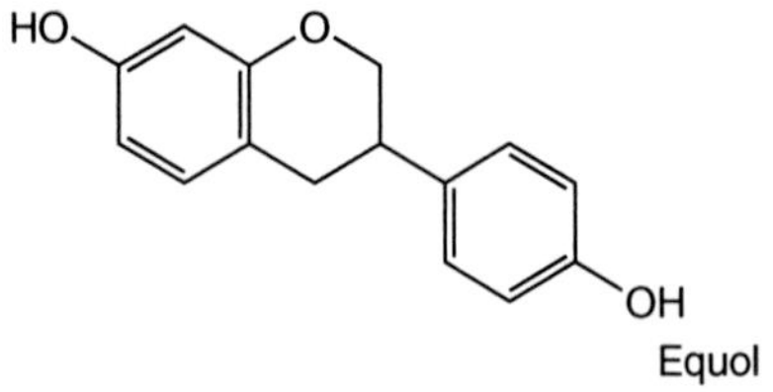

Equol

Figure 2.25 The structure of equol.

daidzein and genistein to the non-acylated form,[75] allowing absorption in the gut. Once in the plasma, the compounds can be taken up by the liver and excreted in the bile as conjugates, mainly as 7-O-β-glucuronide.[73]

The isoflavones become highly bound to proteins in the plasma, and less than 3% will circulate as the free aglycone form.[76] A study conducted on subjects fed a soy beverage for two weeks reported plasma levels of genistein and daidzein to range between 0.55 and 0.96 μmol, mostly as glucuronide and sulfate conjugates.[77]

The metabolism of genistein and daidzein occurs mainly in the liver, and these metabolites are excreted via the biliary, urinary or faecal routes. Only 1–2% of genistein is excreted faecally, the biliary and urinary routes are of greater significance when considering clearance.[78] Genistein and daidzein both undergo extensive first-pass metabolism, removing them from the plasma.[77] The genistein 7-O-β-glucuronide can be excreted in the bile duct, where reabsorption may occur. It was suggested that daidzein is less bioavailable than genistein due to its more rapid excretion in the urine. This may be due, however, to the less hydrophobic nature of daidzein.[71]

> Therapeutic areas: Cardiovascular, mental, bone, women's and skin health, cancer prevention (antioxidant and oestrogenic)
> Legal classification: No restriction
> Recommended dose: 30–50 mg/day
> Formulations available: Tablet, powder

Tea

Structure and properties

Tea is obtained from *Camellia sinensis*, an evergreen shrub native to South-East Asia but cultivated in over 30 countries worldwide.[79] Tea is derived from the leaves of the plant, with the top two leaves and the bud producing the finest tea.[80] The leaves contain polyphenols (approximately a third of the dry weight)[81] together with an enzyme called polyphenol oxidase.

Approximately 3 billion kg of tea are produced and consumed each year[82] and of the three main types of tea produced – black, green and oolong – black tea accounts for approximately 78% of the total consumed worldwide, with green tea representing 20% and oolong tea less than 2%.[79]

Green tea is produced by steaming or heating the freshly harvested leaves; this inactivates the enzyme polyphenol oxidase, and prevents

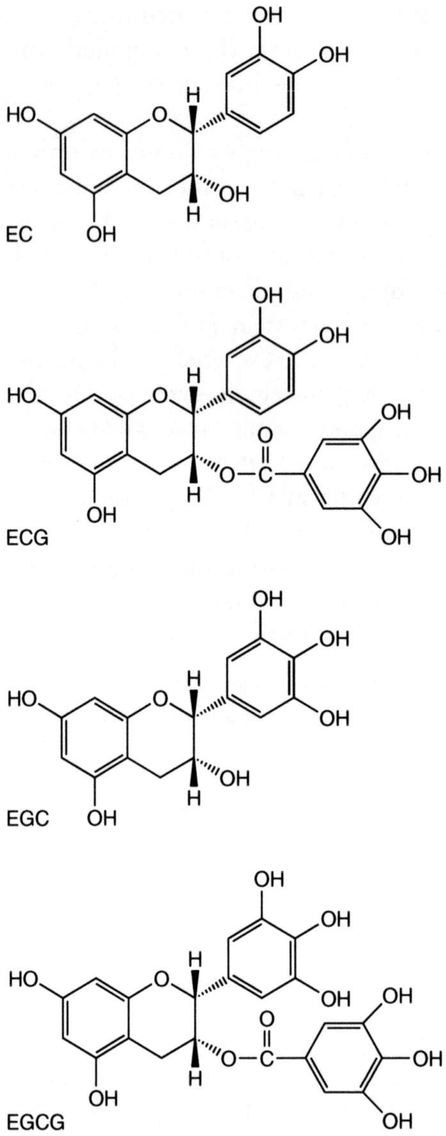

Figure 2.26 The major catechins in tea: (—)-epicatechin (EC), (—)-epicatechin gallate (ECG), (—)-epigallocatechin (EGC) and (—)-epigallocatechin gallate (EGCG).

fermentation of the polyphenols such as catechins. To produce black tea the leaves are left to wither, which allows the moisture content to decrease. The leaves are then rolled and crushed, which permits the release of polyphenol oxidase and the oxidation of the polyphenols. The catechins (polyphenols) are converted into theaflavins and thearubigins. After 60–90 minutes the product is dried using a stream of hot air.[79,83–85] Oolong tea is produced via the same process as black tea but the leaves are dried with hot air after only 30 minutes, and therefore only partial fermentation occurs.[81]

The polyphenols (proanthocyanidins) include catechins, quercetin, myricetin and kaempferol and they account for 30–42% of the dry weight of tea. Catechins are the main components and the four principal ones found in tea are (—)-epicatechin (EC), (—)-epicatechin gallate (ECG), (—)-epigallocatechin (EGC) and (—)-epigallocatechin gallate (EGCG),[86] of which EGCG is the most abundant, accounting for 50–80% of the catechins.[83] A typical brewed cup of green tea, approximately 240 mL, can contain up to 200 mg of EGCG.[79] Figure 2.26 shows the structures of the major catechins in tea.

In addition to gallic acids and theanine, green tea contains approximately 3–6% of caffeine, and theophylline and theobromine.[83] Black tea also contains catechins but to a lesser extent – only 3–10% of the dry weight compared with 30–42% in green tea. Black tea also contains theaflavins, including: theaflavin, theaflavin-3-gallate, theaflavin-3'-gallate and theaflavin-3,3'-digallate. Theaflavins only account for 2–6% of the dry weight of black tea; thearubigins are the major components accounting for over 20% of the dry weight.[85] Thearubigins have a higher molecular weight than theaflavins and are presently poorly defined chemically.[85] Black tea contains slightly less caffeine than green tea, on average 2–4% of the dry weight. Oolong tea also contains thearubigins, theaflavins and catechins.[83] Figure 2.27 shows the basic structures of theaflavins.

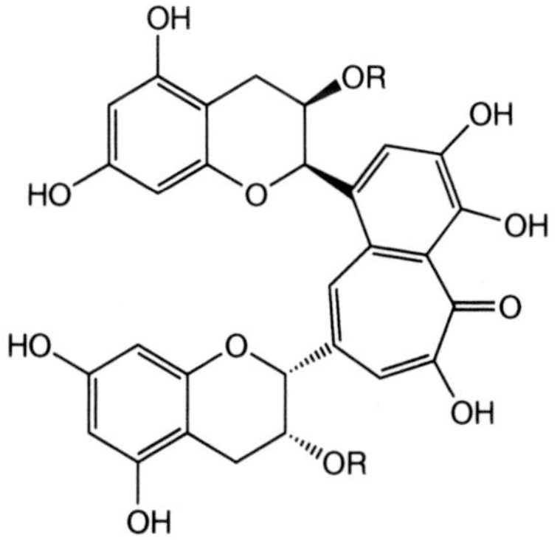

Theaflavins (R = H or gallate–all combinations possible)

Figure 2.27 The structure of the theaflavins.

Catechins are the main polyphenolic component of green tea and EGCG has been claimed to be the most biologically active.[87]

Metabolism and pharmacokinetics

Following the administration of decaffeinated green tea (1.5, 3.0 and 4.5 g tea solids) to human volunteers, peak plasma concentrations of 326, 550 and 190 µg/L were observed for EGCG, EGC and EC, respectively 1.4–2.4 hours after ingestion. The half-life of EGCG (5.0–5.5 hours) was higher than the half-lives of EGC or EC (2.5–3.4 hours). Over 90% of total EGC and EC were excreted in the urine within 8 hours, but EGCG was not, only appearing in faeces.[88]

Following consumption of 2–3 cups of green tea, peak saliva levels of 4.8–22, 11.7–43.9 and 1.8–7.5 mg/L were observed respectively for EGCG, EGC and EC. After volunteers held a solution of EGCG in their mouths for a few minutes, both EGCG and EGC were detected in saliva. EGCG was converted to EGC via an enzyme, catechin esterase, and both compounds were absorbed through the oral mucosa.[88] These results suggest that drinking tea slowly is very effective in delivering high concentrations of catechins to the oral cavity and oesophagus.[85]

In another study in humans, single oral doses of 200–800 mg EGCG were administered, and the mean area under the plasma concentration time curves of EGCG was from 22.5 to 167.1 min $\times$ µg/mL for the 200–800 mg doses. EGC and EC were not detected in the plasma, and the availability of EGCG increased over the dosage range, possibly due to the presence of saturable presystemic elimination.[89] Later work using multiple-dose administration of EGCG revealed a >60% increase in the plasma concentration time curves after four weeks of administration at the 800 mg doses.[90] A study using 195 mg EGCG found similar pharmacokinetic data, but considerable interindividual variability was noted.[91]

Catechin bioavailability from 28 studies has been reviewed.[92] It was noted that the bioavailability differed markedly between the different catechins. EGCG was seen to be methylated in a number of studies, at either the 4'-O- or 4',4''-di-O-positions, and these were often the major metabolites of EGCG. EGCG is also the only polyphenol present in plasma as a major proportion of the ingested dose. Other catechins have been found as glucuronide and sulfate conjugates.[92] A range of hydroxyphenyl valerolactone analogues have been identified in plasma and urine, mainly as conjugates, and these account for high levels

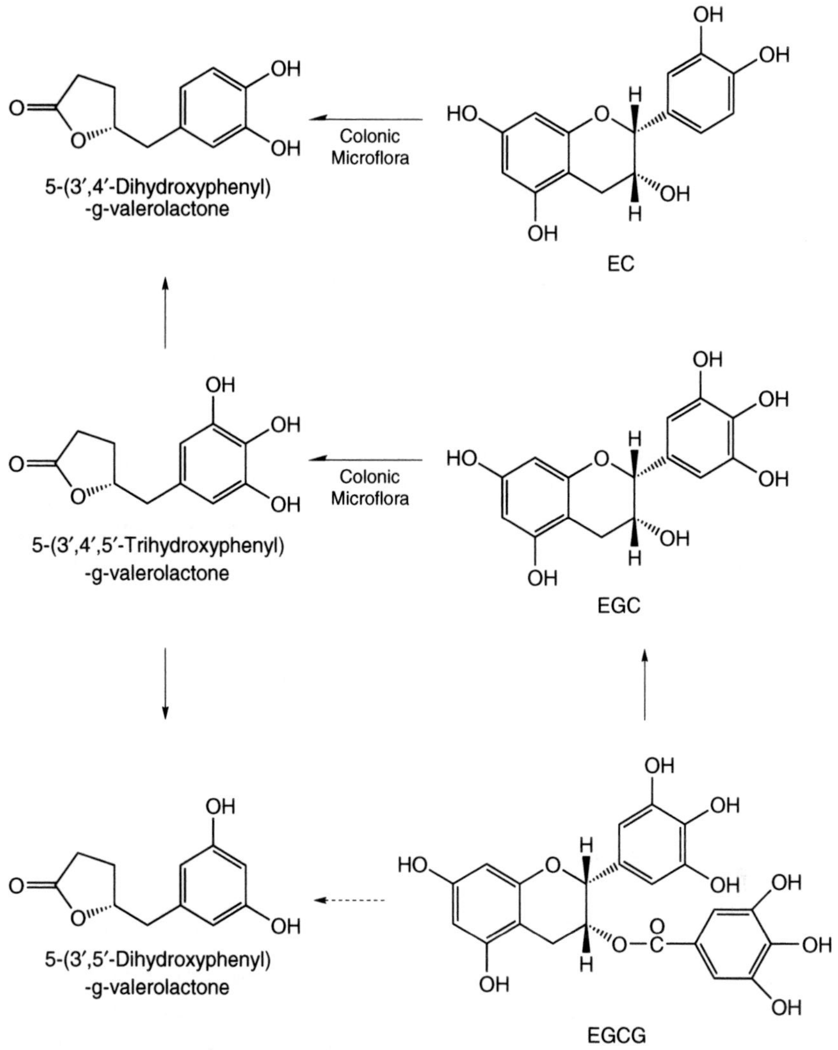

Figure 2.28 Biotransformation of catechins. Reprinted from Lambert J D, Yang Chung S. Cancer chemopreventive activity and bioavailability of tea and tea polyphenols. *Mutat Res* 2003; 523–524: 201–208, with permission.

of EGC and EC, 8–25 times the levels detected of the unchanged compounds.[92]

Tea polyphenols have low bioavailability due to their high molecular weights and polarity. The large number of hydroxyl substituents may hinder absorption of the compounds across the gut lumen.[93]

Figure 2.28 outlines a number of human metabolites from catechins catalysed by colonic microflora. A number of methylations of EC, EGC and EGCG catalysed by catechol-O-methyltransferase (COMT) have also been shown to give rise to mono- and di-methyl forms.[93]

Human colonic microflora, *in vitro*, have also been shown to degrade exogenous catechin polymers into monohydroxylated phenylacetic, phenylpropionic and phenylvaleric acids, over 48 hours of incubation in anoxic conditions.[94] Catechins themselves are rapidly eliminated, but galloylated catechins such as ECG and EGCG have not been detected in the urine, due to their preferential excretion in the bile.[91]

Tea polyphenols have low bioavailability due to their high molecular weights and a high number of hydroxyl substituents. This makes them susceptible to phase II enzymes, resulting in their biotransformation. Also, the hydroxyl groups may hinder absorption of the compounds across the gut lumen.[95] The theaflavins are still less bioavailable.[84]

> Therapeutic areas: Cardiovascular, bone, skin and oral health, cancer prevention and weight management (antioxidant)
> Legal classification: No restriction
> Recommended dose: 5–100 mg/day of tea polyphenols
> Formulations available: Tablet, capsule, powder, tea

Creatine

Structure and properties

Creatine (Figure 2.29) is distributed throughout the human body, with 95% found in skeletal muscle.[96] It occurs naturally in the human diet, as red meat and fish contain 4–10 g/kg. It is also synthesised in the kidney, liver and pancreas. Creatine supplementation gives rise to higher levels of phosphocreatine, which is used to produce and regenerate ATP, resulting in cells being better able to deal with energy requirements in health and disease.[96]

Metabolism and pharmacokinetics

Creatine and phosphocreatine are catabolised to creatinine, which is eliminated in the urine. Creatine pharmacokinetics are non-linear, as skeletal muscle which acts as a depot for creatine, has a finite capacity

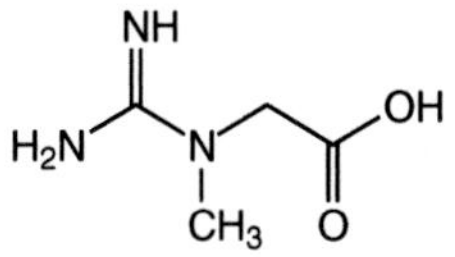

Figure 2.29 The structure of creatine.

for its storage. When this capacity is taken up, the volume of distribution and clearance can decrease, which causes complex pharmacokinetics.[96]

Therapeutic areas: Mental health, sport enhancement
Legal classification: No restriction
Recommended dose: 5–25 g/day
Formulations available: Tablet, capsule, effervescent tablet, liquid

References

1. Briffa J. Glucosamine sulphate in the treatment of osteoarthritis. *J Altern Complement Med* 1997; 15: 15–16.
2. Muller-Fabbender H, Bach G L, Haase W *et al.* Glucosamine sulphate compared to ibuprofen in osteoarthritis of the knee. *Osteoarthritis Cartilage* 1994; 2: 61–69.
3. Setnikar I, Rovati L C. Absorption, distribution, metabolism and excretion of glucosamine sulfate. A review. *Arzneimittel-Forschung* 2001; 51: 699–725.
4. Conte A, Volpi N, Palmieri L, Bahous I, Ronca G. Biochemical and pharmacokinetic aspects of oral treatment with chondroitin sulfate. *Arzneimittel-Forschung* 1995; 45: 918–925.
5. Volpi N. Oral absorption and bioavailability of ichthyic origin chondroitin sulfate in healthy male volunteers. *Osteoarthritis Cartilage* 2003; 11: 433–441.
6. Conte A, De Bernardi M, Palmieri L *et al.* Metabolic fate of exogenous chondroitin sulfate in man. *Arzneimittel-Forschung* 1991; 41: 768–772.
7. Ely A, Lockwood B. What is the evidence for the safety and efficacy of dimethyl sulphoxide and methylsulphonylmethane in pain relief ? *Pharm J* 2002; 269: 685–687.
8. Jacob S W, Lawrence D M, Zucker M. *The Miracle of MSM: The Natural Solution for Pain.* New York: Putnam's, 1999.
9. Kolb K H, Janicke G, Kramer M, Schulze P E, Raspe G. Absorption, distribution and elimination of labelled diemethylsulfoxide in man and animals. *Ann N Y Acad Sci* 1967; 141: 85–95.
10. Mason P. *Dietary Supplements,* 2nd edn. London: Pharmaceutical Press, 2001.
11. Weber C, Bysted A, Holmer G. Coenzyme Q10 in the diet – daily intake and relative bioavailability. *Mol Asp Med* 1997; 18: s251–s254.
12. Grunler J, Dallner G. Investigation of regulatory mechanisms in coenzyme Q metabolism. *Method Enzymol* 2004; 378: 3–17.
13. Birdsall TC. The biological effects and clinical uses of the pineal hormone melatonin. *Altern Med Rev* 1996; 1: 94–101.

14. Brzezinski A. Melatonin in humans. *N Engl J Med* 1997; 336: 186–195.
15. Lamberg L. Melatonin potentially useful but safety, efficacy remain uncertain. *JAMA* 1996; 276: 1011–1014.
16. Moss J. Melatonin revisited – what is it? *Altern Ther Clin Pract* 1996; 3: 11–14.
17. Garfinkle D, Laudon M, Nof D, Zisapel N. Improvement of sleep quality in elderly people by controlled-release melatonin. *Lancet* 1995; 346: 541–544.
18. Gladwin C. Time capsule. *Chemist and Druggist* 1997; 2 Aug.
19. Kletzmayr J, Mayer G, Legenstein E *et al.* Anemia and carnitine supplementation in hemodialyzed patients. *Kidney Int* 1999; 55: S93–S106.
20. Kelly G S. L-Carnitine: therapeutic applications of a conditionally essential amino acid. *Altern Med Rev* 1998; 3: 345–360.
21. Walter P, Schaffhauser A O. L-Carnitine, a 'vitamin-like substance' for functional food. Proceedings of the Symposium on L-Carnitine, April 28 to May 1, 2000, Zermatt, Switzerland. *Ann Nutr Metab* 2000; 44: 75–96.
22. Li Wan Po A. Carnitine: a scientifically exciting molecule. *Pharm J* 1990; 245: 388–389.
23. Rodriguez-Benitez P, Perez-Garcia R, Arenas J, Valderrabano F. L-Carnitine in dialysis, more than a commercial affair. *Nephrol Dial Transplant* 2000; 15: 1477–1478.
24. Brass E P, Hiatt W R. The role of carnitine and carnitine supplementation during exercise in man and in individuals with special needs. *J Am Coll Nutr* 1998; 3: 207–215.
25. Grandi M, Perderzoli S, Sacchetti C. Effect of acute carnitine administration on glucose insulin metabolism in healthy subjects. *Int J Clin Pharmacol Res* 1997; 17: 143–147.
26. Etzioni A, Levy J, Nitzan M, Erde P, Benderly A. Systemic carnitine deficiency exacerbated by a strict vegetarian diet. *Arch Dis Childhood* 1984; 59: 177–179.
27. Rebouche C J, Chenard C A. Metabolic fate of dietary carnitine in human adults: identification and quantification of urinary and fecal metabolites. *J Nutr* 1991; 121: 539–546.
28. Anon. Carnitine deficiency. *Lancet* 1991; 335: 631–633.
29. Inoue F, Terada N, Nakajima K *et al.* Effect of sports activity on carnitine metabolism. *Nippon Iyo Masu Supekutoru Gakkai Koenshu* 1998; 23: 169–172.
30. Spagnoli A, Lucca U, Menasce G *et al.* Long-term acetyl-L-carnitine treatment in Alzheimer's disease. *Neurology* 1991; 41: 1726–1732.
31. Carta A, Calvani M, Bravi D, Bhuachalla S N. Acetyl-L-carnitine and Alzheimer's disease: pharmacological considerations beyond the cholinergic sphere. *Ann N Y Acad Sci* 1993; 695: 324–326.
32. Pettegrew J W, Klunk W E, Panchalingam K, Kanfer J N, McClure R J. Clinical and neurochemical effects of acetyl-L-carnitine in Alzheimer's disease. *Neurobiol Aging* 1995; 16: 1–4.
33. Kato S, Karino K, Hasegawa S *et al.* Octacosanol affects lipid metabolism in rats fed on a high-fat diet. *Br J Nutr* 1995; 73: 433–441.
34. Saint-John M, McNaughton L. Octacosanol ingestion and its effects on

metabolic responses to submaximal cycle ergometry, reaction time and chest and grip strength. *Int Clin Nutr Rev* 1986; 6: 81–87.

35. Lin Y, Rudrum M, van der Wielen R P J *et al.* Wheat germ policosanol failed to lower plasma cholesterol in subjects with normal to mildly elevated cholesterol concentrations. *Metab Clin Exp* 2004; 53: 1309–1314.

36. Gouni-Berthold I, Berthold H K. Policosanol: clinical pharmacology and therapeutic significance of a new lipid-lowering agent. *Am Heart J* 2002; 143: 356–365.

37. Stramentinoli G. Pharmacologic aspects of S-adenosylmethionine. Pharmacokinetics and pharmacodynamics. *Am J Med* 1987; 83: 35–42.

38. Fetrow C W, Avila J R. Efficacy of the dietary supplement S-adenosyl-L-methionine. *Ann Pharmacother* 2001; 35: 1414–1425.

39. Linko Y-Y, Hayakawa K. Docosahexaenoic acid: a valuable nutraceutical? *Trends Food Sci Technol* 1996; 7: 59–63.

40. Marsen T A, Pollok M, Oette K, Baldamus C A. Pharmacokinetics of omega-3-fatty acids during ingestion of fish oil preparations. *Prostaglandins Leukot Essent Fatty Acids* 1992; 46: 191–201.

41. Martens-Lobenhoffer J, Meyer F P. Pharmacokinetic data of γ-linolenic acid in healthy volunteers after the administration of evening primrose oil (Epogam). *Int J Clin Pharmacol Ther* 1998; 36: 363–366.

42. Erasmus U. *Fats that Heal, Fats that Kill: The Complete Guide to Fats, Oils and Cholesterol*, 2nd edn. Burnaby BC, Canada: Alive Books, 1993.

43. Simopoulos A P. Essential fatty acids in health and chronic disease. *Am J Clin Nutr* 1999; 70: 560S–569S.

44. Cunnane S C, Zhen-Yu C, Yang J *et al.* α-Linoleic acid in humans: direct functional role or dietary precursor? *Nutrition* 1991; 7: 437–439.

45. Kelly G S. Conjugated linoleic acid: a review. *Altern Med Rev* 2001; 6: 367–382.

46. Rowland I, Faughnan M, Hoey L *et al.* Bioavailability of phyto-oestrogens. *Br J Nutr* 2003; 89: S45–S58.

47. Heinonen S, Nurmi T, Liukkonen K *et al.* In vitro metabolism of plant lignans: new precursors of mammalian lignans enterolactone and enterodiol. *J Agric Food Chem* 2001 49: 3178–3186.

48. Rohdewald P. A review of the French maritime pine bark extract (Pycnogenol), a herbal medication with a diverse clinical pharmacology. *Int J Clin Pharmacol Ther* 2002; 40: 158–168.

49. Duweler K G, Rohdewald P. Urinary metabolites of French maritime pine bark extract in humans. *Die Pharmazie* 2000; 55: 364–368.

50. Wolter F, Stein J. Biological activities of resveratrol and its analogs. *Drugs of the Future* 2002; 27: 949–959.

51. Sovak, M. Grape extract , resveratrol, and its analogs: a review. *J Med Food* 2001; 4: 93–105.

52. Haslam E. *Plant Polyphenols: Vegetable Tannins Revisited.* Cambridge: Cambridge University Press, 1989.

53. Ward N C, Croft K D, Puddey I B, Hodgson J M. Supplementation with grape seed polyphenols results in increased urinary excretion of 3-hydroxyphenyl-propionic acid, an important metabolite of proanthocyanidins in humans. *J Agric Food Chem* 2004; 52: 5545–5549.

54. Bramley P M. Is lycopene beneficial to human health? *Phytochemistry* 2000; 54: 233–236.

55. Hughes D A, Wright A J, Finglas P M *et al.* Effects of lycopene and lutein supplementation on the expression of functionally associated surface molecules on blood monocytes from healthy male nonsmokers. *J Infect Dis* 2000; 18: S11–S15.

56. Bohm V, Bitsch R. Intestinal absorption of lycopene from different matrices and interactions to other carotenoids, the lipid status, and the antioxidant capacity of human plasma. *Eur J Nutr* 1999; 38: 118–125.

57. Rao A V, Agarwal S. Role of antioxidant lycopene in cancer and heart disease. *J Am Coll Nutr* 2000; 19: 563–569.

58. Rao A V, Agarwal S. Role of lycopene as antioxidant carotenoid in the prevention of chronic diseases: a review. *Nutr Res* 1999; 19: 305–323.

59. Schwedhelm E, Maas R, Troost R, Boeger R H. Clinical pharmacokinetics of antioxidants and their impact on systemic oxidative stress. *Clin Pharmacokinet* 2003; 42: 437–459.

60. Khachik F, Carvalho L, Bernstein P S *et al.* Chemistry, distribution, and metabolism of tomato carotenoids and their impact on human health. *Exp Biol Med* 2002; 227: 845–851.

61. Alves-Rodrigues A, Shao A. The science behind lutein. *Toxicol Lett* 2004; 150: 57–83.

62. Hartmann D, Thuermann P A, Spitzer V, Schalch W, Manner B, Cohn W. Plasma kinetics of zeaxanthin and 3'-dehydro-lutein after multiple oral doses of synthetic zeaxanthin. *Am J Clin Nutr* 2004; 79: 410–417.

63. Wadsworth F, Lockwood B. Combined alpha-lipoic acid and acetyl-L-carnitine supplementation. *Pharm J* 2003; 270: 587–589.

64. Teichert J, Hermann R, Ruus P, Preiss R. Plasma kinetics, metabolism, and urinary excretion of alpha-lipoic acid following oral administration in healthy volunteers. *J Clin Pharmacol* 2003; 43: 1256–1267.

65. Biewenga G Ph, Haenen G R M M, Bast A. The pharmacology of the antioxidant lipoic acid. *Gen Pharmacol* 1997; 29: 315–331.

66. Pepping J. DHEA: Dehydroepiandrosterone. *Am J Health-Syst Pharm* 2000; 57: 2048, 2050, 2053–2054, 2056.

67. Yamamoto S, Sobue T, Kobayashi M *et al.* Soy, isoflavones and breast cancer risk in Japan. *J Natl Cancer Inst* 2003; 95: 906–913.

68. Murphy P A, Song T, Buseman G *et al.* Isoflavones in retail and institutional soy foods. *J Agric Food Chem* 1999; 47: 2697–2704.

69. Cornwell T, Cohick W, Raskin I. Dietary phytoestrogens and health. *Phytochemistry* 2004; 65: 995–1016.

70. Setchell K D, Cassidy A. Dietary isoflavones: biological effects and relevance to human health. *J Nutr* 1999; 129: 758S–767S.

71. Senior H, Lockwood B. Soy isoflavones – their role in cancer prevention. *Nutrafoods* 2005; 4: 5–17.

72. Kirk C J, Harris R M, Wood D M *et al.* Do dietary phytoestrogens influence susceptibility to hormone-dependent cancer by disrupting the metabolism of endogenous oestrogens? *Biochem Soc Trans* 2001; 29: 209–216.

73. Makela S, Poutanen M, Kostian M L *et al.* Inhibition of 17 beta-hydroxysteroid oxidoreductase by flavonoids in breast and prostate cancer cells. *Proc Soc Exp Biol Med* 1998; 217: 310–316.

74. Le Bail J C, Champavier Y, Chulia A J, Habrioux G. Effects of phytoestrogens on aromatase, 3β and 17β-hydroxysteroid dehydrogenase activities and human breast cancer cells *Life Sci* 2000; 66: 1281–1291.

75. Dixon R A, Ferreira D. Molecules of interest: genistein. *Phytochemistry* 2002; 60: 205–211.

76. Vermeulen A. Metabolic effects of obesity in men *Koninkl Acad Geneesk Belgie* 1993; 55: 393–397.

77. Steensma A, Noteborn H P J M, Van der Jagt R C M *et al.* Bioavailability of genistein, daidzein, and their glycosides in intestinal epithelial Caco-2 cells. *Environ Toxicol Pharmacol* 1999; 7: 209–212.

78. Adlercreutz H, Honjo H, Higashi A *et al.* Urinary excretion of lignans and isoflavonoid phytoestrogens in Japanese men and women consuming a traditional Japanese diet. *Am J Clin Nutr* 1991; 54: 1093–1100.

79. Mukhtar H, Ahmad N. Tea polyphenols: prevention of cancer and optimizing health. *Am J Clin Nutr* 2000; 71: 1698S–1702S.

80. Weisburger J H. Prevention of coronary heart disease and cancer by tea. A review. *Environ Health Prevent Med* 2003; 7: 283–288.

81. Weisburger J H, Chung F-L. Mechanisms of chronic disease causation by nutrtional factors and tobacco products and their prevention by tea polyphenols. *Food Chem Toxicol* 2002; 40: 1145–1154.

82. Yang C S, Landau J M. Effects of tea consumption on nutrition and health. *J Nutr* 2000; 130: 2409–2412.

83. Siddiqui I A, Afaq F, Adhami V M *et al.* Antioxidants of the beverage tea in promotion of human health. *Antiox Redox Signal* 2004; 6: 571–582.

84. Lambert J D, Yang C S. Mechanisms of cancer prevention by tea constituents. *J Nutr* 2003; 133: 3262S–3267S.

85. Yang C S, Chung J Y, Yang G *et al.* Tea and tea polyphenols in cancer prevention. *J Nutr* 2000; 130: 472S–478S.

86. Hakim I A, Harris R B, Brown S *et al.* Effect of increased tea consumption on oxidative DNA damage among smokers: a randomized controlled study. *J Nutr* 2003; 133: 3303S–3309S.

87. Fujiki H. Two stages of cancer prevention with green tea. *J Cancer Res Clin Oncol* 1999; 125: 589–597.

88. Yang C S, Chen L, Lee M J, Balentine D. Blood and urine levels of tea catechins after ingestion of different amounts of green tea by human volunteers. *Cancer Epidemiol Biomarkers Prev* 1998; 7: 351–354.

89. Chow H-H S, Cai Y, Alberts D S *et al.* Phase I pharmacokinetic study of tea polyphenols following single-dose administration of epigallocatechin gallate and polyphenon E. *Cancer Epidemiol Biomarkers Prev* 2001; 10: 53–58.

90. Chow H-H S, Cai Y, Hakim I A, Crowell J A. Pharmacokinetics and safety of green tea polyphenols after multiple-dose administration of epigallocatechin gallate and polyphenon E in healthy individuals. *Clin Cancer Res* 2003; 9: 3312–3319.

91. Lee M-J, Maliakal P, Chen L, Meng X. Pharmacokinetics of tea catechins after ingestion of green tea and (—)-epigallocatechin-3-gallate by humans: formation of different metabolites and individual variability. *Cancer Epidemiol Biomarkers Prev* 2002; 11: 1025–1032.

92. Manach C, Williamson G, Morand C *et al.* Bioavailability and bioefficacy of

polyphenols in humans. I. Review of 97 bioavailability studies. *Am J Clin Nutr* 2005; 81: 230S–242S.

93. Lambert J D, Yang Chung S. Cancer chemopreventive activity and bioavailability of tea and tea polyphenols. *Mutat Res* 2003; 523–524, 201–208.

94. Deprez S, Brezillon C, Rabot S *et al*. Polymeric proanthocyanidins are catabolized by human colonic microflora into low-molecular-weight phenolic acids. *J Nutr* 2000; 130: 2733–2738.

95. Lipinski C A., Lombardo F, Dominy B W, Feeney P J. Experimental and computational approaches to estimate solubility and permeability in drug discovery and development settings. *Adv Drug Deliv Res* 2001; 46: 3–26.

96. Persky A M, Brazeau G A. Clinical pharmacology of the dietary supplement creatine monohydrate. *Pharmacol Rev* 2001; 53: 161–176.

3

Source, manufacture and analysis of major nutraceuticals

Table 3.1 summarises information on the source, manufacturer, GRAS (Generally Recognized As Safe) status and representative analytical techniques available for a selection of major nutraceuticals.

Most nutraceuticals are natural products, being derived roughly equally from plants and animals. Some are endogenous human metabolites, while others are common dietary constituents that appear in human metabolism, for example lycopene. A number of entities exist in higher plants, and are commercially extracted from them, although some are present in insufficient levels for commercial exploitation, such as methyl-sulfonylmethane (MSM) and dehydroepiandrosterone (DHEA), and consequently are produced commercially by chemical synthesis. Similarly, those of animal origin may be produced by chemical synthesis, such as carnitine, creatine and the carotenoids, but may also be produced by fermentation, such as coenzyme Q10 (Co Q10) and S-adenosyl methionine (SAMe). Soy isoflavones which occur naturally in the glycoside form are available as both glycosides and their aglycones, and are invariably complex mixtures, as are green tea extracts, grape seed proanthocyanidin extract (GSPE) and pycnogenol. The n-3 fatty acids such as docosahexaenoic acid (DHA)/eicosapentaenoic acid (EPA) and α-linolenic acid are usually available as complex mixtures, containing supradietary levels of the active constituents, and often partial purification from the other fatty acids is not carried out. However, enrichment of these entities is increasingly being carried out using sophisticated techniques.[29,30] Microalgal fermentation is also an option for production of DHA/EPA.[31] In certain cases nutraceuticals exist in a number of isomeric forms, which may have varied activities or even be toxic; an example of this latter situation occurs with carnitine, in which the D-form is toxic, and thus chiral synthesis of the L-form is carried out.[18]

Because of their long standing presence in particular foodstuffs, a number of nutraceuticals have GRAS status as defined by the US Food and Drug Administration (FDA), and increasingly manufacturers are

Table 3.1 Major nutraceuticals, their source, manufacture and extraction, and techniques used for their analysis

Nutraceutical	Source	Manufacture/extraction/fermentation	GRAS	Analytical techniques
Glucosamine	Bovine trachea, shellfish[1]	Chitin acid hydrolysis,[2] fish shell enzymic hydrolysis[3]		HPLC[U,R,P 4]
Chondroitin	Bovine trachea/cartilage[1]	Enzymic hydrolysis of beef trachea[5]	✓	HPLC[R 6] Agarose electrophoresis[P 7] CE[R 8]
Methylsulfonylmethane	Meat, milk, capers, etc.[9]	Distillate of peroxide oxidation of DMSO[10]	✓	GC[P,U 11]
Coenzyme Q10	Common foods[12]	MeOH/NaOH digest of hearts/livers after H2S treatment,[13] fermentation[1]	✓	HPLC-Electrochemical detector[R 14] HPLC-Electrochemical detector[P 15]
Melatonin	Bovine pineal glands[16]	Aqueous extraction of defatted beef pineal glands[17]	✓	RIA[P,U 16] GC-MS[R 16] HPLC[P,U 16]
Carnitine	Heart, skeletal muscle[18]	Chiral synthesis from butyrolactone[18]	✓	Chiral HPLC[R 19] HPLC-MS[U 20]
Acetyl-L-carnitine	Brain, liver, kidney[21]	Synthesis from racemic carnitine[22]	✓	HPLC-MS[U 20]
Octacosanol/policosanol	Sugarcane waste, wheatgerm, rice bran[23]	Ultrasound aqueous extraction[24]	✓	GC-MS[R 25]
S-Adenosyl methionine	Meat, yeast, vegetable[26]	Enzymatic synthesis[27]		SPE + HPLC[R,U 28]
Docosahexaenoic acid/eicosapentaenoic acid (DHA/EPA)	Fish, algae, plankton,[29] seal blubber[30]	Oil extraction, lipase-catalysed enrichment,[29] fish oil distillation,[30] microalgal oil[31]	✓	HPLC[R 32] GC[R 32]

Table 3.1 Continued

Nutraceutical	Source	Manufacture/extraction/fermentation	GRAS	Analytical techniques
γ-Linolenic acid	Oenothera biennis, Borago officinalis	Whole oil used		FAME-GC[P 33] GLC[34] FTIR[35]
α-Linolenic acid	Linum usitatissimum	Pressed oil/solvent extraction[36]		As for DHA/EPA FTIR[35]
Conjugated linoleic acid	Beef, dairy products[37]	Microbiological fermentation, extraction from soy/sunflower[38]		Reversed phase HPLC[39]
Flax lignans	Linum usitatissimum	Supercritical extraction CO_2[40]		CCC[41]
Pycnogenol	Pinus pinaster	Aqueous/ethanolic extract of pine bark[42]		As for GSPE
Resveratrol	Red wine,[43] Polygonum capsidatum root,[44] Veratrum sp.,[45] Vaccinium macrocarpon[46]	Mid polarity solvent extraction[47]		HPLC[P 48] CE[R 49] GC-MS[R 44] ELISA[R 44]
Grape seed proanthocyanidin extract (GSPE)	Vitis vinifera	Water/ethanol extraction[50]	√	Supercritical extraction[R 51] HPLC[R 52] LC-MS[R 53] HP Gel permeation chromatography[R 54]
Lycopene	Foods, including tomato,[55,56] green algae[57]	Tomato extraction,[38] chemical synthesis[38]	√	HPLC[R 58]

continued

Table 3.1 Continued

Nutraceutical	Source	Manufacture/extraction/fermentation	GRAS	Analytical techniques
Lutein	Tomato, butternut squash[56]	PET ether extraction of *Tagetes* spp.[59]	√	HPLC[60]
Zeaxanthin	Butternut squash[56]	Unsaponifables of methanol extract[61]		HPLC[56]
Astaxanthin	Fish, shellfish[62]	Oil extract from *Haematococcus pluvialis*[62]		HPLC[63]
Lipoic acid	Meat, liver[37]	Isolation from liver,[64] synthesis[65]		HPLC fluorimetric detector[P,U 66]
Dehydroepiandrosterone	Wild yams[67]	Cholesterol oxidation[68]		HPLC[R 69]; GC-MS[P 70]
Soy isoflavones	Soy and fermented soy products	Fermentation–glycoside hydrolysis[71]		HPLC coulometric electrode array detector[R 72]
Green tea extracts	*Camelia sinensis*	Aqueous extraction, synthesis of catechins[73]		1H-NMR[R 74]
Creatine	Skeletal muscle[76]	Synthesis[77]		CE[R 75]; CE[U 78]

[R]Raw material; [P]Plasma; [U]Urine.

√, GRAS status for named products; HPLC, high-pressure liquid chromatography; CE, capillary electrophoresis; GC, gas chromatography; RIA, radioimmunoassay; GC-MC, gas chromatography–mass spectrometry; SPE, solid phase extraction; CCC, counter current chromatography; ELISA, enzyme-linked immunosorbent assay; FAME, fatty acid methyl esters; FTIR, Fourier transform infrared; NMR, nuclear magnetic resonance.

gaining GRAS certification for products not normally ingested (in realistic levels) by consumption of foodstuffs, such as MSM and octacosanol/policosanol. This certification is thought to enhance the product, by gaining a cachet that denotes that a product is of natural origin, even if it is produced by other means.

A list of GRAS entities is published on the Internet[79] and manufacturers of many consumed constituents often choose to incorporate these constituents as opposed to non-GRAS constituents, as they appear to convey a suggestion of safety to the end product. Nutraceutical manufacturers not only use these products, but also actively press for GRAS status of existing products, and products produced by a new manufacturing process.

As with pharmaceuticals, the analytical procedures used for identification and quantification of nutraceuticals are becoming increasingly sophisticated, reflecting the analytical advances being made, and the desire by manufacturers to produce detailed information about levels of active constituents, both in the natural materials, and in formulated products, but also in biological fluids which are increasingly being investigated both in clinical trials and *in vivo* research in an attempt to determine the fate of ingested entities. Traditional solvent extraction techniques, although still widely used, are often supplanted by solid phase extraction (SPE), and more recently by supercritical fluid extraction, which removes/reduces levels of solvents used, and is particularly beneficial for thermolabile constituents.

Non-polar molecules such as MSM are most easily analysed by gas chromatography (GC)[11] due to their volatility, and polar molecules are widely separated and quantified using high-pressure liquid chromatography (HPLC). A number of detection systems are used in HPLC, such as ultraviolet (UV) and electrochemical detectors, and as with GC, increasingly systems are being linked to mass spectroscopy (MS), to allow detailed elucidation of individual molecular structures. This latter area is now increasingly being used for the identification of metabolites in biological fluids, such as urine and blood plasma, and chromatographic systems are now widely available for the identification and quantification of most nutraceuticals at the low levels found in these matrices.

Agarose electrophoresis has been used for the analysis of chondroitin, and the relatively recent development of capillary electrophoresis (CE) has allowed analysis of a number of extremely complex nutraceuticals such as green tea, and grape and wine products containing GSPE and resveratrol. The phytoestrogens from soy and flax, *n*-3 polyunsaturated fatty acids (PUFAs) and conjugated linoleic acid (CLA), carotenoids, lycopene, zeaxanthin, astaxanthin and lutein, and tea catechins have been the subject of a recent edited book on the subject, in which monographs list techniques for sample preparation and extraction, chromatographic separation, detection methods and quantitation methods.[80]

Particularly in investigation of entities and their metabolites, radioimmunoassays and enzyme-linked immunosorbent assay (ELISA) are now being used for detection at extremely low levels.

References

1. Challener C. Speciality dietary supplements are the hot spot. *Chem Market Report* 2000; 25 Sept.
2. Reginster J Y, Deroisy R, Rovati L C *et al.* Long-term effects of glucosamine sulphate on osteoarthritis progression: a randomised, placebo-controlled clinical trial. *Lancet* 2001; 357: 251–256.
3. Jarvis L. BEI to launch US-based glucosamine production. *Chem Market Report* 2002; 11 March.
4. Liang Z, Leslie J, Adebowale A, Ashraf M, Eddington N D. Determination of the nutraceutical, glucosamine hydrochloride, in raw materials, dosage forms and plasma using pre-column derivatization with ultraviolet HPLC. *J Pharm Biomed Anal* 1999; 20: 807–814.
5. Solabia Product Data – Sulfate de Chondroitin (2004). Solabia, Paris.
6. Way W K, Gibson K G, Breite A G. Determination of chondroitin sulfate in nutritional supplements by liquid chromatography. *J Liq Chromatogr Relat Technol* 2000; 23: 2851–2860.
7. Volpi N. Oral absorption and bioavailability of ichthyic origin chondroitin sulfate in healthy male volunteers. *Osteoarthritis Cartilage* 2003; 11: 433–441.
8. Payan E, Presle N, Lapicque F *et al.* Separation and quantification by ion-association capillary zone electrophoresis of unsaturated disaccharide units of chondroitin sulfates and oligosaccharides derived from hyaluronan. *Anal Chem* 1998; 70: 4780–4786.
9. Ely A, Lockwood B. What is the evidence for the safety and efficacy of dimethyl sulphoxide and methylsulphonylmethane in pain relief ? *Pharm J* 2002; 269: 685–687.
10. Jacob S W, Appleton J. *MSM – The Definitive Guide*. Topanga, CA: Freedom Press, 2003.
11. Mehta A C, Peaker S, Acomb C, Calvert R T. Rapid gas chromatographic determination of dimethyl sulfoxide and its metabolite dimethyl sulfone in plasma and urine. *J Chrom* 1986; 383: 400–404.
12. Weber C, Bysted A, Holmer G. Coenzyme Q10 in the diet-daily intake and relative bioavailability. *Mol Asp Med* 1997; 18: s251–s254.
13. Morimoto H, Imada I, Sugihara H. Coenzyme Q. *Jpn Tokkyo Koho* 1975.
14. Mattila P, Lehtonen M, Kumpulainen J. Comparison of in-line connected

diode array and electrochemical detectors in the high-performance liquid chromatographic analysis of coenzymes Q9 and Q10 in food materials. *J Agric Food Chem* 2000; 48: 1229–1233.

15. Menke T, Niklowitz P, Adam S *et al.* Simultaneous detection of ubiquinol-10, ubiquinone-10, and tocopherols in human plasma microsamples and macrosamples as a marker of oxidative damage in neonates and infants. *Anal Biochem* 2000; 282: 209–217.

16. Sanders D C, Chaturvedi A K, Hordinsky J R. Melatonin: aeromedical, toxicopharmacological, and analytical aspects. *J Anal Toxicol* 1999; 23: 159–167.

17. Lerner A B, Case J D, Takahashi Y, Lee T H, More W. Isolation of melatonin, the pineal-gland factor that lightens melanocytes. *J Am Chem Soc* 1958; 80: 2587.

18. Held U, Siebrecht S. L-Carnitine: a biological route to a key nutraceutical. *Speciality Chemicals Magazine* 2003; 23: 28–29.

19. Freimuller S, Altorfer H. A chiral HPLC method for the determination of low amounts of d-carnitine in l-carnitine after derivatization with (+)-FLEC. *J Pharm Biomed Anal* 2002; 30: 209–218.

20. Vernez L, Hopfgartner G, Wenk M, Krahenbuhl S. Determination of carnitine and acylcarnitines in urine by high-performance liquid chromatography-electrospray ionization ion trap tandem mass spectrometry. *J Chromatogr A* 2003; 984: 203–213.

21. Wadsworth F, Lockwood B. Combined alpha-lipoic acid and acetyl-L-carnitine supplementation. *Pharm J* 2003; 270: 587–589.

22. Ding T-B, Wang Z, Weng L, *et al.* Chemical synthesis of acetyl-L-carnitine and its enzymatic resolution. *Jilin Daxue Xuebao, Lixueban* 2003; 41: 399–401.

23. Rapport L, Lockwood B. Nutraceuticals (3) Octacosanol. *Pharm J* 2000; 265: 170–171.

24. Cravotto G, Binello A, Merizzi G, Avogadro M. Improving solvent-free extraction of policosanol from rice bran by high-intensity ultrasound treatment. *Eur J Lipid Sci Technol* 2004; 106: 147–151.

25. Jimenez J J, Bernal J L, Aumente S *et al.* Quality assurance of commercial beeswax II. Gas chromatography-electron impact ionization mass spectrometry of alcohols and acids. *J Chromatogr A* 2003; 1007: 101–116.

26. Stramentinoli G. S-Adenosyl-L-methionine: the healthy joint product. *Oxidat Stress Dis* 2001; 6: 63–73.

27. Cantoni G L. The nature of the active methyl donor formed enzymically from L-methionine and adenosine triphosphate. *J Am Chem Soc* 1952; 74: 2942–2943.

28. Luippold G, Delabar U, Kloor D, Muhlbauer B. Simultaneous determination of adenosine, S-adenosylhomocysteine and S-adenosylmethionine in biological samples using solid-phase extraction and high-performance liquid chromatography. *J Chromatogr B* 1999; 724: 231–238.

29. Linko Y-Y, Hayakawa K. Docosahexaenoic acid: a valuable nutraceutical? *Trend Food Sci Technol* 1996; 7: 59–63.

30. Wanasundara U N, Wanasundara J, Shahidi F. Omega-3 fatty acid concentrates: a review of production technologies. In: *Seafoods – Quality, Technology and Nutraceutical Applications (Biennual European Conference*

on Fish Processing), 3rd, Grimsby, UK, 29 June–1 July 1999. Berlin: Springer-Verlag, 2002: 157–174.

31. Kyle D J. The large-scale production and use of a single-cell oil highly enriched in docosahexaenoic acid. In: Shahidi F and Finley J W, eds. *Omega-3 Fatty Acids – Chemistry, Nutrition, and Health Effects.* Washington DC: American Chemical Society, 2001: 92–107.

32. Baty J D, Willis R G, Tavendale R. A comparison of methods for the high-performance liquid chromatographic and capillary gas-liquid chromatographic analysis of fatty acid esters. *J Chromatogr* 1986; 353: 319–328.

33. Liebich H M, Wirth C, Jakober B. Analysis of polyunsaturated fatty acids in blood serum after fish oil administration. *J Chromatogr* 1991; 572: 1–9.

34. Christie W W. The analysis of evening primrose oil. *Indust Crops Products* 1999; 10: 73–83.

35. Ozen B F, Weiss I, Mauer L J. Dietary supplement oil classification and detection of adulteration using Fourier transform infrared spectroscopy. *J Agric Food Chem* 2003; 51: 5871–5876.

36. Reichert R D. Oilseed medicinals: in natural drugs, dietary supplements and in new functional foods. *Trend Food Sci Technol* 2002; 13: 353–360.

37. Mason P. *Dietary Supplements*, 2nd edn. London: Pharmaceutical Press, 2001.

38. Mirasol F. Synthetic lycopene offers new supplement growth for Roche. *Chem Market Reporter* 1999; 16 Aug.

39. Murru E, Angioni E, Carta G *et al.* Reversed-phase HPLC analysis of conjugated linolenic acid and its metabolites. *Adv Conjugated Linoleic Acid Res* 2003; 2: 94–100.

40. Pihlava J-M, Hyvaerinen H, Ryhaenen E-L, Hietaniemi V. Process for isolating and purifying secoisolariciresinol diglycoside from flaxseed. *PCT Int Appl* 2002; 1–17.

41. Degenhardt A, Habben S, Winterhalter P. Isolation of the lignan secoisolariciresinol diglucoside from flaxseed (*Linum usitatissimum* L.) by high-speed counter-current chromatography. *J Chromatogr A* 2002; 943: 299–302.

42. Rohdewald P. A review of the French maritime pine bark extract (Pycnogenol), a herbal medication with a diverse clinical pharmacology. *Int J Clin Pharmacol Ther* 2002; 40: 158–168.

43. Goldberg D M, Yan J, Ng E *et al.* A global survey of trans-resveratrol concentrations in commercial wines. *Am J Enol Viticult* 1995; 46: 159–165.

44. Soleas G J, Diamandis E P, Goldberg D M. Resveratrol: a molecule whose time has come? and gone? *Clin Biochem* 1997; 30: 91–113.

45. Pervaiz S. Resveratrol. From grapevines to mammalian biology. *FASEB J* 2003; 17: 1975–1985.

46. Wang Y, Catana F, Yang Y *et al.* An LC–MS method for analyzing total resveratrol in grape juice, cranberry juice, and in wine. *J Agric Food Chem* 2002; 50: 431–435.

47. Sovak M. Grape extract, resveratrol, and its analogs: a review. *J Med Food* 2001; 4: 93–105.

48. Juan M E, Lamuela-Raventos R M, de la Torre-Boronat M C, Planas J M. Determination of trans-resveratrol in plasma by HPLC. *Anal Chem* 1999; 71: 747–750.

49. Gu X, Creasy L, Kester A, Zeece M. Capillary electrophoretic determination of resveratrol in wines. *J Agric Food Chem* 1999; 47: 3223–3227.

50. Bagchi D, Bagchi M, Stohs S J *et al*. Free radicals and grape seed proanthocyanidin extract: importance in human health and disease prevention. *Toxicology* 2000; 148: 187–197.

51. Palma M, Taylor L T, Zoecklein B W, Douglas L S. Supercritical fluid extraction of grape glycosides. *J Agric Food Chem* 2000; 48: 775–779.

52. Revilla E, Ryan J-M. Analysis of several phenolic compounds with potential antioxidant properties in grape extracts and wines by high-performance liquid chromatography-photodiode array detection without sample preparation. *J Chromatogr A* 2000; 881: 461–469.

53. Wu Q, Wang M, Simon J E. Determination of proanthocyanidins in grape products by liquid chromatography/mass spectrometric detection under low collision energy. *Anal Chem* 2003; 75: 2440–2444.

54. Kennedy J A, Taylor A W. Analysis of proanthocyanidins by high-performance gel permeation chromatography. *J Chromatogr A* 2003; 995: 99–107.

55. Lugasi A, Biro L, Hovarie J *et al*. Lycopene content of foods and lycopene intake in two groups of the Hungarian population. *Nutr Res* 2003; 23: 1035–1044.

56. Khachik F, Carvalho L, Bernstein P S *et al*. Chemistry, distribution, and metabolism of tomato carotenoids and their impact on human health. *Exp Biol Med* 2002; 227: 845–851.

57. Denery J R, Dragull K, Tang C S, Li Q X. Pressurized fluid extraction of carotenoids from *Haematococcus pluvialis* and *Dunaliella salina* and kavalactones from *Piper methysticum. Anal Chim Acta* 2004; 501: 175–181.

58. Feifer A H, Fleshner N E, Klotz L. Analytical accuracy and reliability of commonly used nutritional supplements in prostate disease. *J Urol* 2002; 168: 150–154.

59. Karrer P, Jucker E, Steinlin K. Rubichrome, a new carotenoid with a furanoid ring system, occurring in nature. *Helv Chim Acta* 1947; 30: 531–535.

60. Maoka T, Fujiwara Y, Hashimoto K, Akimoto N. Isolation of a series of apocarotenoids from the fruits of the red paprika *Capsicum annuum* L. *J Agric Food Chem* 2001; 49: 1601–1606.

61. Chen J P, Tai C Y, Chen B H. Improved liquid chromatographic method for determination of carotenoids in Taiwanese mango (*Mangifera indica* L.). *J Chromatogr A* 2004; 1054: 261–268.

62. Lignell A, Wood V. Astaxanthin: the radical defense behind the cell. *Innovations Food Technol* 2004; 23: 78–80.

63. Osterlie M, Bjerkeng B, Liaaen-Jensen S. Plasma appearance and distribution of astaxanthin E/Z and R/S isomers in plasma lipoproteins of men after single dose administration of astaxanthin. *J Nutr Biochem* 2000; 11: 482–490.

64. Reed L J, Gunsalus I C, Schnakenberg G H F *et al*. Isolation, characterization, and structure of α-lipoic acid. *J Am Chem Soc* 1953; 75: 1267–1270.

65. Bullock M W, Brockman J A, Patterson E L *et al*. Synthesis of DL-thioctic acid. *J Am Chem Soc* 1952; 74: 1868–1869.

66. Haj-Yehia A I, Assaf P, Nassar T, Katzhendler J. Determination of lipoic acid and dihydrolipoic acid in human plasma and urine by high-performance liquid

chromatography with fluorimetric detection. *J Chromatogr A* 2000; 870: 381–388.

67. Brown G A, Vukovich M D, Sharp R L *et al.* Effect of oral DHEA on serum testosterone and adaptations to resistance training in young men. *J Appl Physiol* 1999; 87: 2274–2283.

68. Petrow V. A history of steroid chemistry: some contributions from European industry. *Steroids* 1996; 61: 473–475.

69. Thompson R D, Carlson M. Liquid chromatographic determination of dehydroepiandrosterone (DHEA) in dietary supplement products. *J AOAC Int* 2000; 83: 847–857.

70. Zemaitis M A, Kroboth P D. Simplified procedure for measurement of serum dehydroepiandrosterone and its sulfate with gas chromatography-ion trap mass spectrometry and selected reaction monitoring. *J Chromatogr B* 1998; 716: 19–26.

71. Hendrich S, Murphy P A. Isoflavones: source and metabolism. In: Wildman R E C, ed. *Handbook of Nutraceuticals and Functional Foods.* Boca Raton: CRC Press, 2001; 55–75.

72. Nurmi T, Mazur W, Heinonen S *et al.* Isoflavone content of the soy based supplements. *J Pharm Biomed Anal* 2002; 28: 1–11.

73. Challener C. Speciality supplements are the bright spot in US dietary supplement market. *Chem Market Report* 2003; 6–8.

74. Le Gall G, Colquhoun I J, Defernez M. Metabolite profiling using (1)H NMR spectroscopy for quality assessment of green tea, Camellia sinensis (L.). *J Agric Food Chem* 2004; 52: 692–700.

75. Aucamp J P, Hara Y, Apostolides Z. Simultaneous analysis of tea catechins, caffeine, gallic acid, theanine and ascorbic acid by micellar electrokinetic capillary chromatography. *J Chromatogr A* 2000; 876: 235–242.

76. Persky A M, Brazeau G A, Hochhaus G. Pharmacokinetics of the dietary supplement creatine. *Clin Pharmacokinet* 2003; 42: 557–574.

77. Kessel K, Scherr G, Kluge M *et al.* Process for the preparation of creatine or creatine monohydrate by the reaction of sodium or potassium sarcosinate with cyanamide. Eur Pat Appl 2000; 1–5.

78. Burke D G, MacLean P G, Walker R A *et al.* Analysis of creatine and creatinine in urine by capillary electrophoresis. *J Chromatogr B* 1999; 732: 479–485.

79. US Food and Drug Administration. Center for Food Safety and Applied Nutrition. *Summary of All GRAS Notices.* http://www.cfsan.fda.gov/~rdb/opa-gras.html (accessed 12 June 2006).

80. Hurst W J. *Methods of Analysis for Functional Foods and Nutraceuticals.* Boca Raton: CRC Press, 2002.

4

Metabolism, bioavailability and pharmacokinetics of nutraceuticals

The metabolism, bioavailability and pharmacokinetics of many nutraceuticals have been reported, particularly over the previous 10 years. Results have been presented for both physiological and dietary compounds after supplementation, which may cause problems in interpreting the data.

Metabolism data

Metabolites have now been identified for the majority of nutraceuticals, and a number of these may be responsible for the activity of particular nutraceuticals. The evidence is discussed in later chapters. Table 4.1 lists the physiological and dietary levels of some major nutraceuticals and their metabolites. Rarely do available dietary levels impact on physiological levels. Except for excessive intake of foods containing coenzyme Q10 (Co Q10), carnitine, soy and tea phenolics, and creatine, there is little chance of normal dietary supplementation substantially increasing physiological levels. With some nutraceuticals there are no physiological levels, and no realistic dietary sources. With others any physiological levels are caused by consumption of specific foods, for example those containing lycopene, tea catechins or soy isoflavones. Although metabolites have been identified for many entities, detailed lists have still not been collated for others.

Bioavailability data

Studies on the bioavailability of a number of nutraceuticals have been carried out, revealing wide differences. These data give an insight into the possible effectiveness of the different entities following consumption. Table 4.2 lists reported levels from a variety of studies, from which a rough comparison can be made. Nevertheless, as in the case of serum levels, a number of variable circumstances were involved in deriving these figures and any conclusions should be treated with caution. The

Table 4.1 Physiological and dietary levels of nutraceuticals and their metabolites

Nutraceutical	Physiological level	Dietary level	Metabolites
Glucosamine[1]	No data	N/A	Glucosaminic acid
Chondroitin[2]	N/A	–	Lower molecular weight polysaccharide
Chondroitin[3]	N/A	–	Chondroitin-4-sulfate
Methylsulfonylmethane[4]	4 mg/person	Minimal	DMS
Methylsulfonylmethane[5]	4 mg/person	Minimal	Methionine?
Coenzyme Q10[6]	0.5 μg/mL	3–5 mg/day	Coenzyme Q9
Coenzyme Q10[7]	0.5 μg/mL	3–5 mg/day	6-(5′ and 6′) Carboxylated derivatives
Melatonin[8]	10–50 pg/mL plasma (day–night)	Minimal	6-Hydroxymelatonin
Carnitine[9]	9 mg/L	3–97 mg/100 g meats	Acetylcarnitine, C-4/C-8 acetyl carnitines, propionylcarnitine
Carnitine[10]	9 mg/L	3–97 mg/100 g meats	γ-Butyrobetaine, acetylcarnitine
Acetyl-L-carnitine[11]	No data, present	No data, present	Carnitine
Octacosanol/ policosanol[12]	Present in central nervous system	N/A	Fatty acids
Octacosanol/policosanol[13]	See above	N/A	Myristic, palmitic, stearic, oleic, and palmitoleic acids
Octacosanol/policosanol[14]	See above	N/A	See above
S-Adenosyl methionine[15]	30–40 ng/mL	–	Methylthioadenosine, S-adenosylhomocysteine, adenosine, putrescine, polyamines
S-Adenosyl methionine[16]	30–40 ng/mL	0.1–10 mg/kg food	Taurine
n-3-Fatty acids[17]	1–3% total body fat	≤10% total fat	ALA→EPA/DHA
n-3-Fatty acids[18]	1–3% total body fat	≤10% total fat	ALA→EPA/DHA
γ-Linolenic acid[19]	4–6 μg/mL	Minimal	
γ-Linolenic acid[20]	–	Minimal	DGLA Arachidonic acid

Table 4.1 Continued

Nutraceutical	Physiological level	Dietary level	Metabolites
Flaxseed/α-linolenic acid[18]	10–30 μg/mL	–	ALA→DHA
Flaxseed/α-linolenic acid[21]	–	1.5 g/day	
Conjugated linoleic acid[22]	–	–	Elongated and desaturated CLA metabolites
Conjugated linoleic acid[23]	–	350–430 mg/day	
Flax lignans[24]	Diet dependent	Diet dependent	SDG→enterolactone
Pycnogenol[25]	N/A	N/A	Ferulic acid, taxifolin, δ-(3,4-dihydroxyphenyl) and (3-methoxy 4-hydroxy phenyl) gamma-valerolactones
Resveratrol[26]	N/A	0.1–2.3 mg/L wine	Piceatanol
Resveratrol[27]	N/A	0.1–2.3 mg/L wine	–
Resveratrol[28]	N/A	0.1–2.3 mg/L wine	Piceatanol, plus another tetrahydroxystilbene
Resveratrol[29]	N/A	0.1–2.3 mg/L wine	Dihydroresveratrol
Grape seed proanthocyanidin extract[30]	N/A	N/A	Catechin/proanthocyanidin metabolites, mainly 3-hydroxyphenylpropionic acid
Lycopene[31]	N/A	2–5 mg/day	5,6-Dihydroxy-5,6-dihydrolycopene
Lycopene[32]	N/A	–	Lycopene epoxides, cyclocopene diols, cyclocopene epoxides
Lutein[33]	10–12 μg/g, testes, adrenal	–	–
Zeaxanthin[34]	N/A	5–26 ng/day	Zeaxanthin→lutein
Zeaxanthin[35]	N/A	5–26 ng/day	Zeaxanthin→lutein
Lipoic acid[36]	Minimal	Minimal	Dihydrolipoic acid, 3-ketolipoic acid, bisnorlipoic acid, 3-methoxylipoic acid

continued

Table 4.1 Continued

Nutraceutical	Physiological level	Dietary level	Metabolites
Lipoic acid[37]	Minimal	Minimal	Bisnorlipoic acid, hydroxybisnorlipoic acid, tetranorlipoic acid, 4,6-bismethylthio-hexanoic acid, 6,8-bismethylthio-octanoic acid, 2,4-bismethylthio-butanoic acid
Dehydroepiandrosterone[38]	–	–	Testosterone, 5-androstenediol
Dehydroepiandrosterone[39]	1–5 µg /L	0.2–1% in foods	Oestradiol, oestrone
Soy isoflavones, daidzein/genistein[40]	N/A	Diet dependent	Unidentified
Soy isoflavones[41]	N/A	15–20 mg/day by specific consumers	18 demethylated and hydroxylated metabolites
Soy isoflavones[25]	N/A	15–20 mg/day by specific consumers	Daidzein→equol and intermediates
Green tea catechins, EGCG, EGC, EC, ECG[42]	N/A	Diet dependent, minimal in low dose green tea	4-O-Methyl-epigallocatechin, valerolactones
Green tea catechins, EGCG, EGC, EC, ECG[43]	N/A	–	3 and 4-O-methyl-EC, EGC and EGCG, valerolactones
Green tea catechins, EGCG, EGC, EC, ECG[44]	N/A	18–50 mg/day	–
Creatine[45]	1 g/day produced	Present 5 g/kg meat	Creatinine, phosphocreatine

N/A, not available endogenously.

ALA, α-linolenic acid; EPA, eicosapentaenoic acid; DHA, docosahexaenoic acid; CLA, conjugated linoleic acid; SDG, secoisolariciresinol diglucoside; DHEA, dehydroepiandrosterone; EC, (−)-epicatechin; ECG, (−)-epicatechin gallate; EGC, (−)-epigallocatechin; EGCG, (−)-epigallocatechin gallate.

Table 4.2 Oral bioavailability in humans after single-dose administration of nutraceuticals (except where stated)

Nutraceutical	Dose	Bioavailability	Increased serum levels
Glucosamine[46]	7.5 g	26%, 44% incorporation into globulin	–
Chondroitin[4]	3 g	13%	–
Coenzyme Q10[6]	30 mg	–	35% increase in serum levels at 6 hours
Coenzyme Q10[48]	30 mg	–	2.7–6 times normal level
Melatonin[27]	2–4 mg	15%	–
Melatonin[49]	250 μg	10–56%	240–620 pg/mL
Melatonin[50]	1–6 g	5–18%	–
Carnitine[51]	2 g/12 hours	14–16%	–
Carnitine[11]	0.5–0.6 g	14–18%	–
Acetyl-L-carnitine[11]	2 g/day		43% increase
Octacosanol/policosanol[12]	–	5–12% (rats)	–
S-Adenosyl methionine[15]	2 × 200 mg	–	3.5–6 times
Docosahexaenoic acid[52]	11.6% of 9 g fresh oil	–	2 times normal levels
Eicosapentaenoic acid[52]	18.2% of 9 g fresh oil	–	5–6 times normal levels
Resveratrol[53]	50 mg/kg	38% (rats)	
Resveratrol[29]		Almost zero	–
Lycopene, lutein, zeaxanthin, astaxanthin[34]	1 mg	4%	–
Lipoic acid[37]	10 mg	20%	–
Lipoic acid[36]	600 mg/day for 4 days	30%	–
Dehydroepiandrosterone[54]	1 g	20–38%	5–6 times normal
Green tea extracts[42]	200 mg	Low	
EGC	20 mg/kg body weight	0.8%	179 ng/mL peak serum level
EC	15.5 mg	0.7%	
EGCG	36.5 mg	0.1%	
ECG[55]	16.7 mg	0.09% 1.7% in total	
Creatine[56]	31.1 mg		5–6 times normal
	2–3 g		

EC, (−)-epicatechin; ECG, (−)-epicatechin gallate; EGC, (−)-epigallocatechin; EGCG, (−)-epigallocatechin gallate.

absence of data for some major nutraceuticals, such as methylsulfonyl-methane (MSM), γ-linolenic acid (GLA) and grape seed proantho-cyanidin extract (GSPE), means that there is no guidance for optimal dosage levels.

Further evidence for the different bioavailability of different formulations and complex mixtures only allows the individual consumer/patient/clinician to use the most detailed/only available published data. Detailed comparative data for some individual nutraceuticals have been published (e.g. Co Q10,[57] creatine[45]), and in these cases comparison of a range of studies is possible. In the study on the bioequivalence of Co Q10 formulated products, 180 mg doses of four products were evaluated in nine individuals. Although the absolute bioavailability of Co Q10 is not known, it has been found to be strongly lipophilic, practically insoluble in aqueous solution, and has poor bioavailability. A range of products have been formulated with emulsifying agents and oil-based vehicles, as well as fully solubilised formulations, in an attempt to improve bioavailability. An increased serum concentration and area under the curve (blood concentration–time profile) (AUC) of about 50% was recorded for the oil suspension in soft gelatin capsule when compared with a standard dry formulation.[58]

Research into the variability of ten Co Q10 products available in New Zealand showed that there was at least fourfold variation in the increase in plasma Co Q10 levels achieved by the different products, and patients showed no increase in levels with the least effective products.[59] Bioequivalence comparison of four products showed the best to be the one containing the reduced form of Co Q10, ubiquinol, which was even superior to solubilised formulations.[57]

In a review of the pharmacokinetics of 17 formulated creatine products taken from six published studies, accumulated data allow direct comparison of the data on single dose use of 5 mg formulated products.[45] There is a wide variation in the levels of quoted pharmacokinetic parameters: the maximum concentration (blood concentration–time profile) (C_{max}) varies from 67 to 160 mg/L, AUC from 183 to 340 mg h/L, half-life ($t_{\frac{1}{2}}$) from 0.89 to 1.7 hours, clearance from 14 to 27 L/hour, and the volume of distribution from 18 to 47 L. Overall, these levels show variations of the order of 100%, and even comparable data from a single study using different volunteer groups (young or elderly) exhibited variations of up to 50%.

In addition to formulation differences, it has been reported that various dietary factors also affect the bioavailability of certain nutraceuticals. The absorption of lycopene has been reported to improve following ingestion of a combined dose of β-carotene and lycopene, instead of lycopene alone.[60] Optimal intestinal uptake of lutein esters has been reported to require higher dietary fat levels than other carotenoids, and with concomitant intake of high fat supplementation, plasma lutein uptake more than doubled.[61] Lutein-containing yellow carrots caused significantly increased lutein concentrations in humans, and did not result in the decrease of β-carotene concentrations that normally accompanies administration of lutein.[62] Further evidence of the effect of the food matrix on the bioavailability of lutein was shown when present in spinach.[63] Dietary fat levels have also been shown to affect absorption of lutein beneficially, high levels resulting in five times higher absorption.[64]

Pharmacokinetic data

Pharmacokinetic data for a number of nutraceuticals have been reported. This is of great importance in deciding optimum dosage levels and frequency of administration of the particular entities. Comparison of data available for different nutraceuticals is extremely difficult due to the wide range of possible parameters available and published. Table 4.3 lists some of the major pharmacokinetic parameters for many of the major nutraceuticals. Some of the most important parameters (C_{max}, time of C_{max} (t_{max})), $t_{\frac{1}{2}}$, maximum AUC at ∞ (AUC_{∞})) have been reported, but only rarely is the whole pharmacokinetic picture available. Comparisons between nutraceuticals, even nutraceuticals of similar type, are extremely difficult due to lack of data, different dosage levels (different dimensions and units in published works) and wide variations between different volunteer/patient groups involved. C_{max} gives an idea of maximal serum concentration after dosing. The half-life, $t_{\frac{1}{2}}$, is sometimes available, but this varies if above saturation dose. AUC_{∞} is often quoted, but not invariably, sometimes AUC_{24h} or another timescale is used. AUC_{∞} is an acccepted indicator of bioavailability, but takes no account of dosing level used.

From Table 4.3 it would appear that glucosamine, chondroitin, eicosapentaenoic acid (EPA), GLA and creatine have far better bioavailability (as seen from AUC values) than other nutraceuticals. However, the dosages used were usually far greater as well, although they were in the normal therapeutic range. Bioavailability appears to be very low for carnitine, lipoic acid, dehydroepiandrosterone (DHEA) and tea catechins. The t_{max} and $t_{\frac{1}{2}}$ values indicate a comparatively low retention for melatonin and lipoic acid. The n-3 fatty acids docosahexaenoic acid

Table 4.3 Pharmacokinetic profiles of major nutraceuticals after single dose oral supplementation to healthy individuals (unless otherwise stated)

Nutraceutical	Number of subjects	Dose	C_{max}	t_{max} (h)	$t_{\frac{1}{2}}$ (h)	AUC_∞
Glucosamine[65]	8 beagles	1500 mg	12.7 µg/mL	1.5	1.52	178.1 µg.h/mL
Chondroitin[66]	20	4 g (bovine)	4.87 µg/mL	2.4		179.1 µg.h/mL (48 h)
Chondroitin[3]	20	4 g (ickthyc)	1.03 µg/mL	8.7		141.4 µg.h/mL (48 h)
Coenzyme Q10[57]	9	180 mg	125 pg/mL	6.2		51.67 µg.h/mL
Melatonin[49]	12	250 µg		0.38		255 pg.h/mL
Melatonin[67]	16	0.5 µg/kg	12.4 µg/mL		0.79	377 pg.h/mL
Carnitine[51]	15	2 g every 12 h				0.12 µg.h/mL
S-Adenosyl methionine[68]	6	100 mg i.v.			1.35	78 µg.h/mL
	6	500 mg i.v.			1.68	425 µg.h/mL
Docosahexaenoic acid[69]	12	1200 mg	131 µg/mL			645 µg.h/mL
Eicosapentaenoic acid[69]	12	1140 mg	126 µg/mL			674 µg.h/mL
Eicosapentaenoic acid[70]	10	1 g	50 µg/mL	4.7		137.1 µg.h/mL
γ-Linolenic acid[70]	10	1.5 g	73 µg/mL	3.4		280 µg.h/mL
γ-Linolenic acid[19]	6	240 mg	21.7 µg/mL	3.6	4.4	525 µg.h/mL
Flax lignans[71]	12	0.9 mg/kg SDG			12.6	2.74 µg.h/mL
	12	0.9 mg/kg SDG	0.04 µg/mL	16.6	28.1	9.70 µg.h/mL
Lycopene[72]	25	10 mg	0.11 µg/mL	32.6	40.9	1.6 µg.h/mL
	25	120 mg	1 µg/mL	15	13	42 µg.h/mL
Zeaxanthin[34]	10	10 mg	1.3 mg/mL	6.7	21	1.35 µg.h/mL
Astaxanthin[73]	3	100 mg	55 µg/mL	8	16.7	0.66 µg.h/mL
Astaxanthin[74]	8	40 mg	70.8 µg/mL	1.8	0.66	2.8 µg.h/mL
Lipoic acid[36]	12	200 mg	7.6 µg/mL	0.5	0.7	
Lipoic acid[11]	4	600 mg daily				

Table 4.3 Continued

Nutraceutical	Number of subjects	Dose	C_{max}	t_{max} (h)	$t_{\frac{1}{2}}$ (h)	AUC_{∞}
Dehydroepiandrosterone[38]	12 Men	25 mg/day for 8 days		27.7	26	0.16 µg.h/mL
	12 Women	25 mg/day for 8 days		27.7	26	0.20 µg.h/mL
Daidzein[40]	10	(20 g soybean) 13 mg daidzein	214 000 µg/mL			2.6 µg.h/mL
Daidzein[75]	10	7.47 mg SR	0.05 µg/mL	7.4	11.4	1.07 µg.h/mL
Genistein[40]	10	(20 g soybean) 20 mg genistein	0.31 µg/mL			4.4 µg.h/mL
Genistein[75]	10	22.3 mg SR	0.04 µg/mL	6.7	10.2	0.97 µg.h/mL
Green tea extracts[76]	5	400 mg epigallolocatechin gallate	0.11 µg/mL	1.8	2.7	2124 µg.h/mL
Green tea catechins[77]	12	910 mg total catechin derivatives	159 500 µg/mL	2.3	4.8	0.64 µg.h/mL
Black tea catechins[77]	12	300 mg total catechin derivatives	49 300 µg/mL	2.2	6.9	0.15 µg.h/mL
Black tea catechins (with milk)[77]	12	300 mg total catechin derivatives	52 200 µg/mL	2	8.6	0.17 µg.h/mL
Creatine[45]	1	10 g	120 µg/mL	1.25	0.94	360 µg.h/mL

SR, sustained release; SDG, secoisolariciresinol diglucoside.

(DHA) and EPA exhibit comparable data in the same study, but astaxanthin shows widely different data (C_{max}, AUC) from the two studies quoted. As one would expect, hydrophobic substances often exhibit longer half-lives, and the data shown for DHEA and carotenoids confirm this.

Half-lives are available for some of the published nutraceuticals, which should allow dosage regimens to be designed. Comparative data[45] published for creatine show a wide variation in half-life values, both within single studies, of the order of 2.5 times, and also between different studies using the same dosage regimen. If pharmacokinetic experimentation was available from similarly designed studies, derived data may be useful in comparing the effectiveness of nutraceuticals used for the same therapeutic application (e.g. in the case of glycoaminoglycans (GAG)), and one should be able to compare dosing of individual compounds and thereby select the best individual entity for the application.

Recently, the comparable bioavailability of a number of polyphenols has been studied.[44] Comparable data from 28 studies on catechin bioavailability were reported, and there are marked differences between different individual entities. When supplementation with single pure catechins was studied it was found that galloylation of catechins reduces their absorption. It was also shown that 77–90% of (—)-epigallocatechin gallate (EGCG) is present in plasma in the free form, although other catechins are highly conjugated with glucuronic acid and/or sulfate groups. The valerolactone metabolites of the catechin derivatives are of microbiological origin, and were mainly found in plasma and urine in conjugated forms. These metabolites represented 6–39% of (—)-epigallocatechin (EGC) and (—)-epicatechin (EC), and were present in concentrations 8–25 times higher than those of the free compounds. It is likely that as these appear later than the catechins in plasma, and have long half-lives, they may prolong the action of the catechins. Very limited absorption of polymeric proanthocyanidins has been shown to occur, but their activity may be via direct action on the intestinal mucosa, protecting it from oxidative stress or carcinogens. Alternatively, these polymers usually occur in conjunction with their monomers at levels of 5–25%, and these may be responsible for the activity.

Similar comparative bioavailability studies have also been carried out on soy phytoestrogens, using 15 published studies.[78] Unfortunately, contradictory results were obtained: one particular study had indicated that there was greater bioavailability for the glucoside forms, another that there was greater bioavailability for the aglycone form, and two showed no differences in the absorption rates for the two forms. Production of the metabolite equol was shown to be greater for daidzin than for daidzein, and the bioavailability of genistein was higher than that of daidzein, but glycitein was higher still.

Overall, data for metabolites produced from most nutraceuticals are now available, and bioavailability data have been published for the majority. Detailed pharmacokinetic data have not been published for MSM, octacosanol/policosanol, CLA, Pycnogenol, resveratrol, GSPE, and any of the isolated components from complex products such as CLA, Pycnogenol or GSPE.

Dosage levels that have been used for collection of the data are largely intuitive, and more studies involving greater dosage ranges are needed.

It needs to be borne in mind that dosage regimens used in reported clinical trials and pharmacokinetic work may not have been the most effective for treating symptoms, and also that different researchers have often used different regimens. Pharmacokinetic data from trials involving wide dosage levels and regimens may supply extremely worthwhile information for planning future clinical trials of nutraceuticals, particularly in cases where there is a possibility of side-effects, for example with the caffeine content of green tea.[79]

Some scientists would question the validity of carrying out pharmacokinetic evaluation of those nutraceuticals which are themselves endogenous constituents of living tissue. A number are also possible or probable components of individual diets, for example soy products, green tea and *n*-3 fatty acids, and may either be consumed at variable levels or not at all, thus compromising other data.

References

1. Imanaga Y, Yoshifuji K, Momose N *et al*. Metabolism of D-glucosamine. *Koso Kagaku Shinpojumu* 1960; 14: 183–189.
2. Davidson E A, Riley J G. Chondroitin sulfate B metabolism. *Biochim Biophys Acta* 1960; 42: 566–567.
3. Volpi N. Oral absorption and bioavailability of ichthyic origin chondroitin sulfate in healthy male volunteers. *Osteoarthritis Cartilage* 2003; 11: 433–441.
4. Ely A, Lockwood B. What is the evidence for the safety and efficacy of dimethyl sulphoxide and methylsulphonylmethane in pain relief ? *Pharm J* 2002; 269: 685–687.
5. Otsuki S, Qian W, Ishihara A, Kabe T. Elucidation of dimethylsulfone metabolism in rat using a 35S radioisotope tracer method. *Nutr Res* 2002; 22: 313–322.

6. Weber C, Bysted A, Holmer G. Coenzyme Q10 in the diet-daily intake and relative bioavailability. *Mol Asp Med* 1997; 18: s251–s254.
7. Grunler J, Dallner G. Investigation of regulatory mechanisms in coenzyme Q metabolism. *Method Enzymol* 2004; 378: 3–17.
8. Benes L, Claustrat B, Horriere F *et al.* Transmucosal, oral controlled-release, and transdermal drug administration in human subjects: a crossover study with melatonin. *J Pharm Sci* 1997; 86: 1115–1119.
9. Inoue F, Terada N, Nakajima K *et al.* Effect of sports activity on carnitine metabolism. *Nippon Iyo Masu Supekutoru Gakkai Koenshu* 1998; 23: 169–172.
10. Evans A M, Fornasini G. Pharmacokinetics of L-carnitine. *Clin Pharmacokinet* 2003; 42: 941–967.
11. Rebouche C J. Kinetics, pharmacokinetics, and regulation of L-carnitine and acetyl-L-carnitine metabolism. *Ann N Y Acad Sci* 2004; 1033: 30–41.
12. Gouni-Berthold I, Berthold H K. Policosanol: clinical pharmacology and therapeutic significance of a new lipid-lowering agent. *Am Heart J* 2002; 143: 356–365.
13. Kabir Y, Kimura S. Tissue distribution of ($^{8-14}$C)-octacosanol in liver and muscle of rats after serial administration. *Ann Nutr Metab* 1995; 39: 279–284.
14. Menendez R, Marrero D, Mas R *et al.* In vitro and in vivo study of octacosanol metabolism. *Arch Med Res* 2005; 36: 113–119.
15. Stramentinoli G. Pharmacologic aspects of S-adenosylmethionine. Pharmacokinetics and pharmacodynamics. *Am J Med* 1987; 83: 35–42.
16. Stramentinoli G. S-Adenosyl-L-methionine: the healthy joint product. *Oxidat Stress Dis* 2001; 6: 63–73.
17. Linko Y-Y, Hayakawa K. Docosahexaenoic acid: a valuable nutraceutical? *Trend Food Sci Technol* 1996; 7: 59–63.
18. Kurowska E M, Dresser G K, Deutsch L *et al.* Bioavailability of omega-3 essential fatty acids from perilla seed oil. *Prostaglandins Leukot Essent Fatty Acids* 2003; 68: 207–212.
19. Martens-Lobenhoffer J, Meyer F P. Pharmacokinetic data of γ-linolenic acid in healthy volunteers after the administration of evening primrose oil (Epogam). *Int J Clin Pharmacol Ther* 1998; 36: 363–366.
20. Curtis C L, Harwood J L, Dent C M, Caterson B. Biological basis for the benefit of nutraceutical supplementation in arthritis. *Drug Discovery Today* 2004; 9: 165–172.
21. Burdge G C. α-Linolenic acid metabolism in men and women: are there implications for dietary recommendations? *Lipid Technol* 2004; 16: 221–225.
22. Emken E A, Adlof R O, Duval S *et al.* Effect of dietary conjugated linoleic acid (CLA) on metabolism of isotope-labeled oleic, linoleic, and CLA isomers in women. *Lipids* 2002; 37: 741–750.
23. Berven G, Bye A, Hals O *et al.* Safety of conjugated linoleic acid (CLA) in overweight or obese human volunteers. *Eur J Lipid Sci Technol* 2000; 102: 455–462.
24. Rowland I, Faughnan M, Hoey L *et al.* Bioavailability of phyto-oestrogens. *Br J Nutr* 2003; 89: S45–S58.

25. Duweler K G, Rohdewald P. Urinary metabolites of French maritime pine bark extract in humans. *Die Pharmazie* 2000; 55: 364–368.
26. Zhu Y, Chiang H, Zhou J, Kissinger P T. In vitro metabolism study of resveratrol and identification and determination of its metabolite piceatannol by LC/EC and LC/MSMS. *Curr Separation* 2003; 20: 93–96.
27. Schwedhelm E, Maas R, Troost R, Boeger R H. Clinical pharmacokinetics of antioxidants and their impact on systemic oxidative stress. *Clin Pharmacokinet* 2003; 42: 437–459.
28. Piver B, Fer M, Vitrac X *et al.* Involvement of cytochrome P450 1A2 in the biotransformation of trans-resveratrol in human liver microsomes. *Biochem Pharmacol* 2004; 68: 773–782.
29. Wenzel E, Somoza V. Metabolism and bioavailability of trans- resveratrol. *Mol Nutr Food Res* 2005; 49: 472–481.
30. Ward N C, Croft K D, Puddey I B, Hodgson J M. Supplementation with grape seed polyphenols results in increased urinary excretion of 3-hydroxyphenyl-propionic acid, an important metabolite of proanthocyanidins in humans. *J Agric Food Chem* 2004; 52: 5545–5549.
31. Khachik F, Beecher G R, Smith J. C Jr. Lutein, lycopene, and their oxidative metabolites in chemoprevention of cancer. *J Cell Biochem* 1995; 22(Suppl): 236–246.
32. Khachik F, Carvalho L, Bernstein P S *et al.* Chemistry, distribution, and metabolism of tomato carotenoids and their impact on human health. *Exp Biol Med* 2002; 227: 845–851.
33. Kaplan L A, Lau J M, Stein E A. Carotenoid composition, concentrations, and relationships in various human organs. *Clin Physiol Biochem* 1990; 8: 1–10.
34. Hartmann D, Thuermann P A, Spitzer V *et al.* Plasma kinetics of zeaxanthin and 3′-dehydro-lutein after multiple oral doses of synthetic zeaxanthin. *Am J Clin Nutr* 2004; 79: 410–417.
35. Khachik F, Bertram J S, Huang M-T *et al.* Dietary carotenoids and their metabolites as potentially useful chemoprotective agents against cancer. *Antioxidant Food Supplements in Human Health* Kaminoyama-city, Japan, 1999; 203–229.
36. Hermann R, Niebch G, Borbe H O *et al.* Enantioselective pharmacokinetics and bioavailability of different racemic α-lipoic acid formulations in healthy volunteers. *Eur J Pharm Sci* 1996; 4: 167–174.
37. Teichert J, Hermann R, Ruus P, Preiss R. Plasma kinetics, metabolism, and urinary excretion of alpha-lipoic acid following oral administration in healthy volunteers. *J Clin Pharmacol* 2003; 43: 1256–1267.
38. Legrain S, Massien C, Lahlou N *et al.* Dehydroepiandrosterone replacement administration: pharmacokinetic and pharmacodynamic studies in healthy elderly subjects. *J Clin Endocrinol Metab* 2000; 85: 3208–3217.
39. Milewich L, Catalina F, Bennett M. Pleiotropic effects of dietary DHEA. *Ann N Y Acad Sci* 1995; 774: 149–170.
40. Setchell K D R, Brown N M, Desai P B *et al.* Bioavailability, disposition, and dose-response effects of soy isoflavones when consumed by healthy women at physiologically typical dietary intakes. *J Nutr* 2003; 133: 1027–1035.
41. Heinonen S-M, Waehaelae K, Adlercreutz H. Metabolism of isoflavones in human subjects. *Phytochem Rev* 2002; 1: 175–182.

42. Lee M-J, Maliakal P, Chen L et al. Pharmacokinetics of tea catechins after ingestion of green tea and (—)-epigallocatechin-3-gallate by humans: formation of different metabolites and individual variability. Cancer Epidemiol Biomarker Prev 2002; 11: 1025–1032.

43. Lambert J D, Yang C S. Cancer chemopreventive activity and bioavailability of tea and tea polyphenols. Mutat Res 2003; 523–524, 201–208.

44. Manach C, Williamson G, Morand C et al. Bioavailability and bioefficacy of polyphenols in humans. I. Review of 97 bioavailability studies. Am J Clin Nutr 2005; 81: 230S–242S.

45. Persky A M, Brazeau G A, Hochhaus G. Pharmacokinetics of the dietary supplement creatine. Clin Pharmacokinet 2003; 42: 557–574.

46. Setnikar I, Rovati L C. Absorption, distribution, metabolism and excretion of glucosamine sulfate. A review. Arzneimittel-Forschung 2001; 51: 699–725.

47. Conte A, De Bernardi M, Palmieri L et al. Metabolic fate of exogenous chondroitin sulfate in man. Arzneimittel-Forschung 1991; 41: 768–772.

48. Chopra R K, Goldman R, Sinatra S T, Bhagavan H N. Relative bioavailability of coenzyme Q10 formulations in human subjects. Int J Vitamin Nutr Res 1998; 68: 109–113.

49. Fourtillan J B, Brisson A M, Gobin P et al. Bioavailability of melatonin in humans after day-time administration of D7 melatonin. Biopharm Drug Disp 2000; 21: 15–22.

50. Evans A M, Fornasini G. Pharmacokinetics of L-carnitine. Clin Pharmacokinet 2003; 42: 941–967.

51. Sahajwalla C G, Helton E, Purich E D et al. Multiple-dose pharmacokinetics and bioequivalence of L-carnitine 330-mg tablet versus 1-g chewable tablet versus enteral solution in healthy adult male volunteers. J Pharm Sci 1995; 84: 627–633.

52. Liebich H M, Wirth C, Jakober B. Analysis of polyunsaturated fatty acids in blood serum after fish oil administration. J Chromatogr 1991; 572: 1–9.

53. Marier J-F, Vachon P, Gritsas A et al. Metabolism and disposition of resveratrol in rats: extent of absorption, glucuronidation, and enterohepatic recirculation evidenced by a linked-rat model. J Pharmacol Exp Ther 2002; 302: 369–373.

54. Frye R F, Kroboth P D, Kroboth F J et al. Sex differences in the pharmacokinetics of dehydroepiandrosterone (DHEA) after single- and multiple-dose administration in healthy older adults. J Clin Pharmacol 2000; 40: 596–605.

55. Warden B A, Smith L S, Beecher G R et al. Catechins are bioavailable in men and women drinking black tea throughout the day. J Nutr 2001; 131: 1731–1737.

56. Harris R C, Soderlund K, Hultman E. Elevation of creatine in resting and exercised muscle of normal subjects by creatine supplementation. Clin Sci 1992; 83: 367–374.

57. Miles M V, Horn P, Miles L et al. Bioequivalence of coenzyme Q10 from over-the-counter supplements. Nutr Res 2002; 22: 919–929.

58. Weis M, Mortensen S A, Rassing M R et al. Bioavailability of four oral coenzyme Q10 formulations in healthy volunteers. Mol Asp Med 1994; 15: S273–S280.

59. Molyneux S, Florkowski C, Lever M, George P. The bioavailability of coenzyme Q10 supplements available in New Zealand differs markedly. *N Z Med J* 2004; 117: U1108.

60. Johnson E J, Qin J, Krinsky N I, Russell R M. Ingestion by men of a combined dose of β-carotene and lycopene does not affect the absorption of β-carotene but improves that of lycopene. *J Nutr* 1997; 127: 1833–1837.

61. Roodenburg A J C, Leenen R, Van het Hof K H *et al*. Amount of fat in the diet affects bioavailability of lutein esters but not of α-carotene, β-carotene, and vitamin E in humans. *Am J Clin Nutr* 2000 71: 1187–1193.

62. Molldrem K L, Li J, Simon P W, Tanumihardjo S A. Lutein and β-carotene from lutein-containing yellow carrots are bioavailable in humans. *Am J Clin Nutr* 2004; 80: 131–136.

63. Castenmiller J J M, West C E, Linssen J P H *et al*. The food matrix of spinach is a limiting factor in determining the bioavailability of β-carotene and to a lesser extent of lutein in humans. *J Nutr* 1999; 129: 349–356.

64. Unlu N Z, Bohn T, Clinton S K, Schwartz S J. Carotenoid absorption from salad and salsa by humans is enhanced by the addition of avocado or avocado oil. *J Nutr* 2005; 135: 431–436.

65. Adebowale A, Du J, Liang Z, Leslie J L, Eddington N D. The bioavailability and pharmacokinetics of glucosamine hydrochloride and low molecular weight chondroitin sulfate after single and multiple doses to beagle dogs. *Biopharm Drug Disp* 2002; 23: 217–225.

66. Volpi N. Oral bioavailability of chondroitin sulfate (Condrosulf) and its constituents in healthy male volunteers. *Osteoarthritis Cartilage* 2002; 10: 768–777.

67. Cavallo A, Ritschel W A. Pharmacokinetics of melatonin in human sexual maturation. *J Clin Endocrinol Metab* 1996; 81: 1882–1886.

68. Giulidori P, Cortellaro M, Moreo G, Stramentinoli G. Pharmacokinetics of S-adenosyl-L-methionine in healthy volunteers. *Eur J Clin Pharmacol* 1984; 27: 119–121.

69. Marsen T A, Pollok M, Oette K, Baldamus C A. Pharmacokinetics of omega-3-fatty acids during ingestion of fish oil preparations. *Prostaglandins Leukotr Essent Fatty Acids* 1992; 46: 191–201.

70. Surette M E, Koumenis I L, Edens M B *et al*. Inhibition of leukotriene biosynthesis by a novel dietary fatty acid formulation in patients with atopic asthma: a randomized, placebo-controlled, parallel-group, prospective trial. *Clin Ther* 2003; 25: 972–979.

71. Kuijsten A, Arts I C W, Vree T B, Hollman P C H. Pharmacokinetics of enterolignans in healthy men and women consuming a single dose of secoisolariciresinol diglucoside. *J Nutr* 2005; 135: 795–801.

72. Gustin D M, Rodvold K A, Sosman J A *et al*. Single-dose pharmacokinetic study of lycopene delivered in a well-defined food-based lycopene delivery system (tomato paste–oil mixture) in healthy adult male subjects. *Cancer Epidemiol Biomarker Prev* 2004; 13: 850–860.

73. Osterlie M, Bjerkeng B, Liaaen-Jensen S. Plasma appearance and distribution of astaxanthin E/Z and R/S isomers in plasma lipoproteins of men after single dose administration of astaxanthin. *J Nutr Biochem* 2000; 11: 482–490.

74. Mercke Odeberg J, Lignell A, Pettersson A, Hoglund P. Oral bioavailability

of the antioxidant astaxanthin in humans is enhanced by incorporation of lipid based formulations. *Eur J Pharm Sci* 2003; 19: 299–304.

75. Setchell K D R, Brzezinski A, Brown N M *et al.* Pharmacokinetics of a slow-release formulation of soybean isoflavones in healthy postmenopausal women. *J Agric Food Chem* 2005; 53: 1938–1944.

76. Chow H–H S, Cai Y, Alberts D S *et al.* Phase I pharmacokinetic study of tea polyphenols following single-dose administration of epigallocatechin gallate and polyphenon E. *Cancer Epidemiol Biomarker Prev* 2001; 10: 53–58.

77. Van Het Hof K H, Kivits G A A, Weststrate J A, Tijburg L B M. Bioavailability of catechins from tea: the effect of milk. *Eur J Clin Nutr* 1998; 52: 356–359.

78. Williamson G, Manach C. Bioavailability and bioefficacy of polyphenols in humans. II. Review of 93 intervention studies. *Am J Clin Nutr* 2005; 81: 243S–255S.

79. Pisters K M, Newman R A, Coldman B *et al.* Phase I trial of oral green tea extract in adult patients with solid tumors. *J Clin Oncol* 2001; 19: 1830–1838.

5

Joint health

Prevalence of joint disease

Joint disease is a major cause of disability in the UK, affecting people of all ages, particularly the elderly. Currently, 29% of adults report being affected by arthritis or joint pain, which translates to over 13 million people across the UK.[1] The prevalence of joint disease is higher amongst women, those aged over 55 and those from less affluent populations.[1]

Most sufferers of joint disease describe their condition in terms of 'joint pain' or 'back pain', with fewer reporting having a specific arthritic condition. In fact, it can sometimes be difficult to determine where joint pain ends and arthritis begins. The term arthritis and related conditions can be used to cover a myriad of over 200 different complaints, of which the most common are osteoarthritis, rheumatoid arthritis, juvenile arthritis, gout and ankylosing spondylitis.[1]

Osteoarthritis

Osteoarthritis (OA) is the most common arthritic disorder, affecting 3–6% of the general population and over 10% of those aged over 64 years. This prevalence in the elderly makes arthritis almost a normal part of ageing. OA is characterised by the degenerative damage and loss of the articular cartilage of the joints, and hypertrophy of the underlying bone.[2] This damage is caused by the overexpression of enzymes known as metalloproteinases that degrade the cartilage matrix with the resultant loss of collagen and proteoglycans, the building blocks of this tissue.[3] The synthesis of these enzymes may be induced by the pro-inflammatory cytokine interleukin 1 (IL-1), which also inhibits the synthesis of new cartilage and induces the apoptosis of chondrocytes (the cellular component of cartilage) and the production of nitric oxide and prostaglandins. All of these factors may contribute to the destruction of cartilage that characterises OA.[3]

OA commonly affects the large joints such as those of the knee, hip or hand, and may well be present in a single joint only. The pain suffered by patients tends to be localised and worsens with activity, while early-morning joint stiffness tends to improve throughout the day.[2]

Rheumatoid arthritis

Rheumatoid arthritis (RA) affects 0.5–1% of the world's population and is a chronic systemic inflammatory disease affecting the synovial joints and exhibiting additional non-articular features.[4] RA is an autoimmune disease, initiated by the interaction between an unidentified antigen and the body's T lymphocytes. This causes an inflammatory response in the joints, leading to oedema, manifested as joint swelling and pain. This response also leads to the development of new blood vessels (angiogenesis), and hyperplasia of the synovial membrane lining the joint, with an increase in the number of macrophages and fibroblasts present. Infiltration of immune cells, including T and B lymphocytes, macrophages and plasma cells, into the joint also occurs. The synovial membrane starts to invade the tissue between cartilage and bone, resulting in the formation of a mass of tissue known as a 'pannus', which goes on to cause erosions of the joint.[4]

The proinflammatory cytokines IL-1 and tumour necrosis factor alpha (TNF-α) have been identified as crucial in the pathogenesis of RA, causing an increase in vascular permeability, chemotaxis, angiogenesis, metalloproteinase production and lymphocyte activation.[4]

RA is often symmetrical (affecting both right and left sides of the body) and usually affects multiple joints, particularly those of the hands and wrists, although other body areas may be affected. Pain may move from joint to joint, and increases with immobility. Morning stiffness may remain throughout the day and is relieved by modest activity. Extra-articular features include fatigue, weight loss, dry eyes and cardiovascular symptoms.[2]

Conventional treatment

The two main aims in treating arthritis patients are management of the symptoms, mainly pain and movement limitation, and slowing the disease process. The American College of Rheumatology guidelines for the management of OA[5] propose that the foundation of treatment for OA should be non-pharmacological, including patient education on factors such as exercise, diet and weight loss, physiotherapy, occupational therapy and special footwear. The treatment most commonly offered to people with joint disease of any description is drug therapy, with the most widely used drugs being the non-steroidal anti-inflammatory drugs (NSAIDs), such as ibuprofen or diclofenac.[1]

The widespread use of NSAIDs is a concern as they are associated with a high incidence of side-effects, particularly on the gastrointestinal system. It is estimated that at least 10–20% of patients experience dyspepsia while taking NSAIDs, with 16 500 NSAID-related deaths occurring among patients with RA or OA every year and over 103 000 admissions to hospital each year in the USA alone.[6] The incidence of such effects may be reduced somewhat by the use of cyclooxygenase-2 (COX-2)-selective agents such as celecoxib, which are designed to inhibit the inflammatory COX-2 enzyme without affecting the COX-1 isoform, which is responsible for maintaining normal renal function, gastric mucosal integrity and haemostasis.[7] However there has been some concern over the cardiovascular safety of some of these agents, leading to the withdrawal of rofecoxib from the market. NSAIDs may also precipitate a deterioration in renal function, and they cause asthmatic patients to develop wheezing.[7] Research has also indicated that NSAIDs may even worsen the disease process of OA, which has been linked to their ability to inhibit prostaglandin synthesis.[8]

It would appear, therefore, that none of the existing pharmacological treatments for the most common joint diseases are ideal. In light of this, it is perhaps not surprising that around a quarter of all patients suffering from joint disease have used some form of complementary medicine for their condition, including nutraceuticals.[1]

Glucosamine and chondroitin

Glucosamine is the principal component of the glycosaminoglycans (GAGs), long-chain polymers of repeating disaccharide units, which form the basis of the proteoglycan component of the matrix of all connective tissues, including cartilage. Glucosamine is produced in the body by the addition of an amino group to glucose.[9] This ability declines with age and predisposes the body to arthritis. *In vitro* experiments have shown a dose-dependent increase in proteoglycan after administering glucosamine, and increased synthesis of collagen.[9] Glucosamine is perhaps the most widely marketed supplement for degenerative joint disease, and is available from most pharmacies and health food stores, usually as the hydrochloride or sulfate salt. It is sometimes combined in supplements with the compound chondroitin sulfate, a GAG derived from bovine or calf cartilage. Both these compounds are reported to improve cartilage metabolism and to have anti-inflammatory effects[9] and thus may slow the degenerative process of OA. This has caused them to be referred to as structure-modifying, as well as slow-acting symptomatic drugs for the treatment of OA.[10]

One study investigated the effects of these agents, alone and in a combination including manganese ascorbate, for their ability to retard the progression of cartilage degeneration in a rabbit model of OA.[10] Animals receiving the combined supplement developed no severe lesions in their damaged joints, while 8 of the 11 control animals did. Animals receiving one supplement alone showed a small decrease in the incidence of severe lesions, but these results were not statistically significant.

In an *in vitro* experiment carried out during the above study, glucosamine hydrochloride stimulated GAG synthesis in cultured chondrocytes, but had little inhibitory activity on the collagenase enzyme responsible for breaking down cartilage, while chondroitin sulfate showed both effects. The combination showed a greater stimulatory effect on GAG synthesis than the additive effects of each compound alone, leading the researchers to propose a synergistic effect for glucosamine and chondroitin in stimulating cartilage synthesis.

In order for glucosamine and chondroitin to exert these effects on cartilage in human patients, it is necessary for them first to be absorbed into the body, and then taken up into the joints. However there is some disagreement in the literature over the pharmacokinetics of these agents, with different figures being quoted. Studies using radiolabelled glucosamine sulfate to track the fate of this compound after oral administration have reported that almost 90% of an administered dose is absorbed through the gastrointestinal tract, with around half of this being removed by first-pass metabolism. The absolute oral bioavailability of glucosamine is therefore reported to be 44%, most of which is incorporated into plasma proteins.[11]

The absorption of chondroitin would be expected to be less than that of glucosamine, due to its high molecular weight. One study using radiolabelled chondroitin[12] reported that in rats and dogs more than 70% of the radioactivity orally administered was found in urine and tissues. After 24 hours, radioactivity was higher in the intestines, liver, kidneys, synovial fluid and cartilage than in other tissues, suggesting that chondroitin shows a tropism for joint tissue. After administration of 0.8 g/day to human volunteers, either as a single dose or as two doses of 0.4 g, a significant increase in the plasma concentration of chondroitin was noted, which persisted over a 24-hour period. While the levels of GAGs in the joints did not alter, a change in the size distribution of these compounds was noticed, with a decrease in the number of high molecular mass components (markers of cartilage breakdown) and an increase in the number of low molecular mass compounds. The researchers suggest that part of this material is exogenous chondroitin sulfate, which has been localised to the joint tissue. This study would appear to demonstrate that chondroitin sulfate is both bioavailable and preferentially targeted to the joint tissue.

A recent study examining the pharmacokinetics of glucosamine hydrochloride following oral administration to horses[13] reported a bioavailability of only 5.9%, as determined by fluorophore-assisted carbohydrate electrophoresis of recovered glucosamine from serum. This method, however, would be unable to detect glucosamine bound to plasma proteins, which may explain the discrepancy between this study and those described above.

The same study also examined the levels of glucosamine in the synovial fluid, and found these to be less than 10% of those found in serum at the same time point, and 500 times less than those needed to exert physiological effects on tissue metabolism. These researchers therefore suggested that the beneficial effect of glucosamine on joint health may stem from changes in levels of systemic mediators of disease, rather than a local effect in the joint capsule.

This study used the hydrochloride salt of glucosamine, whereas the previously mentioned studies used glucosamine sulfate. It has been suggested[13] that the sulfate content of these preparations may influence the uptake of glucosamine by glucose transporters in the gut and its utilisation by intestinal cells. This is interesting as it has previously been suggested that the salt ion of glucosamine will make no difference once the nutraceutical reaches the stomach, where the hydrochloric acid naturally present will convert either form to glucosamine hydrochloride.[14] However it has also been hypothesised[15] that sulfate-containing neutraceuticals may exert their chondroprotective effects by overcoming bodily deficiencies of sulfur, in which case the sulfate component would be crucial for therapeutic activity. This suggestion stems from the observation that GAGs require a source of inorganic sulfate for their synthesis. This is supported by a study[16] showing that the oral administration of glucosamine and chondroitin sulfate only increased the urinary excretion of sulfate in individuals following a low-protein diet, which suggests that their sulfate component is retained by the body if a deficiency of sulfate (possibly caused by a dietary lack of sulfur amino acids) exists. However this study used healthy volunteers rather than arthritis patients, and further studies are needed to determine if increasing dietary sulfur can exert a beneficial effect on the symptoms of joint disease.

Glucosamine and chondroitin have been shown in a number of studies to improve various symptoms of OA, while some investigations have also provided evidence for a structure-modifying effect. However, a meta-analysis conducted in 2000 concluded that many studies are of poor quality, are supported by manufacturers and may exaggerate the benefits of these compounds.[17] This analysis included 15 double-blind, randomised, placebo-controlled trials of four or more weeks' duration testing glucosamine or chondroitin for symptomatic benefit in hip or knee OA. To be eligible for analysis studies had to report results for at least one of a number of outcomes validated for trials of OA drugs,[18] including measures of pain on various activities, Western Ontario and McMaster Universities Osteoarthritis Index (WOMAC) or Lequesne Index (LI) scores. The WOMAC and Lequesne Index are both algo functional measures (they assess both pain and function) commonly used in trials of OA drugs. The researchers calculated an effect size for the treatment in each trial and categorised the effects as small (effect size 0.2), medium (effect size 0.5) or large (effect size 0.8). The aggregated effect size for glucosamine was found to be 0.44, while that for chondroitin was 0.78, suggesting a moderate to large effect of these compounds in OA. However when only high-quality studies were included in the analysis the overall effect size decreased for both compounds.

Interestingly, when only four-week outcomes for those studies that had reported them were analysed, effect sizes were also diminished, suggesting that the full therapeutic response to glucosamine or chondroitin may take longer than a month to develop. The researchers concluded that glucosamine and chondroitin are likely to have some benefits in alleviating symptoms of OA and, given the low incidence of side-effects reported in the trials studied, may have considerable usefulness in the treatment of joint disease. However they recommend that further high-quality studies should be conducted in order to assess further their efficacy.

Glucosamine

A similar conclusion was reached by a Cochrane review of glucosamine therapy for the treatment of OA.[19] In this review, 12 out of 13 randomised controlled trials comparing glucosamine to placebo found glucosamine to be superior. However most of the trials included only evaluated a single preparation of glucosamine sulfate, and the reviewers noted that preparations from different manufacturers may not be equally effective.

NSAIDs are widely used in the management of OA, and sometimes their activity is compared with glucosamine in clinical trials.[7] Of the four trials of glucosamine versus NSAIDs included in the Cochrane review[19] two found the treatments equally effective, and two found glucosamine to be superior. A comparative study of glucosamine 1500 mg/day versus ibuprofen 1200 mg/day in 200 patients with OA of the knee[20] concluded that the two treatments were equally effective in relieving symptoms, assessed using the Lequesne Index, although the effect of glucosamine was slower to develop than that of ibuprofen. Additionally, glucosamine was much better tolerated than the NSAID, with 35% of patients on ibuprofen reporting adverse events compared with 6% of the glucosamine group.

It should be noted that this was only a short-term (four-week) study, during which the full therapeutic effect of glucosamine may not have developed. A three-month study[21] compared the effects of glucosamine 2000 mg/day with those of placebo in individuals experiencing regular knee pain. While both groups of patients improved in various clinical and functional tests over the study period, no significant differences were seen between groups. However, the glucosamine group were found to have significantly better quality of life scores at weeks 8 and 12, and at the end of the study period 88% reported improvements in their symptoms as opposed to only 17% of the placebo group.

These results suggest a beneficial effect of glucosamine in knee pain, which becomes apparent after eight weeks of treatment. However, the dose of glucosamine used in this trial was higher than that used in most other trials and in practice (1500 mg). It should also be noted that patients in this study did not have confirmed OA, and that relatively small numbers were used (24 glucosamine, 22 placebo). These factors may affect the validity of the results from this study and their generalisability to the larger patient population. Additionally, patients in the placebo group were found to have a longer history of knee pain than those in the glucosamine group (15.9 and 10.3 years respectively) which may have affected the results as it is possible that the longer an individual has been suffering from knee pain, the less likely any form of treatment is to have a beneficial effect.[21]

The claim that glucosamine is a structure-modifying as well as a symptom-modifying agent in OA has been investigated by two 3-year studies,[22,23] both involving over 200 patients. These studies compared daily doses of 1500 mg glucosamine sulfate to placebo in terms of the ability to modify joint structure and symptom changes in patients with knee OA. In both studies joint space width was measured using radiographic techniques and symptoms were evaluated using the WOMAC index[24] or a combination of WOMAC and the Lequesne Index.[23] After 3 years, the two groups of patients receiving placebo experienced joint space narrowing of between 0.19 mm and 0.31 mm, while glucosamine patients experienced no significant change. In both studies, the differences between groups became more significant over the 3-year period, suggesting that glucosamine needs to be taken continuously if it is to exert a beneficial effect on structural changes in OA.

In terms of the symptom changes in these two studies, both groups of glucosamine patients experienced an improvement in symptoms, measured by the WOMAC and Lequesne Index scores. Despite this, symptomatic relief did not correlate with structural improvements in either study, so a reduction in pain is unlikely to have biased the measurements of joint space width[23] (it is possible that patients experiencing less pain would have adopted a better posture during the joint space width measurements and thus appeared to have a wider joint space than those who were more symptomatic). This lack of correlation suggests that the symptomatic effects of glucosamine may be independent of its structural effects, with a possible explanation being that symptomatic improvement is due to an anti-inflammatory action, while the longer term structural improvements are due to an increase in the synthesis of proteoglycans and decreases in degradative enzyme activity.[22,23]

Importantly, both these studies included an intent-to-treat analysis, whereby patients who did not complete the study are included in the final analysis, reducing bias that may arise as a result of excluding patients from the final analysis who may have had a poor final outcome. Using this approach did not significantly change the results in either study.

In a subgroup analysis from one of these studies[22] the relationship between the baseline severity of OA and long-term joint space narrowing was investigated.[24] This analysis found that patients in the lowest quartile of baseline joint space with (i.e. those with the most severe OA) actually experienced an increase in joint space width over the 3-year study period, irrespective of whether they had received placebo or glucosamine (although the increase in joint space width in the glucosamine group was slightly larger). In patients with the greatest baseline joint space width, both groups experienced joint space narrowing. Glucosamine use was associated with a lesser degree of narrowing, which did not quite reach statistical significance ($P = 0.10$), which could have been due to the low numbers of patients included in the analysis. The researchers concluded that over a 3-year period, patients with less severe OA will experience a greater degree of deterioration than those with severe disease, and that the former group of patients may derive the most benefit from agents such as glucosamine.

Despite these promising results, trials of glucosamine are not uniformly positive. A six-month trial[25] comparing glucosamine sulfate 1500 mg/day with placebo concluded that there was no difference between groups in terms of the global assessment of pain in 80 patients with knee OA. However the patients in this trial had more severe arthritis than those in many other studies involving glucosamine, with 21% suffering from Kellgren and Lawrence grade 4 arthritis (classed as severe disease according to radiographic assessment) which lends support to the view that glucosamine is of more benefit to patients with mild to moderate OA.[24]

Interestingly, this study reported a strong placebo response with 33% of patients classified as responders. This may indicate a selection response, whereby patients who agreed to participate in the trial had a strong affinity for complementary therapies and would thus be inherently more likely to respond.[25] This may have implications for the design of all trials of complementary therapies, in order not to exaggerate effects.

A different approach to assess the efficacy of glucosamine involved a six-month randomised double-blind discontinuation trial, evaluating the effect of continuing or withdrawing glucosamine in 137 patients with knee OA who had been using glucosamine for at least one month and who had experienced at least moderate improvement in pain while taking this supplement.[26] The primary outcome was the proportion of disease flares in the two groups using an intent-to-treat analysis. This study found no difference in the proportion of disease flares between the two groups, and time to and severity of flare, consumption of rescue analgesia, change in pain, stiffness, function and quality of life were also similar.

This trial involved a moderately severely affected patient population, with the glucosamine group having more severe OA. This further supports the view that glucosamine may be of more benefit in mild disease. However after adjustment for radiographic severity, there was still no difference in the risk of disease flare between the two groups in this study, casting a shadow of doubt on this theory.

As this study was designed as a discontinuation trial, any initial benefit derived from glucosamine therapy could not be evaluated, particularly as patients were only enrolled if they had experienced subjective improvement in symptoms while taking this supplement.

However, as the researchers note, even if initial benefit was achieved, their findings suggest that there is no evidence of benefit from continued glucosamine use. They also noted that patients who had derived an initial benefit from glucosamine would be more likely to flare when this treatment was removed, making a trial such as theirs particularly efficient at highlighting any difference between glucosamine and placebo. Thus, their conclusion that there is no evidence of symptomatic benefit from continued use of glucosamine sulfate is strengthened.[26]

In an Internet-based trial involving 205 patients who took either 1500 mg/day glucosamine or placebo for a 12-week period,[27] no difference in the primary outcome (pain subscale of the WOMAC index) between the two groups was observed using either intent-to-treat analysis or analysis only of those patients completing the trial. Conclusions were also the same when scores were stratified by disease severity, casting further doubts on the theory that glucosamine is likely to be of more benefit in less severely affected patients. However, it should be noted that 82% of the patients in this trial suffered from severe disease (as classified by radiography) and so this study may not have had sufficient statistical power to detect a difference in outcome between severely and less severely affected patients.

It is interesting that all of the trials with null findings discussed above have been independently funded,[27] while many previous trials have been funded by industry. Possible bias in such trials cannot be excluded and it is clear that more high-quality, independent clinical trials are required to evaluate more clearly the efficacy of glucosamine as a long-term therapy for OA.

Chondroitin sulfate

As far as chondroitin sulfate is concerned, the picture is even less clear. A meta-analysis of seven clinical trials examining the efficacy of this supplement in the treatment of OA has been reported.[28] Trials had to be conducted over at least three months and the Lequesne Index and pain rating on visual analogue scale were the main outcome measures of interest. Chondroitin was shown to be significantly superior to placebo on both these measures, with relative improvement reaching statistical significance at two months when assessed by the Lequesne Index, and at four months when pain improvement was considered. Pooled results showed at least 50% improvement in the study variables in patients taking chondroitin compared with placebo. Doses of chondroitin sulfate used in the studies range from 800 to 2000 mg daily, but did not correlate with improvements in the outcome measures, indicating that an increase in dosage did not increase efficacy.

No investigation included in the analysis used an intent-to-treat analysis, which may have biased results slightly; however since there were few dropouts, and they were equally distributed between chondroitin and placebo patients, completer analyses may have been sufficiently valid. It should also be noted that only a small number of studies were included in the analysis, each of which only included a relatively small number of patients (700 in total, 372 of whom took chondroitin). Despite this, the included studies were uniformly positive and the results provide some evidence for the efficacy of chondroitin in ameliorating pain and improving function in patients with OA, possibly in combination with analgesics or low-dose NSAIDs.

Interestingly, a later trial[29] that did use an intent-to-treat analysis showed only a non-significant improvement in the Lequesne Index for chondroitin compared with placebo, which became significant when only the completer population was considered. In this study, treatment was continued for three months, followed by a three-month post-treatment period. The benefits associated with chondroitin persisted to one month post treatment, suggesting a sustained effect when this supplement is discontinued. Clearly further long-term studies are required to assess fully the efficacy of chondroitin sulfate in ameliorating symptoms and improving functional handicap in OA.

There is little available research evaluating the effect of chondroitin sulfate on disease progression in OA. Researchers carried out a randomised, double-blind, placebo-controlled trial in which 300 patients with knee OA received either 800 mg chondroitin or placebo daily for 2 years.[30] The primary outcome was joint space loss, with secondary outcomes including assessments of pain and function using the WOMAC index. This study found a significant joint space narrowing (of 0.14 mm) in the placebo group over 2 years, compared with no change in patients receiving chondroitin, representing a significant difference between the groups. Joint space width at baseline was not correlated with radiographic progression, in contrast to what has been found in trials involving glucosamine.[24] WOMAC scores did not show significant improvements for either group, although slightly more improvement was seen in patients taking chondroitin. This may have been due to a relatively low mean pain score at study entry, which left little room for improvement.[30] The results of this study suggest that long-term treatment with chondroitin sulfate may halt structural progression in OA; however further research is needed to confirm this.

In combination

Many supplements containing combinations of glucosamine and chondroitin are available; however it is not clear whether such products offer any benefit over the individual compounds. Recently, the results of the Glucosamine/chondroitin Arthritis Intervention Trial (GAIT),[31] a multicentre trial involving over 1500 patients with knee OA, have been published. GAIT was designed to address the methodological flaws in previous trials of glucosamine or chondroitin, such as failure to adhere to an intent-to-treat analysis, use of small numbers of patients, and possible bias due to sponsorship by manufacturers. Patients received either 1500 mg glucosamine, 1200 mg chondroitin, a combination of the two, 200 mg celecoxib or placebo daily for 24 weeks.

The primary outcome used was a 20% decrease in knee pain over the study period, and neither glucosamine, chondroitin nor the combination was significantly better than placebo in achieving this. However for patients with moderate to severe pain at baseline the rate of response was significantly higher with the combined therapy. In fact, improvements were seen with all treatments in this subgroup of patients, although the relatively small number of patients in this group may have limited the power of the study to detect clinical significance. The authors also note that the high rate of response to placebo and the relatively mild degree of pain among the participants, both of which have been discussed previously, may have limited the ability to detect benefits. Importantly, celecoxib was found to have a much shorter time to effect than the other treatments, with substantial improvements at four weeks. This tallies with the results of other studies indicating that nutraceuticals have a slower onset of action than conventional therapies, and patients considering using the supplements as alternatives to allopathic medicine should be informed of this.

In all the studies reviewed, adverse effects of glucosamine and chondroitin were mild, infrequently reported, and usually consisted of transient effects on the gastrointestinal system. This obviously gives them a huge advantage over the NSAIDs with their frequent and potentially serious side-effects. Of note, there has been some concern among researchers about reports that large concentrations of glucosamine can affect insulin secretion and action in animal and *in vitro* models.[32] However there is no evidence from clinical trials that glucosamine in usual doses affects insulin sensitivity or plasma glucose concentrations, even when administered to diabetic subjects.[32]

It seems, therefore, that these two widely used nutraceuticals are safe and may indeed provide benefit to some patients with OA, particularly in the relief of symptoms and possibly over longer periods slowing down the structural progression of the disease. However it should be noted that higher quality trials have generally shown lower levels of effect, and a substantial placebo response may be involved. Furthermore, benefits in other forms of joint disease have not been demonstrated.

Methylsulfonylmethane

Methylsulfonylmethane (MSM) is the oxidised form of dimethyl sulfoxide (DMSO), a natural organic form of sulfur.[33] Both these compounds have been used in the treatment of pain and inflammation, and MSM is found in many formulated products, often in combination with glucosamine and/or chondroitin.[34] MSM has advantages over DMSO as it is odourless and does not cause skin irritation.[33]

Exactly how MSM may be of benefit in joint disease is not certain, but it may well function by providing a source of sulfur for the formation of the cartilage matrix or the antioxidant systems N-acetylcysteine and glutathione.[33] This parallels the suggestion that compounds such as glucosamine and chondroitin sulfate may function by overcoming dietary deficiencies in sulfur amino acids.[15]

A study of the effect of MSM on a mouse model of RA[35] found that the arthritic score and levels of inflammatory markers were lower in mice that had had MSM added to their drinking water for one week before and eight weeks after immunisation with type II collagen. This result suggests that MSM is able to modify the immune response in mice, resulting in protection from the development of arthritis.

The effects of MSM in humans were evaluated in a study comparing MSM, glucosamine and their combination to placebo on 118 patients with mild to moderate OA of the knee.[33] A number of outcome measures related to pain and function were used, and both MSM and glucosamine were found to decrease significantly the mean pain and swelling indices after 12 weeks of treatment at a dose of 500 mg three times daily. The combination treatment was found to decrease these indices even further, and also to produce a statistically significant decrease in the Lequesne Index. Apart from mild gastrointestinal discomfort (more commonly reported in the glucosamine group), no significant adverse effects were reported.

A pilot scale clinical trial was recently carried out involving 50 subjects aged 40–76 years old with knee OA.[36] Patients took 3 g MSM twice daily for 12 weeks, and significant reductions in WOMAC pain and physical function impairment were reported. No effects were noted on stiffness or total symptom scores.

These two timely trials go some way towards providing evidence for the use of a widely used nutraceutical, previously only backed up with anecdotal evidence.

While these results for MSM seem encouraging, long-term trials involving larger groups of patients with different arthritic conditions are obviously required to provide more evidence regarding its safety and efficacy in the treatment of joint disease.

S-Adenosyl methionine

The potential of *S*-Adenosyl methionine (SAMe) for treatment of OA was accidently discovered when patients involved in clinical trials of SAMe for depression reported great improvements in OA symptoms! The diet alone cannot provide adequate quantities of SAMe, so the body relies on *de novo* synthesis to sustain required levels.[37]

The mechanism by which SAMe exerts an effect in OA is not clear, but may involve an antagonistic effect on cytokine-induced cell damage, an increase in proteoglycan synthesis, an increase in chondrocyte proliferation rate or protection of the anionic proteoglycans of the cartridge matrix by the cationic polyamine molecules synthesised in response to SAMe.[37]

A meta-analysis of 11 randomised controlled trials[38] compared SAMe with NSAIDs or placebo in the treatment of OA. SAMe was found to be effective in reducing functional limitation but not in reducing pain compared with placebo; however these results were calculated based on only two studies. Compared with NSAIDs, SAMe showed similar efficacy in reducing pain and functional limitation, and was associated with significantly fewer side-effects.

A range of doses from 400 mg/day intravenously to 1200 mg/day orally were used in the studies, some of which exceeded the dose recommendations for this supplement at that time (800 mg/day for two weeks followed by 400 mg/day maintenance, or 200 mg/day increased to 1200 mg/day over a 19-day period followed by 400 mg/day thereafter).[38] Despite this, dosage was not related to effect size in studies comparing SAMe to NSAIDs. Additionally, most studies had short follow-up periods (28–30 days) which may not have been long enough for the full effect of SAMe to develop.[38]

The results of this meta-analysis were supported by a more recent crossover study comparing SAMe at a dose of 1200 mg/day to celecoxib

200 mg/day.[39] This study was divided into two phases of two months each, with a one-week washout period in between. The treatments were compared based on a range of measures of pain, functional ability, mood and in terms of their side-effects.

At the end of the first month of phase 1, celecoxib was shown to be significantly more effective in reducing pain then SAMe, but pain reduction with SAMe increased steadily over the treatment period and by the end of the second month, no difference existed between the two groups. At the beginning of phase 2, the group switching from celecoxib to SAMe experienced an increase in pain, which was reversed during the second part of this phase. In contrast, those patients switching from SAMe to celecoxib continued to experience a decrease in pain over the first month of phase 2, which then levelled off so that by the end of the study the two groups were comparable. No differences between the two treatments were detected in terms of the other outcome measures, including side-effects.

These results, as well as providing further evidence for the similarity in efficacy between SAMe and NSAIDs in OA, suggest two things. First, the effect of SAMe takes some time to develop, and second, its effects may be sustained after discontinuation of treatment, possibly indicating an effect on the structural progression of the disease. This highlights the need for long-term studies to assess the effectiveness and safety of SAMe, to elucidate its mechanism of action and establish the optimal dose.[39] Finally, given the similar level of efficacy of SAMe to NSAIDs, could a combination of the two treatments be more effective than either alone in the management of OA?

Fish oils

Fish oils have been used to treat musculoskeletal conditions for over 200 years.[14] Epidemiological evidence supports this use, with studies of the Inuit Eskimo population revealing a relatively low incidence of musculoskeletal disease, which may be attributed to their high dietary intake of fish. The basis for this beneficial effect is believed to be the high concentrations of n-3 polyunsaturated fatty acids (PUFAs) such as eicosapentaenoic acid (EPA) and docosahexaenoic acid (DHA) present in oily fish such as mackerel, sardines and salmon.[14]

The typical Western diet is relatively poor in n-3 PUFAs and rich in n-6 PUFAs such as linoleic acid, which is converted to arachidonic acid, the precursor for the 2-series of prostaglandins and the 4-series of leukotrienes, both have which have strong proinflammatory activity.[14]

Since the metabolism of these two different types of fatty acids is competitive,[40] the balance of *n*-6 and *n*-3 PUFAs in the diet may be crucial in the regulation of the levels of inflammatory compounds in the body. Thus an increased intake of *n*-3 PUFAs leads to their incorporation into macrophage and neutrophil membranes in preference to arachidonic acid,[40] possibly decreasing the production of inflammatory mediators. Interestingly, *n*-9 PUFAs, such as those found in olive oil, are able to replace *n*-6 PUFAs in several aspects of cell metabolism and in doing so reduce the competition between the *n*-6 and *n*-3 PUFAs, leading to increased use and incorporation of *n*-3 PUFAs into cell membranes.[40]

n-3 PUFAs have also been shown to increase the expression and activity of both collagen-degrading enzymes such as metalloproteinases and proinflammatory factors such as IL-1 and TNF-α,[14] which may provide another explanation for any beneficial effects in arthritic disease.

Studies investigating the benefits of fish oils on joint health have concentrated on RA, the likely rationale being the strong inflammatory component of this disease.[4] A number of these studies were evaluated in a meta-analysis of 10 randomised, double-blind, placebo-controlled clinical trials investigating the benefits of fish oil in RA.[41] Statistically significant improvements in the studies were found after three months for tender joint count and duration of morning stiffness in patients receiving fish oil compared with those receiving placebo.

Following this analysis, the researchers gathered together primary data from each study used in the meta-analysis (for a total of 395 patients), re-evaluated it and compared these results with the results of the meta-analysis, a technique they termed 'mega-analysis'. The aim of this was to address the statistical issues of pooling data from studies with slightly different designs or outcome measures, assess bias and variability between studies, and identify outlying studies. Using the complete primary data set also allows researchers to adjust the data included in analyses to make comparisons more valid, to vary the form of the outcome measure used and to analyse subsets of the data, evaluating whether factors such as age, sex, duration of disease and other medications taken could affect the results. Fortin *et al.* concluded that the mega-analysis confirmed the results of their meta-analysis (i.e. that the use of fish oils improved the number of tender joints and duration of morning stiffness at three months in RA patients), and that the effects demonstrated were unaffected when alternative forms of the outcome measure were used (for example absolute change, proportional change or fractional change) or when the analysis was changed to include patient demographic factors.[41]

An overview of the use of *n*-3 PUFAs in RA,[42] which reviews many of the same studies as the previous meta-analysis,[41] makes particular reference to the potential of *n*-3 PUFAs to allow a reduction in the long-term requirements of NSAIDs in RA patients. In one study[43] in which patients were allowed to change their dose of NSAID, a significant decrease in NSAID requirement was observed both at three months and six months. The greater significance noticed at six months may indicate that the effect of fish oils in RA is slow to develop, and questions the validity of trials with short follow-ups.

In two further studies,[44,45] both carried out over the course of 12 months, the use of *n*-3 PUFAs was similarly associated with reduction in NSAID requirements, along with the significant improvements in patients' global assessments and pain score measured by the physician. In one of these studies,[45] the reduction in NSAID usage became significant by the third month of the study and reached its maximum at 12 months. After an additional three-month period, during which all patients received placebo, NSAID usage was still significantly reduced in the fish oil group. This provides further evidence for the slow onset of effect of fish oil supplementation, and also suggests that once established, this effect is sustained for some time even if therapy is discontinued.

In a further study,[46] which recorded significant benefits in terms of physician and patient global assessment, pain score, morning stiffness and painful joint count in patients taking NSAIDs and *n*-3 PUFAs in combination, deterioration was seen in a number of outcome measures when NSAIDs were discontinued. Whether *n*-3 PUFAs constitute a real alternative to NSAIDs in the treatment of RA is therefore open to question.

A recent survey of patients with non-surgical neck or back pain found that 78% were taking 1200 mg, and 22% taking 2400 mg of fish oil daily. 59% had discontinued treatment with NSAIDs as a result of overall pain reduction. This finding appears to demonstrate equivalent effects of these *n*-3 fatty acids to standard NSAID treatment.[47]

One study[48] attempted to evaluate whether using fish oils and olive oil in combination could provide any additional benefit to patients with RA over the use of fish oil alone. Forty-three patients were randomised to one of three groups, with the first (G1) receiving placebo, the second (G2) receiving fish oil *n*-3 PUFAs at a dose of 3 g/day and the third (G3) receiving fish oil plus 9.6 mL of olive oil. Patients were evaluated after 12 and 24 weeks in terms of the number of measures of symptoms and functional ability.

This study found that patients in G2 and G3 showed a statistically significant improvement compared with G1 in pain intensity and grip strength at 12 and 24 weeks, and in duration of morning stiffness, onset of fatigue, Ritchie's articular index and various functional aspects at 24 weeks only. This suggests that ingestion of n-3 PUFAs was able to improve certain clinical parameters in RA, with the benefits experienced increasing over time. Furthermore, patients in G3 experienced additional benefits, including earlier improvements in duration of morning stiffness and a significantly greater in improvement in patient global assessment than those in G2. Patients in G3 also showed a significant reduction in rheumatoid factor after 24 weeks compared with G1, while G2 did not. The researchers therefore concluded that their findings favoured the hypothesis that adding oleic acid (a major constituent of olive oil thought to have anti-inflammatory properties) to the diet of RA patients taking fish oils may lead to an additional improvement in their disease status. They also note that, because of its intrinsic activity, some earlier trials using olive oil as placebo may not be true evaluations of the benefits of n-3 PUFAs in arthritis, thus accounting for the modest effect sizes reported.

Contradicting these results, another trial, in which three groups of patients received either n-3 PUFAs, olive oil or a combination daily, benefits were seen only in the n-3 PUFAs group, suggesting that the benefits of olive oil in the treatment of arthritis are by no means established.[44]

Adverse effects to n-3 PUFAs reported in clinical trials are generally mild and usually related to gastrointestinal disturbances such as nausea, flatulence, diarrhoea, fishy taste and odour.[42] This gives them a further advantage over NSAIDs, with their frequently reported and often serious side-effects.

It therefore appears that the use of fish oils containing n-3 PUFAs, and possibly supplements containing different types of PUFAs may be beneficial in improving certain parameters such as joint tenderness or pain and early morning stiffness, and may also have the potential to reduce the NSAID requirement of patients with RA. However these effects are slow to develop, and at least three months of treatment may be required before benefits are observed.

γ-Linolenic acid

The potential of n-3 PUFAs to improve symptoms of arthritic disease has led researchers to consider whether other types of fatty acids may also exhibit benefits in these conditions. γ-Linolenic acid (GLA) is an *n*-6 PUFA found in evening primrose oil and borage oil, which is metabolised in the body to dihomo γ-linolenic acid (DGLA).[49] DGLA is the precursor of the 1-series of prostaglandins, which, although they are able to induce signs of inflammation, may actually decrease the activity of inflammatory cells. Ingestion of GLA, and its subsequent metabolism to DGLA, may also suppress inflammation through competitive inhibition of the production of leukotrienes and the 2-series prostaglandins[49] and may therefore be of benefit to those with arthritic conditions.

In order to assess the effects of GLA in RA patients, a study was carried out in which 37 patients with RA were treated with either 1.4 g/day GLA in borage seed oil or a cotton seed oil placebo.[50] Patients were assessed in terms of physician and patient global assessment, joint tenderness and swelling, morning stiffness, grip strength and ability to do daily activities. When compared with placebo, the GLA treatment was found to reduce significantly joint tenderness and swelling, physician global assessment and pain score at the end of the 24-week study period. Moreover, seven patients in the GLA group exhibited a meaningful improvement (defined as a 25% improvement or improvement of two levels in at least four measures) over the study period, in contrast to only one in the control group. Adverse reactions were restricted to mild gastrointestinal effects, and no GLA-treated patients withdrew from the study because of adverse reactions.

A further study[51] involved 56 patients who received either 2.8 g/day GLA or a sunflower seed oil placebo for six months in a double-blind trial, followed by a six-month single blind trial where all patients received GLA. During the first six months, significant reductions were seen in signs and symptoms of disease activity in the GLA group, and more patients in this group demonstrated overall meaningful responses (according to criteria similar to those used in the previous study) than in the control group. During the second six months both groups showed improvements, indicating progressive improvement over the entire 12-month period for those patients treated with GLA.

Both these studies involved doses of GLA much greater than those found in over-the-counter supplements containing GLA (for example evening primrose oil). Further studies involving large groups of patients are therefore required in order to evaluate further the positive and adverse effects of GLA, and to define an optimal dosage for use in RA patients.

Cetylated fatty acids

Another group of fatty acids currently undergoing evaluation of their beneficial effects in joint disease are the cetylated, monounsaturated fatty acids (CFA) such as cetyl myristoleate (CMO), which, although their mechanism of action is uncertain, may act to reduce inflammation, possibly due to the inhibition of 5-lipooxygenase.[52]

One study evaluated the benefits of the administration of an oral preparation of a blend of CFA in 64 patients with chronic knee OA.[52] Patients were evaluated after 30 and 68 days of treatment by means of physician assessment, measurement of range of motion of the affected joint, and completion of the Lequesne Index. This study found a significant (P 0.001) improvement in knee flexion in the CFA group compared with the control group at each time point. Minimal improvements were also noted in this group compared with the controls in terms of the physician assessment, but these did not reach statistical significance. In terms of the Lequesne Index, a trend towards improvement in the CFA group compared with the control group was reported, which reached statistical significance when the data were analysed as ordinal.

Following this study, a series of investigations were carried out by Kraemer *et al.*[53–55] to assess the benefits of topical formulations of CFA in OA. The first of these[53] involved a total of 40 patients with OA of the knee who received either a cream consisting of a blend of CFA or a placebo cream which they were to apply twice a day for 30 days. Patients were assessed at baseline, 30 minutes after the first application of cream and at the end of the 30-day treatment period in terms of a variety of functional parameters including knee range of motion, postural stability, balance, and ability to rise from a chair (up and go test), walk and ascend/descend stairs.

Patients receiving the CFA cream performed better in most of the outcome measures at the follow-up assessments than the control group, although it should be noted that the control group also improved their performance in some of these measures. However, these improvements were not as large as those in the CFA group, and were usually only apparent at the second test (30 minutes after initial treatment). Additionally, improvements were noticed in the CFA group after 30 minutes, during which time it would have been unlikely that the CFAs in the cream could have been absorbed across the skin. These results suggest that some of the initial improvements seen may be attributed to the acute, pain-relieving effects of massaging the cream into the knee, rather than to the active ingredients. However, the fact that the CFA group improved more, and continued to improve over the 30-day treatment period supports the researchers' conclusion that the use of the CFA topical cream is effective for improving some aspects of functional performance in patients with OA.

A further study by these researchers[54] evaluated the effects of a cream similar to that used in the above study, but to which menthol had been added, in a group of 28 patients with OA of the knee, or severe pain of the elbow or wrist. Treatment was continued for one week, and no control group was used since the researchers were only looking to compare their results with those from the last trial.[20] For patients with knee OA, similar tests were used to those in the original study, with the addition of the WOMAC index. For patients with upper extremity pain, a range of tests were used to evaluate grip strength, range of motion and muscular endurance, and a pain scale was completed.

This study found functional improvements in the OA patients comparable to those demonstrated in the previous study and a significant improvement in the pain and function subscales of the WOMAC measure were also noticed. In those patients with elbow or wrist pain, improvements were noticed in muscular endurance and in pain perception, but not the other outcome measures. The researchers concluded that the use of a CFA cream in patients with joint disease may be useful for enhancing the potential for exercise training in this population, and may thus be a useful adjunct to other treatments such as physiotherapy. Further research is needed to determine the impact of menthol in such a cream.

The positive outcomes of these studies suggest that CFAs may be beneficial for patients with OA; however the use of short follow-up periods, small groups of patients and, in most cases, failure to use outcome measures validated for the assessment of potential OA drugs,[18] means that further studies are required to assess their effects more fully. In addition, little is known about the mechanism of action of CFAs, which also merits further research. If CFAs work by decreasing inflammation, they may be of more benefit to patients with RA, in whom the disease process involves a larger inflammatory component.

Miscellaneous nutraceuticals

Soy protein has been investigated *in vitro* as an anti-inflammatory agent, and found to be a powerful inhibitor of lipoxygenase and COX-2. A recent clinical trial involving OA patients supplemented with 40 g of soy protein per day over three months was carried out using the same dose of milk protein as placebo. Soy protein was found to improve OA symptoms such as ease of motion and level of pain, and also cartilage metabolism was found to decrease at the same time that growth factor associated with cartilage synthesis was increased.[56]

Green tea has also been investigated *in vitro*, and tea polyphenols, epicatechin gallate and epigallocatechin gallate, were found to be effective in inhibiting proteoglycan and type-II collagen breakdown.[57]

Pycnogenol activity has also been reported following *in vivo* work in human volunteers. Pycnogenol 300 mg was shown to produce a statistically significant increase in inhibition of COX-1 and COX-2, which is consistent with reports of clinical anti-inflammatory effects.[58]

Conclusions

A wide variety of nutraceuticals have been claimed to be of benefit in joint disease, particularly OA and RA. Of these, the current evidence base is perhaps best for the use of *n*-3 PUFAs in RA and glucosamine (and possibly chondroitin) in OA. However, a number of more recently investigated compounds, for example MSM and SAMe, have also shown promise, particularly in OA.

The main attractions of these agents are their lack of side-effects and the possibility that they may be able to affect beneficially the disease course rather than just ameliorating symptoms. However, many of the clinical trials conducted to date have been of low quality and possibly biased by sponsorship from manufacturers, so that their results must be interpreted with care. Furthermore, variations in the quality of formulated products means that supplies must be sourced carefully. Pharmacists advising on the use of nutraceuticals should warn patients of their slow onset of action, and emphasise that as of yet they should be viewed as complementary rather than alternative to conventional therapies for joint disease.

References

1. Arthritis the big picture. *ARC publication* 2002. Available at: http://www.arc.org.uk/about_arth/bigpic.htm#9 (accessed 16 May 2006).
2. Bayrakter A, Hudson S, Watson A, Fraser S. Pharmaceutical care: arthritis. *Pharm J* 2000; 264: 57–68.
3. Osteoarthritis Pathophysiology. *Johns Hopkins Arthritis*. Available at: http://www.hopkins-arthritis.sam.jhmi.edu/osteo/osteo_patho.html (accessed February 2006).

4. Buch M, Emery P. The aetiology and pathogenesis of rheumatoid arthritis. *Hospital Pharm* 2002; 9: 5–9.

5. Recommendations for the medical management of osteoarthritis of the hip and knee: 2000 update American College of Rheumatology Subcommittee on Osteoarthritis Guidelines. *Arthritis Rheum* 2000; 43: 1905–1915.

6. Wolfe M, Lichtenstein D R, Singh G. Gastrointestinal toxicity of nonsteroidal antiinflammatory drugs. *N Engl J Med* 1999; 340: 1888–1896.

7. Parkinson S, Alldred A. Drug regimens for rheumatoid arthritis. *Hospital Pharm* 2000; 9: 11–19.

8. Rashad S, Hemingway A, Rainsford K *et al*. Effect of non-steroidal antiinflammatory drugs on the course of osteoarthritis. *Lancet* 1989; ii: 519–521.

9. Deal C L, Moskowitz R W. Nutraceuticals as therapeutic agents in osteoarthritis. *Osteoarthritis* 1999; 25: 379–396.

10. Lippiello L, Woodward J, Karpman R, Hammad T A. In vivo chondroprotection and metabolic synergy of glucosamine and chondroitin sulfate. *Clin Orthopaed Relat Res* 2000; 381: 229–240.

11. Setikar I, Rovati L C. Absorption, distribution, metabolism and excretion of glucosamine sulfate. *Arzneimittel-Forschung* 2001; 51: 699–725.

12. Conte A, Volpi N. Palmieri L *et al*. Biochemical and pharmacokinetic aspects of oral treatment with chondroitin sulfate. *Arzneimittel-Forschung* 1995; 45: 918–925.

13. Laverty S, Sandy J D, Celeste C *et al*. Synovial fluid levels and serum pharmacokinetics in a large animal model following treatment with oral glucosamine at clinically relevant doses. *Arthritis Rheum* 2005; 52: 181–191.

14. Curtis C L, Harwood J L, Dent C M, Caterson B. Biological basis for the benefit of nutraceutical supplementation in arthritis. *Drug Discovery Today* 2004; 9: 165–172.

15. Parcell S. Sulfur in human nutrition and applications in medicine. *Altern Med Rev* 2002; 7: 22–44.

16. Corboda F, Nimni M E. Chondrotin sulfate and other sulfate containing chondroprotective agents may exhibit their effects by overcoming a deficiency of sulfur amino acids. *Osteoarthritis Cartilage.* 2003; 11: 228–230.

17. McAlindon T E, LaValley M P, Gulin J P, Felson D T. Glucosamine and chondroitin for treatment of osteoarthritis. *JAMA* 2000; 283: 1469–1475.

18. Osteoarthritis Research Society Task Force. Design and conduct of clinical trials in patients with osteoarthritis. *Osteoarthritis Cartilage* 1996; 4: 217–243.

19. Towheed T E, Anastassiades T P, Shea B, *et al*. Glucosamine therapy for treating osteoarthritis (Cochrane Review). In: *The Cochrane Library*, Issue 2, 2001.

20. Muller-Fabbender H, Bach G L, Haase W *et al*. Glucosamine sulfate compared to ibuprofen in osteoarthritis of the knee. *Osteoarthritis Cartilage* 1994; 2: 61–69.

21. Braham R, Dawson B, Goodman C. The effect of glucosamine supplementation on people experiencing regular knee pain. *Br J Sport Med* 2003; 37: 45–49.

22. Reginster JY, Deroisy R, Rovati LC *et al*. Long-term effects of glucosamine sulphate on osteoarthritis progression: a randomised , placebo-controlled clinical trial. *Lancet* 2001; 357: 251–257.

23. Pavelka K, Gatterova J, Olejarva M *et al*. Glucosamine sulfate use and delay of progression of knee osteoarthritis. *Arch Intern Med* 2002; 162: 2113–2123.

24. Bruyere O, Honore A, Ethgen O *et al*. Correlation between radiographic severity of knee osteoarthritis and future disease progression. *Osteoarthritis Cartilage* 2003; 11: 1–5.

25. Hughes R, Carr A. A randomised, double-blind, placebo-controlled trial of glucosamine sulphate as an analgesic in osteoarthritis of the knee. *Rheumatology* 2002; 41: 279–284.

26. Cibere J, Kopec JA, Thorne A *et al*. Randomized, double-blind, placebo-controlled glucosamine discontinuation trial in knee osteoarthritis. *Arthritis Rheum* 2004; 51: 738–745.

27. McAlindon T, Formica M, LaValley M *et al*. Effectiveness of glucosamine for symptoms of knee osteoarthritis: Results from an internet-based randomized double-blind controlled trial. *Am J Med* 2004; 117: 643–649.

28. Leeb B F, Schweitzer H, Montag K, Smolen J S. A metaanalysis of chondroitin sulfate in the treatment of osteoarthritis. *J Rheumatol* 2000; 27: 205–211.

29. Mazieres B, Combe B, Phan Van A *et al*. Chondroitin sulfate in osteoarthritis of the knee: a prospective, double blind, placebo controlled multicenter clinical study. *J Rheumatol* 2001; 28: 173–181.

30. Michel BA, Stucki G, Frey D *et al*. Chondroitins 4 and 6 sulfate in osteoarthritis of the knee. *Arthritis Rheum* 2005; 52: 779–786.

31. Clegg D O, Reda D J, Harris C L *et al*. Glucosamine, chondroitin sulfate and the two in combination for painful knee ostearthritis. *N Engl J Med* 2006; 354: 795–808.

32. Anderson J W, Nicolosi R J, Borzelleca J F. Glucosamine effects in humans: a review of effects on glucose metabolism, side effects, safety considerations and efficacy. *Food Chem Toxicol* 2005; 43: 187–201.

33. Usha P R, Naidu M U R. Randomised, double-blind, parallel, placebo-controlled study of oral glucosamine, methylsulfonylmethane and their combination in osteoarthritis. *Clin Drug Invest* 2004; 24: 353–363.

34. Ely A, Lockwood B. What is the evidence for the safety and efficacy of dimethyl sulfoxide and methylsulfonylmethane in pain relief? *Pharm J* 2002: 269: 685–687.

35. Takashi H, Sugi U, Shoichiro K, Yasunobu Y. Suppressive effect of methylsulfonylmethane on type II collagen-induced arthritis in DBA/1J mice. *Jpn Pharmacol Ther* 2004; 32: 421–427.

36. Kim L S, Axelrod L J, Howard P, Buratovich N, Waters R F. Efficacy of methylsulfonylmethane (MSM) in osteoarthritis pain of the knee: a pilot clinical trial. *Osteoarthritis Cartilage* 2006; 14: 286–294.

37. Bottiglieri T. S-Adenosyl-L-methionine (SAMe): from the bench to the bedside-molecular basis of a pleiotrophic molecule. *Am J Clin Nutr* 2002; 76: 1151s–1157s.

38. Soeken K L, Lee W-L. Bausell R B *et al*. Safety and efficacy of S-adenosylmethionine(SAMe) for osteoarthritis. *J Fam Pract* 2002; 51: 425–430.

39. Najm W I, Reinsch S, Hoehler F, Todis J S, Harvey P W. S-Adenosyl methionine (SAMe) versus celecoxib for the treatment of osteoarthritis symptoms: a double-blind cross-over trial. *BMC Musculoskelet Disord* 2004;5.

40. Darlington L G, Stone T W. Antioxidants and fatty acids in the amelioration of rheumatoid arthritis and related disorders. *Br J Nutr* 2001; 85: 251–269.
41. Fortin P R, Lew R A, Liang M H *et al*. Validation of a meta-analysis: the effects of fish oil in rheumatoid arthritis. *J Clin Epidemiol* 1995; 48: 1379–1390.
42. Ariza-Ariza R, Mestanza-Peralta M, Cardiel M H. Omega-3 fatty acids in rheumatoid arthritis: an overview. *Semin Arthritis Rheum* 1998; 27: 366–370.
43. Skoldseam L, Borjesson O, Kjallman A *et al*. Effect of six months of fish oil supplementation in stable rheumatoid arthritis. A double-blind, controlled study. *Scand J Rheum* 1992; 21: 178–185.
44. Geusens P, Wouters C, Nijs J *et al*. Long-term effect of omega-3 fatty acid supplementation in active rheumatoid arthritis. A 12-month, double-blind controlled study. *Arthritis Rheum* 1994; 37: 824–829.
45. Law C S, Morley K D, Belch J J. Effects of fish oil supplementation on non-steroidal anti-inflammatory drug requirement in patients with mild rheumatoid arthritis-a double blind placebo controlled study. *Br J Rheumatol* 1993; 32: 982–989.
46. Kremer J M, Lawrence D A, Petrillo G F *et al*. Effects of high dose fish oil on rheumatoid arthritis after stopping nonsteroidal anti-inflammatory drugs: clinical and immune correlates. *Arthritis Rheum* 1995; 8: 107–114.
47. Maroon J C, Bost J W. Omega-3 fatty acids (fish oil) as an anti-inflammatory: an alternative to nonsteroidal anti-inflammatory drugs for discogenic pain. *Surg Neurol* 2006; 65: 326–331.
48. Berbert A A, Condo C R M, Almendra C L *et al*. Supplementation of fish oil and olive oil in patients with rheumatoid arthritis. *Nutrition* 2005; 21: 131–136.
49. Belch J J F, Hill A. Evening primrose oil and borage oil in rheumatologic conditions. *Am J Clin Nutr* 2000; 71s: 325s–326s.
50. Lawrence J, Leventhal L J, Borce E G, Zurier R B. Treatment of rheumatoid arthritis with gammalinolenic acid. *Ann Intern Med* 1993; 119: 867–873.
51. Zurier R B, Rossetti R G, Jacobson E W *et al*. Gamma-linolenic acid treatment of rheumatoid arthritis: a randomised, placebo-controlled trial. *Arthritis Rheum* 1996; 39: 1808–1817.
52. Hesslink R, Armstrong D, Nagendran M V *et al*. Cetylated fatty acids improve knee function in patients with osteoarthritis. *J Rheumatol* 2002; 29: 1708–1712.
53. Kraemer W J, Ratamess N A, Anderson J M *et al*. Effect of a cetylated fatty acid topical cream on functional mobility and quality of life of patients with osteoarthritis. *J Rheumatol* 2004; 31: 767–774.
54. Kraemer W J, Ratamess N A, Maresh C M *et al*. A cetylated fatty acid topical cream with menthol reduces pain and improves functional performance in individuals with arthritis. *J Strength Cond Res* 2005; 19: 475–480.
55. Kraemer W J, Ratamess N A, Maresh C M *et al*. Effects of treatment with a cetylated fatty acid topical cream on static postural stability and plantar pressure distribution in patients with knee osteoarthritis. *J Strength Cond Res* 2005; 19: 115–121.
56. Arjmandi B H, Khalil D A, Lucas E A, *et al*. Soy protein may alleviate osteoarthritis symptoms. *Phytomedicine* 2004; 11: 567–575.

57. Adcocks C, Collin P, Buttle D J. Catechins from green tea (*Camellia sinensis*) inhibit bovine and human cartilage proteoglycan and type II collagen degradation in vitro. *J Nutr* 2002; 132: 341–346.
58. Schafer A, Chovanova Z, Muchova J *et al.* Inhibition of COX-1 and COX-2 activity by plasma of human volunteers after ingestion of French maritime pine bark extract (Pycnogenol). *Biomed Pharmacother* 2006; 60: 5–9.

6

Cardiovascular health

Cardiovascular diseases (CVDs), which affect the heart and circulatory system, are known to cause millions of deaths each year worldwide, comprising the largest contribution to mortality in Europe and North America.[1] According to prevalence data from the National Health and Nutrition Examination Survey III, 64.4 million Americans have one or more types of CVD, of whom 25.3 million are aged 65 years or older, and accounted for 38.5% of all deaths in the USA. The cost implications of this, both direct and indirect, have been estimated to be US$368.4 million.[2] Consequently much research has been aimed at developing new treatments and new methods of prevention of CVD.[3]

Known high-risk factors include smoking, diabetes, hypertension and hypercholesterolaemia; eating a diet high in saturated fats accelerates this process. Individuals with a predisposition and those with established CVD are increasingly given advice relating to their dietary habits, particularly relating to their fat and cholesterol intake and the risk of developing coronary heart disease (CHD), which has been linked by both epidemiological studies and clinical trials.[4] Further to this, the National Cholesterol Education Program in the USA, has shown that for every 10% reduction in cholesterol levels, CHD mortality is reduced by 13% and total mortality by 10%.[2]

In CHD, atherosclerotic plaques form on the inner surface of arteries, which narrows the lumen and consequently reduces the blood flow. Low-density lipoprotein (LDL) then deposits at lesion sites in the artery wall and is oxidised, which causes modifications in lipoproteins, stimulates inflammatory reactions, and causes monocytes and macrophages to accumulate, forming foam cells with high lipid levels and atherosclerotic plaques.[5]

Studies of lipid metabolism have shown that it is not the high cholesterol levels that cause atherosclerosis and CHD but rather the oxidised low-density lipoprotein–cholesterol (LDL-C). The use of antioxidants would therefore be expected to reduce the incidence of CHD and this has been shown in epidemiological studies.[6]

Lipids are transported as lipoproteins in the blood. These include very low-density lipoprotein–cholesterol (VLDL-C), LDL-C and high-density lipoprotein–cholesterol (HDL-C). LDL-C is removed from the circulation by binding with both plasma membranes and HDL-C, and is a less concentrated form of cholesterol. An increased level of LDL-C can result from a deficiency in the binding mechanism and is known as type II hypercholesterolaemia. This can be due to a genetic defect (familial hypercholesterolaemia) or multifactorial due to genetics, diet and lifestyle. As well as primary hypercholesterolaemia, increased cholesterol levels may be secondary to diabetes mellitus, hypothyroidism, pregnancy, renal failure, obesity, a high alcohol intake, poor diet and various drugs, such as beta-blockers, diuretics and oral contraceptives. Hypercholesterolaemia is known to be an important risk factor in the development of atherosclerosis and CHD, and studies have shown that a 1% decrease in serum cholesterol can lead to a 2% reduction in mortality. The aims of treatment are to increase HDL-C and decrease total cholesterol and LDL-C.[7,8]

Although diet can be used to lower cholesterol levels, in many cases this is insufficient and pharmacological intervention is required. Although generally safe and well tolerated, some lipid-lowering drugs cause side-effects. The statins, for example pravastatin and lovastatin, which are widely prescribed, have been reported to (rarely) cause hepatotoxicity, reflected by increases in serum transaminases, as well as myopathy leading to renal failure, reflected by increases in creatine phosphokinase.[9] The importance of these side-effects is augmented by the fact that statins are usually taken over a long period.

Myocardial infarctions (MIs) occur in patients who have established CHD where there is severe and/or prolonged impaired supply of oxygenated blood to the cardiac tissue. There are a wide range of risk factors associated with the development of CHD, including family history, hypertension, raised serum cholesterol, diabetes, smoking, poor diet and lack of exercise.[1]

There is evidence that a number of nutraceuticals are beneficial in the prevention or symptom reduction of CHD, including black and green tea and their flavonoids, soy protein and isoflavones, essential fatty acids, flax lignans, coenzyme Q10, lycopene, policosanol and Pycogenol, melatonin, resveratrol, grape seed proanthocyanidin extract (GSPE), lutein, carnitine, and dehydroepiandrosterone (DHEA). The aim of this chapter is to determine what effects these nutraceuticals have on the cardiovascular system and what evidence there is to support their use, both experimentally and clinically. This topic has been the subject of a number of publications, and tea and soy constituents have been researched to a much greater extent than other nutraceuticals.

Black and green tea

Tea is probably the most popular drink in the world, second only to water in terms of average per capita consumption, and annual world-wide per capita consumption of tea has been estimated at 40 L/year.[10] A number of epidemiological surveys have been carried out, in particular in high-consuming populations.

During the production of commercial green teas, varying propor-tions of catechin derivatives are produced, dependent upon the origin of the raw material and treatment conditions.[11] The fermentation process-ing used for black teas results in production of more complex polymeric components in addition,[12] and also produces products of widely varying composition.[13]

Another interesting component of tea is the amino acid theanine (see Chapter 21), which has been shown to significantly reduce blood pressure in hypertensive rats.[14]

Epidemiological studies have been carried out in order to evaluate the effect of tea consumption on the incidence of CVD, but the findings are to some extent contradictory, with beneficial, adverse or no effects being reported.[11] Initially most research was on green tea, but recently research has also included black and oolong teas.

Reduction of plasma lipid levels

One proposed mechanism by which tea may protect from CVD is via its effects on lipid and lipoprotein levels, and a number of epidemio-logical studies have studied the relationship between tea consumption and a possible cholesterol-lowering potential.[15]

In a study on 1371 Japanese men, increased consumption of green tea, from 3 to 10 cups per day, was associated with decreased serum concentrations of total cholesterol and triglyceride and an increased proportion of HDL-C together with a decreased proportion of LDL-C and VLDL-C. The group of subjects consuming the highest level of tea, ten cups daily, showed a significant decrease in the ratio of LDL-C to HDL-C.[16]

A further inverse relationship between green tea consumption and serum cholesterol and triglyceride levels has been identified in another epidemiological study, also conducted in Japan. While ingestion of ten cups of green tea per day (estimated to contain 360–540 mg of epigallocatechin gallate) did not lower total plasma cholesterol levels of postmenopausal women, male subjects were found to have decreased serum levels of both total cholesterol and triglycerides.[17]

One study was conducted to determine the effects of black tea consumption on the blood lipid profiles of a group of mildly hypercholesterolaemic adults, and showed significant reduction in cholesterol levels. Ingestion of five servings of black tea per day during the three weeks of the trial reduced total cholesterol 6.5%, LDL-C 11.1%, apolipoprotein B (apoB) 5% and lipoprotein(a) 16.4%, compared with a caffeine-containing placebo, but less markedly compared with the placebo without caffeine.[18]

In vivo studies with rats have shown that tea catechins reduced the solubility of cholesterol in micelles, which could be linked to reduced intestinal absorption of cholesterol.[15] Also in rats it has been shown that green tea catechins and black tea polyphenols may exert their hypocholesterolaemic activity via a number of mechanisms, including increased faecal excretion of fat and cholesterol, upregulated LDL receptors in liver cells, and reduced hepatic cholesterol concentration.[15] However, it is unknown whether this also occurs in humans.

A randomised controlled trial carried out in China investigated the cholesterol-lowering effect of a theaflavin-enriched (375 mg) green tea extract on adults with mild to moderate hypercholesterolaemia. Patients taking the extract showed an 11.3% reduction in serum total cholesterol and a 16.4% reduction in LDL-C, compared with placebo.[15] However, a study carried out in the USA on patients ingesting 900 mL black tea daily over four weeks found no significant alteration in total cholesterol, LDL-C or HDL-C.[19]

Smoking is a major risk factor for atherosclerotic diseases, as it is known to trigger vascular injury by platelet aggregation. P-selectin is induced by platelet aggregation and is involved in the adhesion of white blood cells to epithelial cells; also plasma concentrations are higher in smokers. A recent study investigated the effects of green tea consumption on atherosclerotic biological markers in smokers. Participants drank 600 mL of green tea per day for four weeks, and there was a significant decrease in P-selectin plasma concentrations, of the order of 55%, and 15% reduction in oxidised LDL.[20]

Activity on endothelial function

As endothelial dysfunction is associated with a state of increased oxidative stress, it follows that ingestion of antioxidants could reverse the associated impaired vascular function.[19] In addition to its importance in the development and progression of atherosclerosis and thrombogenesis, impaired vascular function is associated with CVD, and antioxidant tea flavonoids may mediate improvements in vascular function.[21]

Endothelial cells that line blood and lymphatic vessels and the heart have an integral role in vascular homeostasis, mediating their effects via the production and release of chemical agents such as nitric oxide. Nitric oxide is integral to normal endothelial function, hence vasomotor tone, platelet activity, leukocyte adhesion, and vascular smooth muscle cell proliferation.[11]

If the normal functioning of endothelial cells is disrupted, a loss of nitric oxide is often observed, impairing vasodilator function in conduit arteries and resulting in an increased risk of developing CVD.[22] This situation occurs in atherosclerosis when the production of nitric oxide in the endothelium is reduced, therefore providing antioxidant treatment in response to endothelial dysfunction and atherosclerosis may be able to decrease oxidative stress and improve endothelial health.[11]

Increased antioxidant defences in the body and decreased production of reactive oxygen species may contribute to reduced breakdown and/or enhanced synthesis and release of endothelial-derived nitric oxide, and hence improve vascular function. In studies looking at the beneficial effect of tea flavonoids on endothelial function, brachial artery flow-mediated dilation (FMD) has been used as a marker of vasodilator function, which in turn reflects endothelial function.[21]

The effects of both 2-hour and four-week black tea ingestion on endothelial dysfunction in patients with coronary artery disease have been investigated. Plasma tea flavonoids increased after ingestion during both regimens, and also improved endothelium-dependent FMD of the brachial artery.[19]

Acute consumption of black tea showed a 65% improvement in brachial artery FMD; regular ingestion of black tea over a four-week period was found to improve FMD 56%, while a 77% acute improvement was reported in those subjects who ingested black tea chronically.[19]

Five cups of black tea per day were taken by patients with mild elevations in serum cholesterol or triglyceride concentrations over four weeks. There were insignificant changes in total cholesterol, LDL-C and

HDL-C, but endothelium-dependent FMD improved by approximately 41%.[21]

Effects of tea on atherogenesis

CHD results in the death of over 6.5 million people worldwide each year and atherosclerosis of the coronary arteries is the cause of most incidences.[1] Epidemiological studies have shown that consumption of approximately two cups of black tea per day correlates with a decreased risk of developing CHD, and it is thought that this may be mediated by reduced incidence and degree of progression of atherogenesis in tea-drinking individuals.[23]

Black and green teas have been shown to be equally effective in increasing the total plasma antioxidant status after a single dose, however another study showed green tea to be more effective than black. Epidemiological studies relating tea consumption with lipid levels showed a negative correlation in black tea drinkers in Norway, and no correlation in Japanese green tea drinkers.[10] Animal work using experimentally induced atherosclerosis showed an inverse association between both green and black tea consumption and atherogenesis. Low dose teas, 0.0625%, caused a decrease in atherosclerosis by 26–46%, while the high dose, 1.25% (the 'typical' human level of consumption), caused a decrease of 48–63%. In normal animals, both teas produced some improvement in LDL, LDL/HDL ratios and triglyceride levels.[10] It is thought that the oxidation of both LDL-C and VLDL contributes to the development of atherosclerosis.[10] Consequently, by preventing their oxidation a corresponding reduction in atherogenesis should be seen.

Human trials with both black and green tea have shown a significant increase in plasma antioxidant capacity approximately 1 hour after consumption of 1–6 cups of tea daily.[23] It is thought that this can protect cells and tissues from oxidative damage caused by scavenging oxygen free radicals, after they are absorbed from the gut after ingestion. Significant decrease in foam cell formation, the early form of atherosclerosis, has been reported in animals after consumption of both green and black teas.[10] This may explain how green and black teas have a protective effect against CHD. One recent review of the literature on green tea concluded that green tea possessed stronger cardioprotective activity than black tea, or oolong, simply due to the greater antioxidant capacity.[24] The apparent significance of the antioxidant and other biological activities of the flavonoid metabolites, as demonstrated by *in vivo* activity, shows the importance of investigation into the metabolites themselves.

Effects of tea on hypertension

Hypertension is the most common form of CVD, affecting approximately 20% of the adult population in many countries.[14] It is also one of the major risk factors for cardiovascular mortality, which accounts for 20–50% of all deaths. Some of the evidence was reviewed in 2004[14] and an association was suggested between tea drinking and a reduction in blood pressure in a Chinese population.

An epidemiological study carried out in Norway found that subjects experienced a fall in systolic blood pressure with increased consumption of black tea, while a further study conducted in Japan showed no relation between green tea intake and blood pressure.[14] Clinical trials carried out in both Australia and England failed to show a correlation between short-term consumption of high quantities of green or black tea and a decrease in blood pressure. Animal studies conducted in Japan concluded that a substantial hypotensive effect was observed in rats following short-term supplementation of their diet with green tea extracts.

These variable results have caused some confusion over the possible antihypertensive effect of green and black teas. Further epidemiological work was initiated in 1996, involving the participation of Chinese adult habitual tea drinkers in Taiwan.[14] The long-term effects of tea drinking and various lifestyle and dietary factors were evaluated for the risk of developing hypertension.[14] An inverse relationship was found between consumption of tea and mean blood pressure of individuals. Participants who had consumed at least 120 mL of tea per day for one year had a 46% lower risk of being diagnosed with hypertension than non-habitual tea drinkers. Increased consumption of 600 mL or greater was shown to reduce the risk by 65%. It was suggested that the threshold level of tea consumption likely to reduce the risk of developing hypertension was 120 mL either green or oolong tea per day, for at least one year, as nearly 40% of the 1507 subjects without a history of hypertension consumed tea at this level.[14]

Increased peripheral vascular tone is a characteristic of hypertension, and this could be a result of endothelial dysfunction; a state of oxidative stress is also commonly observed. The presence of superoxide radicals could result in impaired nitric oxide synthesis, or even increased deactivation of nitric oxide, which could explain the increased peripheral vascular resistance observed.[14]

Tea polyphenols are known to act as potent antioxidants, acting as free-radical scavengers and causing chelation of transition metals and inhibition of enzymes.[13,25]

It is thought that green and oolong tea extracts demonstrate anti-hypertensive effects due to their ability to reverse the endothelial dysfunction associated with hypertension, both through their antioxidant activity, and also their capacity to relax vascular smooth muscle.[14]

Effects of tea on myocardial infarction

In addition to the cardiac activities discussed, tea polyphenols are believed to have antiplatelet, antithrombotic and anti-inflammatory properties, and animal studies suggest that they may also improve vascular function. This suggests that ingestion of tea could minimise the risk of developing CHD and of having an MI.[26]

The association between tea consumption and MI has been the subject of a number of epidemiological studies. Both inverse and converse relationships have been found in studies ranging from Saudi to Japan. The Boston Area Health Study reported that consumption at least one cup of black tea per day reduced the risk of suffering an MI by about a half, compared with that of habitual non tea-drinkers.[13] The Zutphen Elderly Study claimed an inverse association between age-adjusted tea polyphenol intake and ischaemic heart disease, but not with MI incidence.[23] Another study on Dutch populations, this time in Rotterdam, found that tea drinkers consuming more than 375 mL/day had a lower relative risk of MI than non tea-drinkers.[26]

A meta-analysis of 17 studies on tea consumption in relation to MI, based on ten cohort studies and seven case–control studies, reported that an increase in tea consumption of three cups per day was associated with an 11% decrease in the incidence rate of MI. However, the authors urged caution as preferential publication of smaller studies appeared to suggest protective effects.[27] A later study in the USA, involving acute MI patients, concluded that post-MI mortality was lower among moderate to heavy tea drinkers, consuming more than 14 cups of tea per week for a year prior to MI, compared with non tea-drinkers.[28]

Unfortunately, not all studies showed that tea consumption reduced the incidence of MI. Two studies conducted within the UK actually identified a positive correlation between tea consumption and CHD risk.[27] Lifestyle factors could have had a profound effect on the findings, and therefore further research needs to be carried out into the effects of tea consumption.

Soy

In 1999, the US Food and Drug Administration (FDA) approved permission for manufacturers of soy foods to state that consumption of at least 25 g of soy protein per day may be beneficial to a reduced risk of developing CHD. It has been claimed that much of the support for this decision was obtained from a meta-analysis published in 1999.[29] The results of this analysis showed that consumption of soy protein instead of animal protein reduced LDL-C levels by 7–24%, depending upon initial cholesterol levels. However, it was not clear whether the benefits reported were due to the soy protein or the constituent isoflavones.[30] This lack of specificity of composition of many of the soy products used in research since that date still causes problems in interpreting the active fraction(s) of the soy tested.

Animal and clinical evidence relating to consumption of soy and soy protein has been published in a number of areas of cardiac health.

Effects of soy consumption on plasma lipids

Over the last 30 years, numerous animal and human studies have indicated that ingestion of isoflavone-rich soy protein is associated with decreased LDL and unchanged or increased HDL-C plasma concentrations,[3] but the results from several clinical trials have been less conclusive.[29] In hypercholesterolaemic men and women, the relationship is particularly evident, but in normocholesterolaemic men and women there is less consistency in results.[31]

One trial involving hypercholesterolaemic postmenopausal women showed increased HDL-C and reduced non-HDL-C in subjects receiving 40 g of soy protein per day for six months. The soy supplements contained either 2.39 mg isoflavones/g protein, or 1.39 mg isoflavones/g protein. Patients in the group taking the low concentration of isoflavones had significantly improved blood lipid profiles before 24 weeks, while the other group did not show improvement until later in the study.[32]

In one previous study by the same authors mildly hypercholesterolaemic men who consumed 50 g of soy protein daily experienced an 11–12% reduction in total and LDL-C concentrations, and in another study subjects showed a 5–6% reduction in total cholesterol after consumption of 25 g of soy protein per day.[32]

Other studies have also compared the effects of isoflavone-rich soy protein and isoflavone-depleted soy protein on the plasma lipid profiles of subjects.[31] One study found that consumption of high isoflavone content soy protein significantly decreased total and LDL-C levels in subjects with the highest baseline LDL-C concentrations.[31] A study of premenopausal women found that subjects taking high isoflavone soy protein had lower LDL-C concentrations and lower ratios of total to HDL-C and of LDL-C to HDL-C than those women taking the low isoflavone soy protein.[31] These studies support the view that the isoflavone content of soy protein is responsible for the cholesterol-lowering capacity of soy products.[28]

In postmenopausal women oestrogen replacement therapy causes a decrease in their plasma cholesterol concentrations.[32] Consequently, the oestrogenic activity of isoflavones, particularly genistein and daidzein, has been hypothesised to cause a reduction of cholesterol levels observed in mild hypercholesterolaemia.[32]

A number of mechanisms implicated in the cholesterol-lowering activity of the isoflavones include altered thyroid status, enhanced bile acid excretion, leading to reduced rates of cholesterol absorption,[28] and upregulation of LDL receptors.[33]

A number of trials have investigated the effects of soy isoflavones on plasma lipid profiles. An eight-week study with healthy middle-aged subjects supplemented with 55 mg of isoflavonoids showed that the isoflavonoids had no significant influence on serum lipid or lipoprotein concentrations.[32] A trial involving healthy individuals taking soy milk for four weeks showed significant increases in plasma genistein and daidzein concentrations, but revealed no significant effect on plasma cholesterol or triglyceride levels.[34]

A recent meta-analysis of 23 trials published between 1995 and 2002 of the effects of soy protein-containing isoflavones on the lipid profile of subjects concluded that soy protein-containing isoflavones significantly reduced serum total cholesterol, LDL-C and triacylglycerol, and significantly increased HDL-C. However, these changes were related to the level and duration of intake, and the gender and initial serum lipid concentrations of the subjects.[35] Compared with the earlier meta-analysis, there was an LDL-C reduction of 5.25%, whereas 7–24% had been found previously. The reductions in total and LDL-C were found to be larger in men than in women, and trials using intakes of >80 mg showed better results. Interestingly, three trials reviewed, in which tablet formulations containing extracted soy isoflavones were investigated, showed no significant effects on total cholesterol reduction.

The metabolism of daidzein results in formation of equol in a wide range of animal species, but is not normally present in humans until soy is ingested. It is not produced by germ-free animals or infants, but is a product of intestinal bacterial metabolism. Adult humans are split into 'equol producers' and 'nonequol producers', the latter making up 50–70% of the population. The perceived benefits of being an 'equol producer' are that equol has enhanced oestrogenic activity *in vivo*, compared with daidzein, and has the greatest antioxidant activity of all the isoflavones when measured *in vitro*. This increased antioxidant activity may provide greater inhibition of lipid peroxidation, and consequently greater reduction in risk of CVD.[36]

In conclusion, further research is necessary to prove that replacement of animal protein in the diet with soy protein could reduce plasma lipid and lipoprotein concentrations, and also establish the relative effects of the protein and isoflavonoid components.

Effects of soy consumption on vascular function

It is possible that phytoestrogens may have a beneficial effect on vascular function by acting directly on vessel walls, perhaps via improved arterial compliance and enhanced FMD.[37] A number of studies have been carried out to investigate the improvement in vascular function after treatment with soy products and isoflavones.

One trial found that dietary soy protein supplementation over three months significantly improved distal pulse wave velocity in normotensive male and postmenopausal female subjects, following reduction in the extent of vasoconstriction in peripheral resistance vessels. Although the trial showed that soy supplementation improved blood pressure and lipid status, it did not improve vascular function, and produced a decline in endothelial function in male subjects.[38]

When atherosclerotic female macaques were fed a diet rich in isoflavones, it was found that administration of acetylcholine dilated their arteries, whereas constriction was reported in those fed a low isoflavone diet. Later intravenous administration of genistein to those animals receiving the low isoflavone diet dilated previously constricted vessels.[39]

Infusion of genistein into the brachial artery of participants in one trial resulted in an increase in blood flow within the microcirculation of subjects' forearms.[33] Another trial reported on arterial compliance in perimenopausal women following administration of 45 mg of genistein (80 mg of total isoflavonoids) over a 5–10 week period and systemic arterial compliance showed a 26% improvement.[40]

Consumption of soy products containing isoflavones may improve vascular function via a variety of mechanisms. Due to their structural similarities to oestrogen, it is thought that they may cause an effect by binding to oestrogen receptor (ER)β receptors present in the vasculature, and protect against atherosclerosis.[33]

After oestrogen therapy postmenopausal women have improved large artery function, enhanced brachial artery FMD and restoration of normal vasomotion.[38,41] Impaired brachial artery FMD is positively associated with coronary artery endothelial dysfunction and with cardiovascular risk factors.[38] Dietary soy could improve vascular function, hence reducing CVD risk, through oestrogenic mechanisms.[38]

Although some studies show beneficial results, others show uncertainty concerning the effects of soy isoflavones on vascular function. The effects of genistein on vascular reactivity show that it may affect development of atherosclerosis, and have some effect on angina, however further trials are necessary to confirm these findings and their possible benefits.[41]

Effects of soy on atherogenesis

One of the major contributing factors implicated in the pathogenesis of CHD is atherogenesis of the coronary arteries, and many experimental studies have shown that diets rich in soy protein may have beneficial effects in preventing the onset and development of atherosclerosis.[41]

After a trial involving male and female macaque monkeys it was found that those fed a diet containing intact soy protein (143 mg/day isoflavonoid human equivalent) had less atherosclerosis than those fed protein from casein–lactalbumin, and those who consumed low isoflavone soy protein isolates (16 mg/day isoflavonoid human equivalent).[41] It was concluded that consumption of soy containing high isoflavonoid content could aid the prevention of atherosclerotic plaque development in monkeys.[41]

A number of *in vitro* studies and human trials have been carried out in order to identify mechanisms involved in the activity of isoflavones in atherogenesis.

LDL oxidation has a major role in the pathogenesis of atherosclerosis, as it acts as the trigger for a cascade of events including accelerated platelet aggregation, injury to arterial endothelial cells, and stimulation of foam cell and fatty streak development. It has been suggested that prevention of this oxidation process could result in an improvement in atherosclerosis, and soy isoflavones are known to have antioxidant properties.[42]

In vitro experiments have indicated that both genistein and daidzein cause inhibition of LDL oxidation in the vascular subendothelium.[42] It is thought that this antioxidative activity of the isoflavones can be attributed to their ability to scavenge free radicals, consequently decreasing oxidative stress.[29]

These data substantiate a widely held view that soy isoflavones exert an antiatherogenic effect in humans through inhibition of LDL oxidation, because of their antioxidant activity. Alternative mechanisms of activity include binding to oestrogen receptors; reduction in hyper-lipidaemia; inhibition of the migration and proliferation of smooth muscle cells by genistein; and inhibition of tyrosine kinase by genistein.[41]

Effects of soy products on blood pressure

Hypertension is the most common form of CVD, and has been the subject of several trials comparing the cardioprotective effects of ingestion of soy protein. As can be seen, conflicting evidence has been collated from these trials. Some of the data concerning the effects of soy on blood pressure in hypertension have recently been reviewed.[43] A trial involving normotensive men and women concluded that soy protein supplementation, involving 40 g protein and 118 mg isoflavonoids daily for three months, resulted in a significant reduction in the systolic, diastolic and mean blood pressures.[38] In one study, consumption of a soy-based diet was found to attenuate the development of hypertension in spontaneously hypertensive rats. Trials in perimenopausal women ingesting soy protein containing 34 mg isoflavonoids per day showed that subjects' diastolic blood pressure was significantly reduced.[43]

A trial involving men and women with mild-to-moderate hyper-tension was carried out in which patients received 500 mL of soy milk twice daily for a three-month period. At the end of the trial, consumers of soy milk were found to have significantly lower systolic, diastolic and mean blood pressures.[43]

This trial also revealed an inverse relationship between the decreases in blood pressure and the daily urinary isoflavonoid excretions, which consisted mainly of genistein, but also of equol, a metabolite of daidzein. Urinary excretion of genistein was found to correlate strongly with reductions in diastolic blood pressure, while lower systolic blood pressures tended to be associated with increased levels of urinary excretion of equol.[43]

The data from another clinical trial, in which patients with essential hypertension received 55 mg of isoflavonoids from red clover per day for eight weeks, showed no significant hypotensive effect. Red clover contained similar isoflavonoids, genistein, daidzein, plus their methylated derivatives, so similar results may have been expected.[43]

A recent review of 22 randomised trials of soy protein and isoflavones concluded that soy products should be beneficial to cardiovascular health because of their high content of polyunsaturated fatty acids (PUFAs), fibre, vitamins and minerals and low content of saturated fat, because studies on the effects of the isoflavones alone were found to have negligible effects.[44]

n-3 and *n*-6 Essential fatty acids

A large amount of research has been carried out into the effects of the so-called 'Mediterranian diet', centred mainly around the fatty acid composition of the diet. The concomitant consumption of a wide range of other constituents may, however, be part of the overall benefits.

A high dietary intake of saturated fat is thought to increase cholesterol levels and increase the risk of atherosclerosis. *n*-3 and *n*-6 PUFAs are believed to be beneficial in preventing or reversing high cholesterol levels.[45] Modern health advice is to reduce cholesterol, saturated fat and *trans* fatty acid intake for reduction of serum cholesterol levels.[46]

The basis of ALA deficiency caused by consumption of a Western diet[47,48] has been dicussed in Chapter 2.

Levels of PUFA intake also need to be maintained to avoid clinical deficiency.[49]

Linoleic acid is the major dietary *n*-6 PUFA, and it is found in vegetable oils including safflower, sunflower and corn oils. It is integrated into phospholipid membranes and lipoproteins and can be elongated and desaturated *in vivo* to form other fatty acids such as arachidonic acid.[4]

Eicosapentaenoic acid (EPA), docosahexaenoic acid (DHA) and ALA are all *n*-3 fatty acids. EPA and DHA are found primarily in fish oils, ALA is found in vegetable oils, particularly flaxseed, but also soybean and canola oil. EPA and DHA can be synthesised from ALA in the liver, but this supplies only a small proportion of the total levels. Eating one or two portions of oily fish per week is recommended to obtain the required dietary amount of *n*-3 PUFAs, as only relatively low doses of *n*-3 PUFAs of the order of 20 mg/kg per day are required.[50]

A large trial carried out in 1994 investigated the effect of an ALA-rich, Mediterranean diet in the survivors of a first MI. The MI survivors were randomly assigned to the experimental diet ($n = 302$), or continued with their normal diets. The experimental diet included a high intake of

ALA, and more bread, root vegetables, green vegetables and fruit. Patients were also advised to eat more fish, less meat and replace butter and cream with margarine supplied by the study, which was canola oil (rapeseed oil)-based and provided about 5% ALA. A reduction of coronary events and cardiac deaths of close to 70% was seen in the experimental group over 5 years and there were significantly fewer deaths in the group on the ALA-rich diet. In the experimental group there were only eight deaths, three from cardiac causes and none were sudden. The high intake of fruits and vegetables in the experimental group led to a significantly higher concentration of antioxidants in the plasma, measured over one year. Although these may well have increased the positive effects of the experimental diet, it was concluded that the increase in ALA in the diet also seemed to have significant consequences for coronary health. However, the number of dietary variables allowed in the diet make assessment of the affect of ALA difficult to judge.

Plant-provided polyunsaturated fatty acids

Low saturated fatty acid diets are thought to be associated with a lower risk of CVD mortality but the majority of trials in this area have shown there to be no beneficial effects. The critical dietary factor appears to be dietary enrichment with PUFAs, which has been positively linked to a decreased risk of CHD mortality.[51]

Linolenic acid is the major dietary fatty acid regulating LDL-C metabolism, by downregulating LDL-C production and improving its hepatic receptor-dependent clearance. One major trial investigated the effect of inclusion of 11.7 g/day linolenic acid in the diet, and revealed that this produced a 39% lower prevalence odds ratio for coronary artery disease.[52] Dietary intake must be above a certain critical threshold, of the order of 12.6 g/day, in order to dictate the hyperlipidaemic effects of the other dietary fat components, including cholesterol, for this action to take place. The corresponding levels of ALA and EPA + DHA are 1.7 g/day and 0.5 g/day respectively, and this level of dietary supplementation results in a *n*-6:*n*-3 fatty acid ratio of approximately 6:1.[45]

Data from a number of human trials suggest that ALA may protect against CHD. In one such study, the National Heart, Lung and Blood Institute Family Heart Study, 1.1 g/day ALA correlated with a 40% reduction in mortality from coronary artery diseases.[52] The mechanism of action of dietary ALA may be related to cardiac function, rather than plasma lipids. ALA is not thought to be as effective as linolenic acid in modulating either LDL-C production and clearance, or in increasing hepatic LDL receptor activity, but ALA has been found to reduce C-reactive protein, interleukin-6 (IL-6) and serum amyloid A, which are inflammatory markers associated with atherogenesis.[45]

It is clear that there are benefits derived from substituting *n*-6 PUFAs for saturated fats, which leads to a reduction in cardiovascular deaths, via reduction in cholesterol levels. It is not known whether the benefits associated with consumption of ALA are independent, or are related to its biotransformation to EPA and DHA.

One study revealed a significant reduction in non-fatal MIs when adipose tissue contained high levels of ALA and low levels of *trans* fatty acids. This association was more marked for individuals with a low dietary fish and hence low EPA and DHA consumption.[53]

Higher consumption of ALA has been found to result in lower prevalence of carotid artery plaques and a reduced intima-media thickness of the carotid arteries. It was thought that this could be caused by the conversion of ALA to EPA and DHA, both of which have been associated with cardioprotective effects.[52] This conversion has been monitored previously in subjects taking 40 g flaxseed oil for 23 days, and the *n*-6:*n*-3 ratios in subjects dropped to 1:2, from a control value of 30:1.[54]

A possible relationship between high intake or blood levels of ALA and prostate cancer has been investigated, by carrying out a meta-analysis of reports on the use of ALA in fatal coronary heart disease. Epidemiological studies have previously shown an increased risk of prostate cancer in men with high intakes of ALA. It was concluded that ALA consumption might be associated with an increased risk of prostate cancer. The dietary sources of the ALA, whether from meat or from vegetables, may be related to the increased risk because of the concomitant intake of many components that are prostate cancer risk factors in high meat diets.[55]

Obesity is one of the main risk factors for CHD. Another risk factor is aortic compliance, or elasticity, which is related to arterial function. A decrease in aortic compliance occurs in advancing age, hypertension, diabetes and atherosclerosis.[56] Middle-aged, obese subjects were supplemented with 20 g of flaxseed oil daily over a four-week study, and improved aortic compliance with a resulting improvement in arterial function was reported. This finding may have significant effects in elderly, diabetic or obese patients, all of whom show a tendency towards decreased aortic elasticity.

The studies involving ALA suggest that it does impart important protection from CVD, however, it is still not certain whether the benefits of ALA are due to its inherent activity, or through its conversion to EPA and DHA.[45]

In a crossover study,[57] flaxseed oil capsules were taken three times daily (20 g oil per day, containing 12 g ALA) and compared with 50 g flaxseed flour per day, containing 12 g ALA. In healthy women the bioavailability of ALA was similar in each case, resulting in lowered blood lipids. Also, there was no weight gain in the subjects, indicating that other energy sources had been displaced from the diet.

In another experiment,[57] flaxseed flour sprinkled on foods was compared with bread made from the flour, both providing 50 g/day of flaxseed for four weeks. The fatty acid profiles of the subjects did not differ significantly between the two groups, and no weight gain was reported. It therefore appears that the form in which flaxseed is consumed, whether flour, oil or in baked goods, does not seem to affect the bioavailability of the ALA.

The optimum intake of ALA is about one or two teaspoons of the oil daily (2–9 g).[58] While still in the seed the oil can keep for years, but once extracted it should be stored carefully and shelf-dated, as it is sensitive to heat and light. Freezing is an alternative way of ensuring that the oil is in prime condition while being stored. Moreover, plant oils are often hydrogenated during processing, which destroys the ALA found in the pure oil. It is therefore important to ensure that flaxseed oil purchased for its therapeutic properties is not in this form.[59]

Polyunsaturated fatty acids from fish oils

The main dietary source of EPA and DHA is fish, and fish consumption has been shown to decrease risk of sudden cardiac death. One investigation into the consumption of fish and heart rate found lower heart rates in men who consumed fish regularly.[60]

Another study found that supplementation with 3 g each of EPA and DHA caused an increase in systemic arterial compliance, and a reduction in pulse pressure and total vascular resistance. Both fatty acids were also found to lower plasma total and VLDL triacylglycerol.[61] The effects of supplementation of 4 g/day of purified EPA or DHA were studied in mildly hyperlipidaemic men over six weeks. Of the two, only DHA, but not EPA, was shown to reduce ambulatory blood pressure and heart rate. DHA supplementation led to a small increase in EPA levels, but EPA supplementation did not change DHA levels, thereby demonstrating the metabolic pathway.[62]

There is growing evidence that EPA and DHA levels are responsible for a decreased risk of ischaemic heart disease mortality. One study revealed that increased plasma levels of combined DHA and EPA and possibly ALA lowered the risk of fatal ischemic heart disease, but not non-fatal heart attacks. A possible explanation for this is that n-3 PUFAs have antiarrhythmic action.[63] A meta-analysis of randomised controlled trials on the effects of n-3 PUFAs in coronary heart disease suggested that both dietary and non-dietary supplementation with n-3 PUFAs may decrease mortality due to myocardial infarction, sudden death and overall mortality in patients with coronary heart disease.[64]

EPA and DHA are antiarrhythmic agents due to their ability to prevent calcium overload in cardiac myocytes during periods of stress, where they have a membrane stabilising effect. The n-6 PUFAs, particularly linolenic acid, are thought to be arrhythmogenic, due to their metabolism to arachidonic acid, prostaglandin and thromboxane.[65]

The decreased blood pressure and vascular resistance are due to an increased arterial compliance. It has also been shown that EPA and DHA produce a dose-dependent reduction in tumour necrosis factor-alpha and IL-6 and hence have an anti-inflammatory effects, which may slow atherogenesis. In addition, EPA and DHA reduced atherosclerotic plaque development through the reduction of vascular adhesion molecules, such as vascular cell adhesion molecule-1 (VCAM-1). EPA and DHA are thought to reduce coronary heart disease mortality through a combination of these mechanisms.[45]

A study involving healthy individuals from three countries looked at the effect of dietary supplementation with 2.4 g of both EPA and DHA. An increase in LDL-C but decrease in VLDL was observed. Triacylglycerol levels were reduced via inhibition of hepatic triglyceride and VLDL apoB secretion. This suggests that other beneficial effects of n-3 PUFAs, rather than just lipid metabolism, are responsible for the decreased risk of coronary mortality.[66] The is opposite to the proposed action of the n-6 fatty acids.

EPA and DHA are also thought to have an antithrombotic effect and to cause a reduction in pro-aggregatory eicosanoids, such as thromboxane B2, which takes place as a result of EPA competing in the arachidonic acid cascade. Reduced platelet aggregation and reduced coagulation factors have been reported, which may reduce CVD.[45]

Comparison of flaxseed and fish oils

Due to the health benefits of *n*-3 fattys acids compared with *n*-6 oils, research has been carried out to see whether flaxseed has the same advantages as fish oils on lipoprotein metabolism. In one review,[67] evaluation of a number of human studies led to the conclusion that ALA was equivalent to *n*-6 fish oils but not as beneficial as *n*-3 fish oils in its effects on lowering serum cholesterol, unless ingested in very large quantities (60 mL oil). This is because long-chain *n*-3 fatty acid production from ALA depends on the amount of *n*-6 fatty acid already present. Fish oils provide long-chain *n*-3 PUFAs – EPA (20:5*n*-3) and DHA (22:6*n*-3) – whereas flaxseed provides an *n*-3 precursor, which must be converted to these beneficial long-chain *n*-3 PUFAs. Since most people have a vast excess of *n*-6 fatty acids, the *n*-6 pathways are preferred and long-chain *n*-6 fatty acids are produced (18:2*n*-6 → 20:4*n*-6). The conversion of the *n*-3 precursor to the long-chain fatty acids from ALA is therefore more significant over a long time period of time or with very large intakes.

In a controlled, randomised, double-blind, crossover study[68] the effect of low-dose flaxseed or fish oils on subjects consuming diets with a high or low polyunsaturated/saturated fatty acid diet was investigated. All subjects took olive oil capsules (consisting mostly of oleic acid, 18:1*n*-9) for three months as a placebo. They were then randomly assigned to take flaxseed oil (35 mg of ALA daily) or fish oil (35 mg of EPA) in capsules for three months, before crossing over to the other supplement. Blood samples and diet records were taken every three months. Neither flaxseed oil nor fish oil capsules significantly altered plasma total, LDL-C or HDL-C. However, it was found that fish oil reduced plasma triacylglycerides in the low polyunsaturated/saturated group. This was not seen in the flaxseed oil subjects but this may have been due to the small dose used.

There is a large body of evidence to suggest that *n*-3 PUFAs contribute to reducing mortality from cardiac diseases via a range of pathways, thereby decreasing the risk factors of raised blood pressure and cholesterol, which are closely related to CVDs. Eating fish regularly maintains a constant input of EPA and DHA, and in non-fish eaters it is clear that taking these in supplement form could be beneficial.[49].

Inexplicable conflicting evidence has been reported from some studies, such as an association of ALA with an increased risk of prostate cancer, but this link has not been investigated with fish oils, and it is possible that these may protect against prostate cancer.[55] In view of these findings supplementation with purified EPA and DHA could be the best course of action.

One study making a direct comparison of the effects of tuna fish oil, evening primrose oil, soy oil and sunflower oil concluded that the fish oil containing 6% EPA and 27% DHA may have significant beneficial effects on cardiovascular health, as it was the only oil tested that produced significant changes in vascular response.[69]

In a number of studies into the effects of dietary fattys acids on cardiac indicators, fatty acid intake is carefully controlled. However, this is not always the case, and personal dietary choices may have conflicted with the aims of the trials. Also, beneficial effects reported may have been caused by either the fatty acid itself or its metabolic products. As a high saturated fat intake is a specified risk factor for CVD, substitution with alternative fatty acids, such as PUFAs, may lower this risk. In all the trials the PUFAs have been well tolerated and no significant side-effects have been reported.

A range of structurally unrelated compounds have also been implicated in beneficial effects on CVD. These include the flax lignans, coenzyme Q10, lycopene, policosanol, Pycnogenol, melatonin and resveratrol, GPSE, lutein and carnitine.

Flax lignans

Flaxseed contains about 35–45% fixed oil, with ALA accounting for at least 50% of the total. Data concerning the effects of ALA have been discussed above in the section '*n*-3 and *n*-6 Essential fatty acids'. In addition to this, flaxseed also contains the lignan secoisolariciresinol diglucoside (SDG) at levels of 10–30 mg/g of defatted flaxseed and fibre.[70]

Understanding of the causes of the beneficial cardiac effects of flax was aided greatly by Canadian researchers who compared the effects of high and low flaxseed diets in rabbits. They found that hypercholesterolaemic atherosclerosis was reduced by 46% in rabbits fed 7.5 g/kg whole flaxseed. Later they showed that there was a 69% reduction in atherosclerosis in subjects given flaxseed oil containing only 3% ALA (to check whether the effects were cause by the lignans or the ALA), with a non-significant decrease in serum total cholesterol and LDL-C. Next they used 15 mg/kg SDG supplementation and found 73% reduction in development of hypercholesterolaemic atherosclerosis. This result clearly shows the involvement of the lignan SDG in the outcome.[70]

In a small human trial the effect of partially defatted flaxseed (low ALA) was investigated in hyperlipidemic men and women.[71] The subjects ate four control muffins (no flaxseed) or four test muffins (defatted flaxseed) daily, for two three-week periods in a randomised, crossover design. There was a two-week washout period between each test period. Serum samples were obtained and analysed for serum lipids. The defatted flaxseed reduced the serum concentrations of total cholesterol and LDL-C in similar amounts to those given full-fat flaxseed in previous experiments, quoted by the authors. However, there was no effect on serum lipoprotein. As well as the lignan effects there are also beneficial effects from the seed coat gum of flaxseed, which may be responsible for the hypolipidaemic action. Additional trials are required in which all the components are isolated, to determine exactly which part of the flaxseed is contributing to these effects.

Recently the outcomes of clinical trials using flaxseed or flaxseed oil in a range of subjects have been compared. Five out of six trials involved the use of flaxseed (38–50 g/day) and showed significant reduction in total cholesterol and LDL-C, and three out of four trials using flaxseed oil showed no reduction in cholesterol parameters. However, one trial using a very high-dose, 60 g/day of flaxseed oil for two weeks showed a decrease in triglyceride levels, and there were also reductions in total cholesterol and LDL-C levels in specific patient groups.[72] Research directed towards the specific involvement of SDG has shown that there is an inverse relationship between serum enterolactone (a major SDG metabolite) levels and risk of acute cardiac events.[73]

The coat of flaxseed contains viscous soluble and insoluble fibre, and the former is thought to be involved in cardiac protection. One meta-analysis has shown that 2–10 g/day, approximately 26–130 g of flaxseed, of viscous soluble fibre produces a small and significant decrease in total cholesterol and LDL-C.[72]

Coenzyme Q10

Coenzyme Q10 (Co Q10) is a powerful antioxidant and free radical scavenger, and is manufactured and used as a medicine in Japan.[65] It occurs naturally in the body and is mainly located in the mitochondria of myocardium, liver and kidney cells. It is an electron carrier in the mitochondrial synthesis of ATP, and has membrane-stabilising effects.[74] It has been used for the treatment of CVDs including heart failure, hypertension, angina and arrhythmias, but the evidence to support its use is contradictory. Significantly reduced levels of myocardium Co Q10, of the order of 50% normal levels, have been reported in heart failure in animals and humans.[75] Contradictory results have been reported in trials using Co Q10 supplementation in heart failure patients, but a meta-analysis of eight clinical trials supported its use.[76] However trials involving doses of less than 100 mg/day produced negative results, and it has been suggested that doses of 150–200 mg/day should be used.[75]

Clinical studies indicate that Co Q10 may be useful as a treatment for hypertension, as it causes a decrease in total peripheral resistance, and is thought to act as an antagonist of vascular superoxide.[77] A number of clinical trials have shown that supplementation causes a fall in blood pressure.[77] A trial involving 109 patients showed when the Co Q10 dose was adjusted to produce a blood concentration above 2 µg/mL, a marked reduction in blood pressure occurred from 159/94 to 147/85 and 51% of patients were able to discontinue their previous antihypertensive medication.[78] Co Q10 may act by decreasing peripheral vascular resistance, or as a superoxide antagonist, and may decrease the cytoplasmic redox potential of the endothelium.[77] It is quite possible that Co Q10 may act via a variety of mechanisms.

Conflicting evidence exists about the benefits for cardiac patients. Other trials noted improvements, but concerns about experimental procedures and small patient numbers has limited the usefulness of the outcomes. Administration of Co Q10 was found to improve the ejection fraction and functional status of the patient and it improved the patient's heart failure classification. In addition, clinical symptoms improved after three months, including arrhythmias in 63% of the patients. However, in another study using 200 mg/day, Co Q10 did not affect ejection fraction, peak oxygen consumption or exercise duration in patients with congestive heart.[79]

The administration of 120 mg/day of Co Q10 for 28 days has been reported to reduce angina, improve ventricular function and reduce total arrhythmias.[80]

A trial using patients with hypertrophic cardiomyopathy supplemented with 200 mg/day Co Q10 reported symptomatic relief of fatigue and dyspnoea, and improvements in measurements of left ventricular thickness and diastolic function. Successful outcomes required blood levels greater than 2 µg/mL. This is thought to be due to an improvement in myocardial bioenergetics and ATP production.[81]

It has been reported that Co Q10 supplementation at a level of 4 mg/kg prior to stress caused by surgery improves the recovery of rats after cardiac operations. Co Q10 apparently improves the efficiency of mitochondrial energy production, therefore more energy is available for contractile function. Reduced troponin I release suggests that Co Q10 reduces myocardial damage. Supplementation in humans may result in increased cardiac recovery and hence reduced hospital stays.[82]

Overall, evidence is available concerning the benefits of Co Q10 in many CVDs, and it has been suggested that supplementation should be sufficient to raise serum blood levels to at least 2.5 µg/mL.[83]

Although Co Q10 is an endogenous compound, and no side-effects or tolerability problems have been reported, beta-blockers may reduce the efficacy of Co Q10 because they interfere with Co Q10-dependent enzymes[84] and statins have been reported to deplete Co Q10.[85] It has been claimed that concomitant Co Q10 supplementation with statins could counteract this reduction in Co Q10 levels.[85]

Co Q10 could possibly be used prior to cardiac surgery to increase cardiac recovery, decrease myocardial damage, prevent arrhythmias, decrease angina, lower blood pressure and overall improve the clinical outlook for the patient. As Co Q10 may reduce hypertension, it may help to prevent more serious complications, such as MI.

Lycopene

High levels of lycopene are present in tomato juice, sauce and other concentrated extracts, plus a number of red fruits and vegetables, for example watermelons, pink grapefruit and pink guava.[86] Lycopene is closely related to beta-carotene and is thought to reduce the risks of coronary heart disease. It is found in blood plasma and other body tissues, and a low level is thought to be associated with many chronic diseases. A recommended daily intake of 35 mg has been suggested,[87] but a review of the lycopene content of tomatoes and tomato products and their contribution to dietary lycopene reported that most people do not obtain sufficient dietary amounts.[88] In lieu of sufficient dietary intake of lycopene, increased intake should be sought from foods or nutraceutical supplements.

The most widely studied carotenoid is beta-carotene. A large, multicentre study showed that a high level of beta-carotene intake from a normal diet, based on adipose tissue concentrations, was associated with a reduced risk of MI, particularly in smokers.[89] However further studies failed to show a reduction in cardiovascular symptoms in smokers receiving beta-carotene supplements, and indeed suggested that supplements of beta-carotene may be harmful in smokers, causing high mortality due to heart disease and lung cancer.[90] It was suggested that there might be other dietary conponents contributing to the antioxidant effect from a diet high in fruits and vegetables, besides the effect of beta-carotene.

One candidate micronutrient for this effect is lycopene, which is often consumed with beta-carotene in the diet. In a large study carried out in ten different countries, the effects of alpha-carotene, beta-carotene and lycopene were studied in a population of men (average age 54 years) from coronary care units, who had undergone a first acute MI.[91] The carotenoid concentration was measured from subcutaneous adipose tissue, since the adipose tissue levels of carotenoids are derived mainly from the diet and provide a better indication of dietary status than serum levels. Lycopene showed the greatest protective effect of the three carotenoids measured, after the results had been corrected for age, obesity, smoking and other risk factors.

Another study was carried out to determine why Lithuanian men have four times higher mortality from coronary heart disease than do Swedish men.[92] One hundred and one Swedish men aged 50, with no serious acute or chronic diseases, were compared with a similar population of 109 men from Lithuania. There were only small differences between the two groups in traditional risk factors (hypertension, smoking, high cholesterol levels), but when the resistance of LDL to oxidation was compared there was a lower resistance to oxidation in the men from Lithuania. There were also lower plasma concentrations of beta-carotene, lycopene and gamma-tocopherol in these men. These lower concentrations of antioxidants are due to the different diets of the two countries. It seems from this study that factors other than the usually cited risk factors are responsible for differences in mortality between Swedish and Lithuanian men. The antioxidant status may well account for these differences and, as already described, lycopene is one of the best dietary antioxidants and may therefore help to prevent CVS.

Oxidation of LDL is also associated with the formation of athero-sclerotic plaques, leading to strokes. Diets containing fruits and vegetables rich in antioxidants may therefore also offer protection against strokes. In a study of 26 593 male smokers, aged 50–69, with no history of stroke in Finland, the subjects were asked to complete a detailed questionnaire about diet.[93] During a 6.1-year follow-up, 736 cerebral infarctions, 83 subarachnoid haemorrhages and 95 intra-cerebral haemorrhages occurred. The associations between these events and dietary intake were found to be significant only for beta-carotene, but not for other nutrients, including flavonols, vitamin C, vitamin E, lutein and lycopene.

Although these reports suggest a beneficial effect of carotenoids and antioxidants on heart disease, and lycopene seems to be responsible for these outcomes, there is not yet conclusive evidence that lycopene itself contributes to the protective effects of fruit and vegetable consumption. A diet rich in fruits and vegetables where many micronutrients are available to act synergistically is therefore recommended at this stage, rather than individual supplements.

Initial research focused on serum cholesterol levels, but more recently oxidative stress induced by reactive oxygen species (ROS) has been highlighted. Lycopene has been shown to significantly lower levels of oxidation of LDL, but it has also been shown to reduce the levels of breath pentane, another biomarker of oxidation.[94] However, other mechanisms of action, including modulation of intracellular gap junction communication, hormonal, immune system and metabolic pathways may also be involved.[87]

ROS and the oxidative damage they cause have been connected with the pathogenesis of atherogenesis and carcinogenesis.[87] Because of its antioxidant and free radical scavenging activity, lycopene is thought to slow the progression of atherosclerosis through the inhibition of the oxidative processes which convert circulating LDL-C to oxidised LDL. The oxidation of LDL is thought to be a key step in the atherogenic process, as oxidised LDL is taken up by macrophages inside the arterial wall which leads to the formation of foam cells and atherosclerotic plaques.[94]

Other mechanisms of action that have been proposed include inhibition of hydroxymethylglutaryl coenzyme A (HMG-CoA) reductase and thereby inhibition of cholesterol synthesis, LDL degradation, alterations in the size and composition of LDL particles, plaque ruptures and altered endothelial functions.[94] More research is needed to determine the exact mechanisms of action of lycopene.

Population-based evidence of the effects of lycopene have been collated from ten European countries. It was found that lycopene levels were most protective against MI when compared with other antioxidants.[91] Only limited research into the effects of lycopene in CVD has been carried out. A clinical trial in Finland, which investigated the relationships between lycopene, atherosclerosis and CHD, concluded that middle-aged men with low levels of serum lycopene had an increased intima-media thickness of the common carotid artery wall and an increased risk of acute coronary event or stroke, demonstrating that lycopene had a significant hypocholesterolaemic effect in men.[95] Another study looking at lycopene and MI risk concluded that low levels of adipose tissue lycopene are associated with an increased risk of heart attacks.[92]

A recent study of the effects of supplementation with 250 mg daily of tomato extract (containing 15 mg of lycopene) demonstrated a reduction in blood pressure in patients with type 1 hypertension over the eight-week treatment period.[96] Work in rats comparing the effects of lycopene with those of tomato juice showed that both reduced the extent of lipid peroxidation, but only tomato juice improved post-ischaemic ventricular function, myocardial infarct size, and cardiomycete apoptosis. The researchers concluded that tomato juice, not lycopene, is responsible for the cardioprotective effects.[97]

Overall, lycopene appears to aid in the prevention of CHD, probably due to its antioxidant properties. More evidence is required before clinical use is made of lycopene in the prevention of CHD.

Octacosanol/policosanol

Policosanol has been claimed to be as effective as the currently available lipid-lowering drugs, such as the statins, in lowering lower plasma cholesterol.[98] Policosanol was first developed in Cuba and used as a major cardiac medicine in the Caribbean region.[99]

It has been postulated that cholesterol levels in people consuming mainly vegetarian diets is lower than in those eating commercially prepared foods, possibly due to the presence of natural alkanols such as octacosanol. To date, policosanol has been used in a number of clinical trials in this area.[100]

During motor endurance experiments on mice, it was noted that octacosanol caused altered hepatic and serum lipid concentrations. This led researchers to investigate the possible role of octacosanol and policosanol on serum lipids and its possible use as a cholesterol-lowering agent. A number of studies have been carried out in a number of animal species and policosanol was shown to reduce total cholesterol and LDL-C in a dose-dependent way, while HDL-C was unchanged.[101]

There have been over 60 clinical trials published, mainly in Cuba, since 1992 concerning the effectiveness of policosanol as a lipid-lowering agent. One double-blind clinical trial investigating the effect in patients with type II hypercholesterolaemia and additional coronary risk factors showed that policosanol 5 mg/day (and 10 mg/day) after

12 weeks of treatment significantly reduced serum LDL-C by 18.2% (and 25.6%) and total cholesterol by 13.0% (17.4%). In addition there was a significant increase in HDL-C by 15.5% (and 28.4%), and triglyceride levels stayed constant up to 12 weeks, but significantly decreased later.[98] A range of other trials produced results with similar benefits. Studies demonstrated that the ability to lower cholesterol was maintained over two years of treatment, but greatest reduction was seen after 6–8 weeks. Studies using higher doses above 20 mg per day have not been undertaken, but may have greater effect. Importantly, no rebound effects have been recorded after stopping the treatment.[99] Details from a large number of clinical trials on patients with both primary and type II hypercholesterolaemia appear to confirm that policosanol causes reduction in LDL-C and total cholesterol, while HDL-C usually rises.[101]

In non-insulin-dependent diabetes mellitus (NIDDM), hyperglycaemia may induce atherosclerosis, leading to CHD, which is a main cause of death in these patients. It is therefore important to maintain low cholesterol levels in NIDDM patients by using glycaemic control, dietary measures and medication. In a double-blind study patients with stable glycaemic control were given policosanol 5 mg twice a day for 12 weeks.[102] Both total cholesterol and LDL-C were significantly reduced in the test group. Side-effects were mild and at week 12 no side-effects were reported in the policosanol group and the treatment did not affect glycaemic control.

Conflicting evidence has been published, however, from a trial using 20 mg daily of wheatgerm policosanol in patients with normal to mildly elevated plasma cholesterol concentrations. Although the composition of this source of policosanol is very similar to that from sugarcane, no beneficial effects were seen.[103]

A comparative study was carried out to compare 10 mg/day policosanol and 20 mg/day lovastatin in patients with hypercholesterolaemia and NIDDM.[104] Patients received either policosanol or lovastatin daily for 12 weeks. Both treatments were effective in lowering LDL-C and total cholesterol, without affecting glucose control. Policosanol was found to be safe and well tolerated, whereas lovastatin caused increased serum values of aspartate aminotransferase, creatine phosphokinase and alkaline phosphatase as well as causing more frequent adverse effects (including in five patients who withdrew from the study).

In an animal study, the effect of oral pretreatment with policosanol 2 hours before isoprenaline-induced MI was investigated. Policosanol reduced the size of the myocardial injury and also decreased the number of polymorphonuclear neutrophils (PMNs) and mast cells in the damaged areas. The clinical value of these findings is unclear.[105]

Policosanol is not thought to act like the statins in causing inhibition of HMG-CoA reductase. It has been shown that policosanol inhibits cholesterol biosynthesis, probably at a stage prior to mevalonate formation, but direct inhibition of HMG-CoA reductase is considered unlikely.[99] Polycosanol is also possibly involved in increasing LDL-C uptake in the liver by increasing the numbers of LDL receptors, and is also thought to increase the rates of breakdown of serum LDL.[98]

Further effects of policosanol that may be indirectly beneficial to cardiac health have been reported. Both animal experiments and human studies have shown that it has an effect on platelets, brought about by lowering thromboxane B2 and elevating serum prostacyclin levels.[98] Anti-ischaemic effects reported in animal studies may be responsible for this. It has been claimed that the antiplatelet effect of 20 mg is equal to that of 100 mg aspirin, but it acts by an alternative route. Very few side-effects have been reported in clinical trials.[98,99] During long-term use weight loss, polyuria and headaches have been described on rare occasions. Healthy volunteers reported no adverse effects after single doses of 1000 mg, and 500 mg/kg has been given orally to rats, with no reports of adverse effects. No drug interactions have been reported with other medicines in concomitant use during trials.[99] Policosanol has shown no adverse effects in NIDDM patients with hypercholesterol-aemia,[102] but it should not be used in pregnant or breastfeeding women, or in children until the possibility of adverse effects has been investi-gated.[99]

Overall, policosanol may have a use in a number of CVDs. The search for safe lipid-lowering agents continues, and the low incidence of side-effects makes it a promising choice. Safety needs further investi-gation and possible long-term side-effects or serious drug interactions, for example with the statins, need to be evaluated. A standardised alkanol content of the product needs to be agreed, allowing precise comparison of published work. It has been claimed that most clinical trials have been carried out by only one group, in Cuba, and also that the origin of most policosanol on sale in the USA is beeswax, not sugarcane, which may account for the contradictory results.[106]

Pycnogenol

Pine bark has been used traditionally to treat inflammatory diseases, which gives some credence to the use of the pine bark extract

Pycnogenol. A range of cardiovascular effects have also been reported, including vasorelaxant effects, inhibition of angiotensin-converting enzyme (ACE) and increase in the microcirculation by increasing capillary resistance.[107]

One clinical trial using Pycnogenol (150 mg/day for six weeks) increased the plasma polyphenol levels and antioxidant activity in subjects and also lowered LDL-C and increased HDL-C.[108]

Pycogenol has been investigated for its activity in hypertensive patients and found to improve endothelial function. A dose of 100 mg daily for 12 weeks allowed reduction of the dose of nifedipine, a calcium channel antagonist, used for control of hypertension. This antihypertensive effect may be caused by a number of factors. Endothelin 1, which is a potent endogenous vasoconstrictor, levels decreased by 20% after dosing with Pycnogenol. There was also a reduction in thromboxane B2 levels, and an increase in nitric oxide, which is an endothelial relaxing factor. There was no evidence to suggest that Pycogenol acted as an ACE inhibitor,[109] as had been claimed in an earlier publication.[107]

Chronic venous insufficiency results in swelling, particularly of the lower legs. It has a prevalence of 10–15% in men and 20–25% in women, and is usually treated with compression therapy. Although not life-threatening, if untreated it may progress to static oedema and ulcerations. One study investigating the effect of Pycogenol at a dose of 360 mg/day over four weeks on chronic venous insufficiency showed a significant reduction in the circumference of the lower limbs and improvement of subjective symptoms such as pain, cramps and feelings of heaviness. This activity is thought to be caused by stimulation of nitric oxide synthesis and by Pycogenol acting as a free radical scavenger, leading to the relaxation of constricted blood vessels. Pycogenol is thought to counteract oedema by sealing leaky capillaries as a result of its high affinity for proteins. In addition, it significantly decreased cholesterol and LDL-C values in blood, and HDL levels remained unaffected.[110]

Pycnogenol has recently been investigated for prophylaxis of deep vein thrombosis in long-haul flights of 8 hours 15 minutes average duration. One hundred and ninety-eight subjects were treated with 200 mg Pycnogenol 2–3 hours before the flight, followed by 200 mg 6 hours later, and 100 mg the following day. In the control group there were five thrombotic events, one deep vein thrombosis (DVT) and four superficial thromboses, while the treatment group showed only symptoms of localised phlebitis.[111] Later work on oedema reduction during long-haul flights reported significant reduction in oedema by passengers receiving the same dosage regimen.[112] A further trial by the same group investigated the effects on 18 patients with venous ulcers over six weeks. In this pilot study, using a combination of both oral and topical Pycnogenol treatment, a faster reduction in the ulcerated area was observed, than that seen using oral treatment alone.[113]

The possibility that Pycogenol may be useful in the inhibition of platelet aggregation induced by cigarette smoking has been investigated. The activity may be due to nitric oxide synthesis inhibiting thromboxane A2 production. The adverse effect on bleeding time produced by aspirin is not shared by Pycnogenol. It has been shown that 100 mg Pycnogenol has the same activity as 500 mg aspirin.[107]

It can be seen that Pycogenol has a wide range of activities with beneficial effects on many CVD risk factors, including DVT. As yet there is no clear evidence as to dosage levels, and safety data, including drug interactions, need to be studied.

Melatonin

In vivo research on animals has shown that melatonin overcomes cardiac injury after arterial occlusion followed by reperfusion. It appears that melatonin is more powerful than other antioxidants tested, in terms of ameliorating hypoxia and reoxygenation damage.[114] Intraperitoneal doses of 150 μg/kg were found to be most effective.[115] Humans dosed with 3 mg oral melatonin showed dramatic increase in plasma melatonin concentrations, at 1830 ± 848 pg/mL, compared with 14 ± 11 pg/mL before ingestion, with maximal levels at 75 minutes after ingestion. This shows that in humans melatonin attenuates the reflex sympathetic increases that occur in response to orthostatic stress.[116]

Resveratrol

There is evidence to suggest that resveratrol acts as an antioxidant and inhibits LDL oxidative susceptibility *in vivo*, by both chelating and free radical scavenging mechanisms. Cardioprotection is thought to result from its ability to inhibit platelet aggregation. At a physiological concentration of 1.2 μg/L, resveratrol was shown to reduce platelet aggregation by ~41% in healthy subjects, and this was raised to 78.5% by increasing the dose.[117] Cardioprotective effects of resveratrol may also be contributed to by inhibition of endogenous cholesterol biosynthesis, by inhibition of squalene monooxygenase, which is the rate-limiting enzyme in cholesterol biosynthesis.[118] This may explain the protective effects on CVD.

Grape seed proanthocyanidin extract

Grape seed proanthocyanidin extract (GSPE) is often considered along-side resveratrol as one of the main reasons for the apparent health of the French population, who have a low mortality from cardiac diseases despite being both high wine and fat consumers (the 'French paradox'). GSPE is a potent antioxidant, with activity levels above those of vitamins C and E.[101]

Recent studies performed on isolated rat hearts treated with red wine extract before ischaemic arrest have provided evidence that GSPEs from red wine are effective cardioprotective agents.[119] The red wine extract reduced myocardial infarct size as well as improving post-ischaemic ventricular functions. In another study by the same group,[119] rats given oral GSPE for three weeks were resistant to subsequent ischaemic injury to the isolated hearts.

Other research has shown that as well as acting as a cardiopro-tective agent directly, GSPE also prevents atherosclerosis, which is a major risk factor for heart disease. It has been shown that oxidation of the polyunsaturated lipid components of LDL damages arteries and it is only this oxidised form of cholesterol that leads to atherosclerosis.[58] To determine whether the 'French paradox' was due to the antioxidant properties of red wine, an *in vitro* study was carried out.[120] De-alcoholised Californian red wine was used to prepare the proantho-cyanidin extract, and LDL from the blood of normolipidaemic, non-smoking volunteers was used for the investigation. The extract caused an inhibition of 60% and 98% of the oxidation of LDL seen in the controls at concentrations of 3.8 mmol/L and 10 mmol/L respectively.

A similar experiment was carried out in humans using samples of de-alcoholised red and white wine which were tested for antioxidant activity. The red wine samples were 20 times more active than the white wine samples.[121]

However, not all red wines have the same protective effect. It has been shown from research on more than 60 different red wines from 11 different countries that the GSPE content and therefore the antioxidant properties vary greatly between different wines.[122] Red wines from Chile have a higher flavonol content than those from France, Italy, Australia and California. It has been suggested that the climate in the grape-growing regions, the thickness of the grape skins, the time of grape harvesting and the actual winemaking process could all affect the flavonoid content.

It is interesting that many by-products of the wine industry are now being used in the nutraceutical industry. The industry produces the grape seeds and grape skins from winery waste and develops them as dietary supplements.[123]

Although it has been presumed that GSPEs protect against CVD by their antioxidant activity, most studies did not measure atherosclerosis directly. One *in vivo* study, however, did determine the effect of a GSPE extract from grape seeds directly on atherosclerosis.[124] In this study, an extract containing 73.4% GPSE was obtained by freeze-drying an aqueous solution of grape seeds. The serum lipid profile did not change dramatically in the GSPE-fed rabbits, but serum LDL-C and the LDL/HDL ratio decreased at six weeks in the 1% GPSE group and HDL-C decreased at eight weeks in the 0.1% GPSE group. There was a lower amount of aortic plaque in the GPSE group. The activity of the GSPE was thought to be related to prevention of LDL oxidation in the arterial cell wall.

Another use for GSPE that has been widespread in Europe is in the treatment of vascular disorders. These include varicose veins, venous insufficiency and microvascular problems such as retinopathies. In France GPSE is the active ingredient in a proprietary product used for microcirculatory disorders, called Endotelon. The antioxidant properties of the GPSE are largely responsible for their vascular properties.[125]

A number of actions on the tissues of the arterial wall have been reported for GPSE, including inhibition of histidine decarboxylase involved in the atheromatous process, vascular relaxation by increasing endothelial nitric oxide production, and inhibition of endothelin-1 formation.[126] Recent research using the atherosclerotic hamster model found approximately 49% and 63% reduction in foam cells, which is a biomarker of the early stage of atherosclerosis, following administration of 50 and 100 mg/kg GSPE, respectively. In a human trial, GSPE supplementation of 100 mg twice daily significantly reduced oxidised LDL.[127]

One human study using GSPE supplementation in conjunction with a novel niacin chromium was shown to yield favourable effects on cholesterol and LDL. It was also shown to improve cardiac functional assessment, including post-ischaemic left ventricular function, reduced myocardial infarct size, reduced ventricular fibrillation and tachycardia, and reduced the levels of ROS.[127]

Although research has shown that antioxidants are beneficial to most people and prevent many different diseases, some trials have not produced the expected results. Some antioxidants act as pro-oxidants, depending on the timing of administration during oxidation processes and the individuals involved. It has been suggested that some individuals have higher rates of lipid peroxidation and are therefore at higher risk of diseases such as atherosclerosis and CVD, but in other individuals very high levels of antioxidants may actually cause pro-oxidation, worsening the damage. It may therefore be useful for populations to be screened to determine which people are at high risk and would benefit from antioxidants, rather than making a general recommendation for everyone to increase their antioxidant intake.[128] However, the trials reviewed here indicate that in general antioxidants can be recommended, as such cases are rare.

Lutein

There is increasing scientific evidence that the incidence of CHD is inversely related to consumption of fruits and vegetables. A comparative study of fruit and vegetable consumption and antioxidant status in Belfast, Northern Ireland (low fruit and vegetable consumption, high rate of heart disease) and Toulouse, France (high fruit and vegetable consumption, low rate of heart disease), showed only one difference, namely that the plasma concentrations of lutein and cryptoxanthin were twice as high in the Toulouse population.[129] Another epidemiological study reported that individuals with the highest serum lutein plus zeaxanthin had a significantly reduced risk of CHD, and a further study showed a significant inverse relationship between lutein intake and the risk of stroke.[130] An *in vivo* study on middle-aged men and women showed that in an *in vitro* artery cell wall system, lutein inhibited LDL-induced migration of monocytes to human artery cell walls, and further that this effect was more pronounced if the cells were pretreated with lutein. There was also an inverse relationship between serum lutein levels and the progression of intima-media thickness (IMT) in the carotid arteries. Using an *in vivo* mouse model, progression of IMT was found to decline with increasing levels of plasma lutein.[131]

Carnitine

Carnitine is found in high concentrations in heart muscle, where it has important functions, including the prevention of lactic acid formation, which is damaging to the myocardium. It has been shown that in the failing heart there is a reduction of up to 50% of both free and total carnitine.[132]

During myocardial ischaemia, blood flow to the heart is reduced, and carnitine levels in myocardial muscle decrease by as much as 40%.[133] This results in an increase of free fatty acids and their metabolites within the cell cytoplasm, and a reduction of the oxidative processes necessary for energy production.[134] Supplementation with carnitine may be of use in patients with ischaemic heart disease.

In a study of patients suffering from exercise-induced stable angina with classical onset and improvement with rest or after the use of sublingual glyceryltrinitrate,[134] the patients were treated with 2 g/day carnitine orally for six months, added to their normal therapy. Medication being used by the patients included nitro-compounds, calcium channel blockers, beta-blockers, antihypertensives, diuretics, cardiac glycosides, antiarrhythmics, anticoagulants and hypolipidaemics. Results showed significant and progressive improvements in cardiac function and quality of life. Although there were no differences in glycaemia or HDL-C, there was a small but significant decrease in total cholesterol and triglycerides. There was also a significant reduction of cardioactive drug consumption.

These results indicate that carnitine may be of importance in the control of exercised-induced stable angina, either alone or in combination with other heart medication. In the year following an MI, patients are prone to cardiac complications, which often result in death. Patients who had had recent acute MI received 2 g carnitine twice daily, for one year, in addition to the standard cardioactive medication. Positive results were seen in terms of cardiac events and life expectancy, with significant differences for nearly all the parameters studied. Particularly striking were the differences in mortality of 1.2% in the carnitine group compared with 12.5% in the control group receiving no carnitine. This study clearly showed that the addition of carnitine had benefits for the patients in the year following MI.[135]

In a similar study, patients with suspected acute MI were supplemented with 2 g carnitine daily, in three divided doses. After 28 days of treatment, the mean infarct size was significantly reduced in the carnitine group, as were cardiac events, including angina pectoris, left ventricular failure and arrhythmias. No side-effects were noted and the use of other heart medication was reduced.[133]

Carnitine 50 mg/kg daily for 15 days has also been used to shorten recovery time in children with heart failure. The children in the test group showed a marked improvement over the controls and decreased recovery time.[136]

In conclusion, the role of carnitine in heart disease seems promising. The reduction in mortality in post-MI patients is very encouraging, as are the many other significant improvements to cardiac parameters seen with carnitine supplementation.

Some individuals may be genetically predisposed to carnitine deficiency, and this is associated with cardiomyopathy and skeletal muscle dysfunction, both of which can be treated with carnitine supplementation. Carnitine deficiency may also be acquired and can result in failing myocardium.[132] One clinical trial has shown a significant beneficial effect when treating MI patients with carnitine at a dose of 9 g/day for 5 days, followed by 6 g/day for the next 12 months.[137]

Carnitine supplementation has also used in patients with a range of arrhythmias.[65]

Short-term administration of carnitine supplements to patients with CHD did not increase cardiac ejection fraction, but did increase skeletal muscle phosphocreatine and led to improvements in muscle strength, endurance and metabolism.[132]

Dehydroepiandrosterone

Several epidemiological studies have found significant inverse relationships between serum dehydroepiandrosterone sulfate (DHEAS) and cardiovascular morbidity and mortality of men, suggesting that dehydroepiandrosterone (DHEA) is a risk factor for CHD. However, DHEAS level was not linked to cardiovascular risk in postmenopausal women, and DHEA supplementation in women caused decreased HDL-C levels.[138] Another study found that plasma levels of DHEAS were decreased in patients with congestive heart failure in proportion to its severity, and that oxidative stress was associated with decreased levels of DHEAS.[139]

Conclusions

The published data outlined from a wide variety studies and clinical trials suggest that dietary supplementation with certain nutraceuticals can improve cardiovascular health, both for healthy individuals and for those with cardiac problems. High-quality evidence from studies involving soy protein supplementation of subjects' diets was sufficient for the FDA to give their approval to manufacturers of soy foods to use the health claim that 'consumption of at least 25 g of soy protein per day is related to a reduced risk of developing CHD'.[30]

Meta-analyses of trials on a number of nutraceuticals used in this area have been carried out. Teas have been found to have produced conflicting results to date,[27] while those for soy variably show decrease in total cholesterol and LDL-C, sometimes demonstrating significant decrease,[30,35] sometimes no benefits [140]. Even analyses showing benefits suggest that the effects may be caused by other factors.[141] Fish oil and EPA/DHA meta-analyses appear to confirm positive effects on blood pressure,[142,143] and also beneficial effects on levels of cardiac morbidity.[64,144] Co Q10 appears well established as a treatment for congestive heart failure, and two analyses confirm this.[76,145] Policosanol appears to be more effective than plant sterols/stanols in reducing LDL-C.[146]

There are many green tea and soy nutraceutical products for consumers to purchase and now a number of formulated nutraceutical supplements have become available. In addition, a number of other nutraceuticals are also available, with claims for improvements in cardiovascular health. A number of these entities are able to reduce various risk factors associated with CVDs, such as cholesterol or hypertension, others are antiarrhythmic and therefore can reduce CHD mortality. However it is difficult to accurately define a recommended dosage, due to the fact that many of these nutraceuticals may be obtained as part of a healthy diet, resulting in some people having higher levels in their body than others. For effective cardiovascular protection, monitoring of plasma levels may be required before these products can be safely and effectively used to reduce CVD.[4]

References

1. Walker R, Edwards C. *Clinical Pharmacy and Therapeutics*, 3rd edn. London: Churchill and Livingstone, 2003.
2. Juturu V, Gormley J J. Nutritional supplements modulating metabolic syndrome risk factors and the prevention of cardiovascular disease. *Curr Nutr Food Sci* 2005; 1: 1–11.
3. Merz-Demlow B E, Duncan A M, Wangen K E *et al.* Soy isoflavones improve plasma lipids in normocholesterolemic, premenopausal women. *Am J Clin Nutr* 2000; 71: 1462–1469.
4. Payne E, Potts L, Lockwood B. Nutraceuticals for cardiovascular protection. In: Starks T P, ed. *Focus on Nutrition Research*. Hauppauge, NY: Nova Science, 2006.
5. Dufresne C J, Farnworth E R. A review of latest research findings on the health promotion properties of tea. *J Nutr Biochem* 2001; 12: 404–421.

6. Sanders T A B, Dean T S, Grainger D *et al.* Moderate intakes of intact soy protein rich in isoflavones compared with ethanol-extracted soy protein increase HDL but do not influence transforming growth factor β_1 concentrations and hemostatic risk factors for coronary heart disease in healthy subjects. *Am J Clin Nutr* 2002; 76: 373–377.

7. Castano G, Mas R, Fernandez L *et al.* Effects of policosanol on postmenopausal women with type II hypercholesterolemia. *Gynecol Endocrin* 2000; 14: 187–195.

8. Craig C R, Stitzel R E. *Modern Pharmacology*, 4th edn. Boston, MA: Little, Brown & Co, 1994.

9. Farnier M, Davignon J. Current and future treatment of hyperlipidemia: the role of statins. *Am J Cardiol* 1998; 82: 3J–10J.

10. Vinson J A, Teufel K, Wu N. Green and black teas inhibit atherosclerosis by lipid, antioxidant, and fibrinolytic mechanisms. *J Agric Food Chem* 2004; 52: 3661–3665.

11. Kris-Etherton P M, Keen C L. Evidence that the antioxidant flavonoids in tea and cocoa are beneficial for cardiovascular health. *Curr Opin Lipidol* 2002; 13: 41–49.

12. Mukhtar H, Ahmad N. Tea polyphenols: prevention of cancer and optimizing health. *Am J Clin Nutr* 2000; 71: 1698S–1702S.

13. Siddiqui I A, Afaq F, Adhami V M *et al.* Antioxidants of the beverage tea in promotion of human health. *Antiox Redox Signal* 2004; 6: 571–582.

14. Yang Y C, Lu F H, Wu J S *et al.* The protective effect of habitual tea consumption on hypertension. *Arch Intern Med* 2004; 164: 1534–1540.

15. Maron D J, Lu G P, Cai N S *et al.* Cholesterol-lowering effect of a theaflavin-enriched green tea extract. A randomized controlled trial. *Arch Intern Med* 2003; 163: 1448–1453.

16. Imai K, Nakachi K. Cross sectional study of effects of drinking green tea on cardiovascular and liver diseases. *BMJ* 1995; 310: 693–696.

17. Nakachi K, Matsuyama S, Miyake S *et al.* Preventive effects of drinking green tea on cancer and cardiovascular disease: epidemiological evidence for multiple targeting prevention. *BioFactors* 2000; 13: 49–54.

18. Davies M J, Judd J T, Baer D J *et al.* Black tea consumption reduces total and LDL cholesterol in mildly hypercholesterolemic adults. *J Nutr* 2003; 133: 3298S–3302S.

19. Duffy S J, Keaney J F Jr, Holbrook M *et al.* Short- and long-term black tea consumption reverses endothelial dysfunction in patients with coronary artery disease. *Circulation* 2001; 104: 151–156.

20. Lee W, Min W-K, Chun S *et al.* Long-term effects of green tea ingestion on atherosclerotic biological markers in smokers. *Clin Biochem* 2005; 38: 84–87.

21. Hodgson J M, Puddey I B, Burke V *et al.* Regular ingestion of black tea improves brachial artery vasodilator function. *Clin Sci* 2002, 102, 195–201.

22. Vita, JA. Tea consumption and cardiovascular disease: effects on endothelial function. *J Nutr* 2003; 133: 3293S–3297S.

23. Rietveld A, Wiseman S. Antioxidant effects of tea: evidence from human clinical trials. *J Nutr* 2003, 133: 3285S–3292S.

24. Cheng T O. All teas are not created equal: the Chinese green tea and cardiovascular health. *Int J Cardiol* 2006; 108: 301–308.

25. Arts I C W, Hollman P C H, Feskens E J M *et al.* Catechin intake might explain the inverse relation between tea consumption and ischemic heart disease: the Zutphen Elderly Study. *Am J Clin Nutr* 2001; 74: 227–232.

26. Geleijnse J M, Launer L J, van der Kuip D A M *et al.* Inverse association of tea and flavonoid intakes with incident myocardial infarction: the Rotterdam study. *Am J Clin Nutr* 2002; 75: 880–886.

27. Peters U, Poole C, Arab L. Does tea affect cardiovascular disease? A meta-analysis. *Am J Epidemiol* 2001; 154: 495–503.

28. Mukamal K J, Maclure M, Muller J E *et al.* Tea consumption and mortality after acute myocardial infarction. *Circulation* 2002; 105: 2476–2481.

29. Lichtenstein A H. Soy protein, isoflavones and cardiovascular disease risk. *J Nutr* 1998; 128: 1589–1592.

30. Anderson J W, Johnstone B M, Cook-Newell M E. Meta-analysis of the effects of soy protein intake on serum lipids. *N Engl J Med* 1995; 333: 276–282.

31. Wangen K E, Duncan A M, Xu X, Kurzer M S. Soy isoflavones improve plasma lipids in normocholesterolemic and mildly hypercholesterolemic post-menopausal women. *Am J Clin Nutr* 2001; 73: 225–231.

32. Potter S M, Baum J A, Teng H *et al.* Soy protein and isoflavones: their effects on blood lipids and bone density in postmenopausal women. *Am J Clin Nutr* 1998; 68: 1375S–1379S.

33. Nestel P. Role of soy protein in cholesterol-lowering. How good is it? *Arterioscl Thromb Vasc Biol* 2002; 22: 1743–1744.

34. Mitchell J H, Collins A R. Effects of a soy milk supplement on plasma cholesterol levels and oxidative DNA damage in men – a pilot study. *Eur J Nutr* 1999; 38: 143–148.

35. Zhan S, Ho S C. Meta-analysis of the effects of soy protein containing isoflavones on the lipid profile. *Am J Clin Nutr* 2005; 81: 397–408.

36. Setchell K D R, Brown N M, Lydeking-Olsen E. The clinical importance of the metabolite equol – a clue to the effectiveness of soy and its isoflavones. *J Nutr* 2002; 132: 3577–3584.

37. Squadrito F, Altavilla D, Morabito N *et al.* The effect of the phytoestrogen genistein on plasma nitric oxide concentrations, endothelin-1 levels and endothelium dependent vasodilation in postmenopausal women. *Athero-sclerosis* 2002; 163: 339–347.

38. Teede H J, Dalais F S, Kotsopoulos D *et al.* Dietary soy has both beneficial and potentially adverse cardiovascular effects: a placebo-controlled study in men and postmenopausal women. *J Clin Endocrinol Metab* 2001; 86: 3053–3060.

39. Honore E K, Williams J K, Anthony M S, Clarkson T B. Soy isoflavones enhance coronary vascular reactivity in atherosclerotic female macaques. *Fertil Steril* 1997; 67: 148–154.

40. Nestel P J, Yamashita T, Sasahara T *et al.* Soy isoflavones improve systemic arterial compliance but not plasma lipids in menopausal and perimenopausal women. *Arterioscl Thromb Vasc Biol* 1997; 17: 3392–3398.

41. Anthony M S, Clarkson T B, Williams J K. Effects of soy isoflavones on athero-sclerosis: potential mechanisms. *Am J Clin Nutr* 1998; 68: 1390S–1393S.

42. Anderson J W, Smith B M, Washnock C S. Cardiovascular and renal benefits of dry bean and soybean intake. *Am J Clin Nutr* 1999; 70: 464S–474S.

43. Rivas M, Garay R P, Escanero J F et al. Soy milk lowers blood pressure in men and women with mild to moderate essential hypertension. *J Nutr* 2002; 132: 1900–1902.

44. Sacks F M, Lichtenstein A, Van Horn L et al. Soy protein, isoflavones, and cardiovascular health: An American Heart Association Science Advisory for Professionals From the Nutrition Committee. *Circulation* 2006; 113: 1034–1044.

45. Wijendran V, Hayes K. Dietary *n*-6 and *n*-3 fatty acid balance and cardiovascular health. *Annu Rev Nutr* 2004; 24: 597–615.

46. Hoffman D R. Fatty acids and visual dysfunction. In: Chow C K, ed. *Fatty Acids in Foods and Their Health Implications*, 2nd edn. New York: Marcel Dekker, 2000: 817–841.

47. Simopoulos AP. Essential fatty acids in health and chronic disease. *Am J Clin Nutr* 1999; 70: 560S–569S.

48. Cunnane S C, Zhen-Yu C, Yang J et al. α-Linoleic acid in humans: direct functional role or dietary precursor? *Nutrition* 1991; 7: 437–439.

49. Uauy R, Valenzuela A. Marine oils: benefits of *n*-3 fatty acids. *Nutrition* 2000; 16: 680–684.

50. Demaison L, Moreau D. Dietary *n*-3 polyunsaturated fatty acids and coronary heart disease-related mortality: a possible mechanism of action. *Cell Mol Life Sci* 2002; 59: 463–477.

51. Bruckner G. Fatty acids and cardiovascular diseases. In: Chow C K, ed. *Fatty Acids in Foods and Their Health Implications*, 2nd edn. New York: Marcel Dekker, 2000: 843–863.

52. Djoussé L, Folsom A, Province M et al. Dietary linolenic acid and carotid atherosclerosis: the National Heart, Lung and Blood Institute Family Heart Study. *Am J Clin Nutr* 2003; 77: 819–825.

53. Baylin A, Kabagambe E, Ascherio A et al. Adipose tissue α-linolenic acid and non-fatal acute myocardial infarction in Costa Rica. *Circulation* 2003; 107: 1586–1591.

54. Allman M A, Pena N M, Pang D. Supplementation with flaxseed oil versus sunflower oil in healthy young men consuming a low fat diet: effects on platelet composition and function. *Eur J Clin Nutr* 1995; 49: 169–178.

55. Brouwer I, Katan M, Zock L. Dietary α-linolenic acid is associated with a reduced risk of fatal coronary heart disease, but increased prostate cancer risk: a meta-analysis. *J Nutr* 2004; 134: 919–922.

56. Nestel P, Pomeroy SE, Sasahara T et al. Arterial compliance in obese subjects is improved with dietary plant *n*-3 fatty acid from flaxseed oil despite increased LDL oxidizability. *Arteriosl Thromb Vasc Biol* 1997; 17: 1163–1170.

57. Cunnane S C, Ganguli S, Menard C et al. High α linoleic acid flaxseed (*Linum usitatissimum*): some nutritional properties in humans. *Br J Nutr* 1993; 69: 443–453.

58. Erasmus U. *Fats that Heal Fats that Kill: the Complete Guide to Fats, Oils and Cholesterol*, 2nd edn. Burnaby BC, Canada: Alive Books, 1993.

59. Cunnane S C. α-Linoleic acid in human nutrition and disease. *Nutrition* 1991; 7: 436.

60. Dallongeville J, Yarnell J, Ducimetière P et al. Fish consumption is associated with lower heart rates. *Circulation* 2003; 108: 820–825.

61.   Nestel P, Shige H, Pomeroy S *et al.* The *n*-3 fatty acids eicosapentaenoic acid and docosahexaenoic acid increase systemic arterial compliance in humans. *Am J Clin Nutr* 2002; 76: 326–330.

62.   Mori T, Bao D, Burke V *et al.* Docosahexaenoic acid but not eicosapentaenoic acid lowers ambulatory blood pressure and heart rate in humans. *Hypertension* 1999; 34: 253–260.

63.   Lemaitre R, King I, Mozaffarian D *et al. n*-3 polyunsaturated fatty acids, fatal ischemic heart disease and non-fatal myocardial infarction in older adults: the Cardiovascular Health Study. *Am J Clin Nutr* 2003; 77: 319–325.

64.   Bucher H, Hengstler P, Schindler C, Meier G. N-3 Polyunsaturated fatty acids in coronary heart disease: a meta-analysis of randomised controlled trials. *Am J Med* 2002; 112: 298–304.

65.   Chung M. Vitamins, supplements, herbal medicines, and arrhythmias. *Cardiol Rev* 2004; 12: 73–84.

66.   Rivellese A, Maffettone A, Vessby B *et al.* Effects of dietary saturated, monounsaturated and *n*-3 fatty acids on fasting lipoproteins, LDL size and post-prandial lipid metabolism in healthy subjects. *Atherosclerosis* 2003; 167: 149–158.

67.   Harris WS. *n*-3 Fatty acids and serum lipoproteins: human studies. *Am J Clin Nutr* 1997; 65(Suppl): 1645S–1654S.

68.   Layne K S, Goh Y K, Jumpsen J A *et al.* Normal subjects consuming physiological levels of 18:3(*n*-3) and 20:5(*n*-3) from flaxseed or fish oils have characteristic differences in plasma lipid and lipoprotein fatty acid levels. *J Nutr* 1996; 126: 2130–2140.

69.   Khan F, Elherik K, Bolton-Smith C *et al.* The effects of dietary fatty acid supplementation on endothelial function and vascular tone in healthy subjects. *Cardiovasc Res* 2003; 59: 955–962.

70.   Westcott N D, Muir A D. Flax seed lignan in disease prevention and health promotion. *Phytochem Rev* 2004; 2: 401–417.

71.   Jenkins D J A, Kendall C W C, Vidgen E *et al.* Health aspects of partially defatted flaxseed, including effects on serum lipids, oxidative measures, and ex vivo androgen and progestin activity: a controlled crossover trial. *Am J Clin Nutr* 1999; 69: 395–402.

72.   Stavro P M, Marchie A L, Kendall C W C *et al.* Flaxseed, fiber, and coronary heart disease: clinical studies. In: Cannane S C, Thompson L U, eds. *Flaxseed in Human Nutrition*, 2nd edn. Champaign, IL: AOCS Press, 2003: 288–300.

73.   Bloedon L T, Szapary P O. Flaxseed and cardiovascular risk. *Nutr Rev* 2004; 62: 18–27.

74.   Witte K, Clark A, Cleland J. Chronic heart failure and micronutrients. *J Am Coll Cardiol* 2001; 37: 1765–1774.

75.   Sole M, Jeejeebhoy K N. Conditioned nutritional requirements and the pathogenesis and treatment of myocardial failure. *Curr Opin Clin Nutr Metab Care* 2000; 3: 417–424.

76.   Soja A M, Mortensen S A. Treatment of congestive heart failure with coenzyme Q10 illuminated by meta-analyses of clinical trials. *Mol Asp Med* 1997; 18: S159–S168.

77. McCarty M. Coenzyme Q versus hypertension: does CoQ decrease endothelial superoxide generation? *Med Hypotheses* 1999; 53: 300–304.
78. Langsjoen P, Langsjoen P, Willis R, Folkers K. Treatment of essential hypertension with coenzyme Q10. *Mol Aspects Med* 1994; 15: S265–S272.
79. Khatta M, Alexander B, Krichten C *et al.* The effect of coenzyme Q10 in patients with congestive heart failure. *Ann Intern Med* 2000; 132: 636–640.
80. Singh R, Wander G, Rastogi A *et al.* Randomised, double-blind placebo-controlled trial of coenzyme Q10 in patients with acute myocardial infarction. *Cardiovasc Drug Ther* 1998; 12: 347–353.
81. Langsjoen P, Langsjoen A, Willis R, Folkers K. Treatment of hypertropic cardiomyopathy with coenzyme Q10. *Mol Aspects Med* 1997; 18: S145–S151.
82. Rosenfeldt F, Pepe S, Linnane A *et al.* Coenzyme Q10 protects the aging heart against stress, studies in rats human tissues and patients. *Ann N Y Acad Sci* 2002; 959: 355–359.
83. Langsjoen P, Folkers K, Lyson K *et al.* Effective and safe therapy with coenzyme Q10 for cardiomyopathy. *Klin Wochenschr* 1988; 66: 583–590.
84. Kishi T, Kishi H, Folkers K. Inhibition of cardiac Co Q10-enzymes by clinically used drugs and possible prevention. In: Folkers K, Yamamura Y, eds. *Biomedical and Clinical Aspects of Coenzyme Q*, Vol. 1. Amsterdam: Elsevier/North Holland Biomedical Press, 1977: 47–62.
85. Preedy V, Mantle D. Adverse effect on coenzyme Q10 levels. *Pharm J* 2004; 272: 13.
86. Rao A, Agarwal S. Role of lycopene as antioxidant carotenoid in the prevention of chronic diseases: a review. *Nutr Res* 1999; 19: 305–323.
87. Rao A, Agarwal S. Role of antioxidant lyopene in cancer and heart disease. *J Am Coll Nutr* 2000; 19: 563–569.
88. Rao A, Waseem Z, Agarwal S. Lycopene content of tomatoes and tomato products and their contribution to dietary lycopene. *Food Res Int* 1998; 31: 737–741.
89. Kardinaal A F, Kok F J, Ringstad J *et al.* Antioxidants in adipose tissue and risk of myocardial infarction: the EURAMIC Study. *Lancet* 1993; 342: 1379–1384.
90. Anon. The effect of vitamin E and beta carotene on the incidence of lung cancer and other cancers in male smokers. The Alpha-Tocopherol, Beta Carotene Cancer Prevention Study Group. *N Engl J Med* 1994; 330: 1029–1035.
91. Kohlmeier L, Kark J D, Gomez-Gracia E *et al.* Lycopene and myocardial infarction risk in the EURAMIC Study. *Am J Epidemiol* 1997; 146: 618–626.
92. Kristenson M, Zieden B, Kucinskiene Z *et al.* Antioxidant state and mortality from coronary heart disease in Lithuanian and Swedish men: concomitant cross sectional study of men aged 50. *BMJ* 1997; 314: 629–633.
93. Hirvonen T, Virtamo J, Korhonen P *et al.* Intake of flavonoids , carotenoids, vitamins C and E, and risk of stroke in male smokers. *Stroke* 2000; 31: 2301–2306.
94. Rao A. Lycopene, tomatoes and the prevention of coronary heart disease. *Exp Biol Med* 2002; 227: 908–913.
95. Rissanen T, Voutilainen S, Nyyssönen K, Salonen J. Lycopene, atherosclerosis and coronary heart disease. *Exp Biol Med* 2002; 227: 900–907.

96. Engelhard Y N, Gazer B, Paran E. Natural antioxidants from tomato extract reduce blood pressure in patients with grade – 1 hypertension: a double-blind, placebo-controlled pilot study. *Am Heart J* 2006; 151: 100.e1–100.e6.

97. Das S, Otani H, Maulik N, Das D K. Lycopene, tomatoes, and coronary heart disease. *Free Radic Res* 2005; 39: 449–455.

98. Más R, Castaño G, Fernandez L *et al.* Effects of policosanol in patients with type II hypercholesterolemia and additional coronary risk factors. *Clin Pharmacol Ther* 1999; 65: 439–447.

99. Gouni-Berthold I, Berthold H. Policosanol: clinical pharmacology and therapeutic significance of a new lipid lowering agent. *Am Heart J* 2002; 143: 356–365.

100. Hargrove J, Greenspan P, Hartle D. Nutritional significance and metabolism of very long chain fatty alcohols and acids from dietary waxes. *Exp Biol Med* 2004; 229: 215–226.

101. Rapport L, Lockwood B. *Nutraceuticals*. London: Pharmaceutical Press, 2001.

102. Torres O, Agramonte A, Illnait J *et al.* Treatment of hypercholesterolemia in NIDDM with policosanol. *Diabetes Care* 1995; 18: 393–397.

103. Lin Y, Rudrum M, van der Wielen R P J *et al.* Wheat germ policosanol failed to lower plasma cholesterol in subjects with normal to mildly elevated cholesterol concentrations. *Metab Clin Exp* 2004; 53: 1309–1314.

104. Crespo N, Illnait J, Mas R *et al.* Comparative study of the efficacy and tolerability of policosanol and lovastatin in patients with hypercholesterolemia and noninsulin dependent diabetes mellitus. *Int J Clin Pharmacol Res* 1999; 19: 117–127.

105. Noa M, Herrera M, Magraner J, Mas R. Effect of policosanol on isoprenaline-induced myocardial necrosis in rats. *J Pharm Pharmacol* 1994; 46: 282–285.

106. Anon. A close look at coenzyme Q10 and policosanol. *Harvard Health Lett* 2002; 13: 1–3.

107. Packer L, Rimbach G, Virgili F. Antioxidant activity and biologic properties of a procyanidin-rich extract from pine (*Pinus maritima*) bark, pycnogenol. *Free Radic Biol Med* 1999; 27: 704–724.

108. Devaraj S, Vega-López S, Kaul N *et al.* Supplementation with a pine bark extract rich in polyphenols increases plasma antioxidant capacity and alters the plasma lipoprotein profile. *Lipids* 2002; 37: 931–934.

109. Liu X, Wei J, Tan F *et al.* Pycogenol, French maritime pine bark extract, improves endothelial function of hypertensive patients. *Life Sci* 2004; 74: 855–862.

110. Koch R. Comparative study of venostasin and pycnogenol in chronic venous insufficiency. *Phytother Res* 2002; 16: S1–S5.

111. Belcaro G, Cesarone M R, Rohdewald P *et al.* Prevention of venous thrombosis and thrombophlebitis in long-haul flights with pycnogenol. *Clin Appl Thrombosis/Hemostasis* 2004; 10: 373–377.

112. Cesarone M R, Belcaro G, Rohdewald P *et al.* Prevention of edema in long flights with pycnogenol. *Clin Appl Thrombosis/Hemostasis* 2005; 11: 289–294.

113. Belcaro G, Cesarone M R, Errichi B M *et al.* Venous ulcers: microcirculatory improvement and faster healing with local use of pycnogenol. *Angiology* 2005; 56: 699–705.

114. Reiter R J, Tan D-X. Melatonin: a novel protective agent against oxidative injury of the ischemic/reperfused heart. *Cardiovasc Res* 2003; 58: 10–19.
115. Chen Z, Chua C C, Gao J et al. Protective effect of melatonin on myocardial infarction. *Am J Physiol* 2003; 284: H1618–H1624.
116. Ray C A. Melatonin attenuates the sympathetic nerve responses to orthostatic stress in humans. *J Physiol* 2003; 551: 1043–1048.
117. Bhat K P L, Kosmeder J W II, Pezzuto J M. Biological effects of resveratrol. *Antiox Redox Signal* 2001; 3: 1041–1064.
118. Laden B P, Porter T D. Resveratrol inhibits human squalene monooxygenase. *Nutr Res* 2001; 21: 747–753.
119. Das D K, Sato M, Ray P S et al. Cardioprotection of red wine: role of polyphenolic antioxidants. *Drugs Exp Clin Res* 1999; 25: 115–120.
120. Frankel E N, Kanner J, German J B et al. Inhibition of oxidation of human low-density lipoprotein by phenolic substances in red wine. *Lancet* 1993; 341: 454–457.
121. Serafini M, Maiani G, Ferro-Luzzi A. Alcohol-free red wine enhances plasma antioxidant capacity in humans. *J Nutr* 1998; 128: 1003–1007.
122. Anon. Not all red wines are equal, new research suggests. *Pharm J* 1999; 262: 213.
123. Shrikhande A J. Wine by-products with health benefits. *Food Res Int* 2000; 33: 469–474.
124. Yamakoshi J, Kataoka S, Koga T, Ariga T. Proanthocyanidin-rich extract from grape seeds attenuates the development of aortic atherosclerosis in cholesterol-fed rabbits. *Atherosclerosis* 1999; 142: 139–149.
125. Fine A M. Oligomeric proanthocyanidin complexes: history, structure, and phytopharmaceutical applications. *Altern Med Rev* 2000; 5: 144–151.
126. Lurton L. Grape polyphenols: the assets of diversity. *Nutracos* September 2003; 39–43.
127. Bagchi D, Sen C K, Ray S D et al. Molecular mechanisms of cardioprotection by a novel grape seed proanthocyanidin extract. *Mutat Res* 2003; 523–524: 87–97.
128. Halliwell B. The antioxidant paradox. *Lancet* 2000; 355: 1179–1180.
129. McClean R, McCrum E, Scally G et al. Dietary patterns in the Belfast MONICA Project. *Proc Nutr Soc* 1990; 49: 297–305.
130. Alves-Rodrigues A, Shao A. The science behind lutein. *Toxicol Lett* 2004: 150: 57–83.
131. Dwyer J H, Navab M, Dwyer K M et al. Oxygenated carotenoid lutein and progression of early atherosclerosis: the Los Angeles atherosclerosis study. *Circulation* 2001: 103: 2922–2927.
132. Sole M J, Jeejeebhoy K N. Conditioned nutritional requirements and the pathogenesis and treatment of myocardial failure. *Curr Opin Clin Nutr Metab Care* 2000; 3: 417–424.
133. Singh R B, Niaz M A, Agaewal P et al. A randomised, double-blind, placebo-controlled trial of L-carnitine in suspected acute myocardial infarction. *Postgrad Med J* 1996; 72: 45–50.
134. Cacciatore L, Cerio R, Ciarimboli M et al. The therapeutic effect of L-carnitine in patients with exercise-induced stable angina: a controlled study. *Drugs Exp Clin Res* 1991; 17: 225–335.

135. Davini P, Bigalli A, Lamanna F, Boem A. Controlled study on L-carnitine therapeutic efficacy in post-infarction. *Drugs Exp Clin Res* 1992; 18: 355–365.

136. Ergur A T, Tanzer F, Cetinkaya O. Serum-free carnitine levels in children with heart failure. *J Trop Pediatr* 1999; 45: 168–169.

137. Iliceto S, Scrutinio D, Bruzzi P *et al*. Effects of L-carnitine administration on left ventricular remodeling after acute anterior myocardial infarction: the L-Carnitine Ecocardiografia Digitalizzata Infarto Miocardico (CEDIM) Trial. *J Am Coll Cardiol* 1995; 26: 380–387.

138. Buvat J. Androgen therapy with dehydroepiandrosterone. *World J Urol* 2003; 21: 346–355.

139. Moriyama Y, Yasue H, Yoshimura M *et al*. The plasma levels of dehydro-epiandrosterone sulfate are decreased in patients with chronic heart failure in proportion to the severity. *J Clin Endocrinol Metab* 2000; 85: 1834–1840.

140. Yeung J, Yu T-F. Effects of isoflavones (soy phyto-estrogens) on serum lipids: a meta-analysis of randomized controlled trials. *Nutr J* 2003; 2: 15.

141. Gardner C D, Newell K A, Cherin R, Haskell W L. The effect of soy protein with or without isoflavones relative to milk protein on plasma lipids in hyper-cholesterolemic postmenopausal women. *Am J Clin Nutr* 2001; 73: 728–735.

142. Morris M C, Sacks F, Rosner B. Does fish oil lower blood pressure? A meta-analysis of controlled trials. *Circulation* 1993; 88: 523–533.

143. Appel L J, Miller E R III, Seidler A J, Whelton P K. Does supplementation of diet with 'fish oil' reduce blood pressure? A meta-analysis of controlled clinical trials. *Arch Intern Med* 1993; 153: 1429–1438.

144. Harper C R, Jacobson T A. Usefulness of omega-3 fatty acids and the prevention of coronary heart disease. *Am J Cardiol* 2005; 96: 1521–1529.

145. Soja A M, Mortensen S A. Treatment of chronic cardiac insufficiency with coenzyme Q10 , results of meta-analysis in controlled clinical trials. *Ugeskrift Laeger* 1997; 159: 7302–7308.

146. Chen J T, Wesley R, Shamburek R D *et al*. Meta-analysis of natural therapies for hyperlipidemia: plant sterols and stanols versus policosanol. *Pharmacotherapy* 2005; 25: 171–183.

7

Eye health

Eye health is an area in which nutraceutical supplements are increasingly used, and they are now widely available at opticians. They are taken to maintain healthy sight, to improve a condition or to delay disease progression. Visual impairment and blindness are common in the elderly. As we age, visual performance decreases. This usually occurs slowly before the age of 50 years and accelerates after reaching 50. One study, carried out to identify the causes of vision loss in a large sample of visually impaired people aged 75 years or over in Britain in 2004,[1] found that in 52.9% of people the main cause of visual loss was age-related macular degeneration (AMD). Another study using pooled findings from three continents found AMD to be present in 0.2% of the combined population aged 55–64 and in 13% of those over 85 years.[2]

Numerous age-related disorders, including visual problems, have been linked to the cumulative effects of oxidative stress. The retina is particularly susceptible to cellular damage by reactive oxygen intermediates.

Age-related macular degeneration

Currently, there is no effective treatment for AMD in most patients. In 1995, the Age- Related Maculopathy Study published an international classification and grading system for AMD.[3] The condition was classified as early or late stage, termed age-related maculopathy (ARM) and AMD, respectively. AMD is further divided into two late-stage lesions: non-neovascular AMD (also termed geographic atrophy or dry AMD) and neovascular (or wet) AMD. ARM can slowly progress to AMD, which leads to rapid and significant loss of central vision and registered blindness within 5–10 years.[4]

As well as increasing age, there is also likely to be a strong hereditary component to AMD.[2] Other proposed risk factors include:

- White ethnicity
- Female gender
- A high dietary saturated fat intake
- Hypertension
- Low antioxidant levels[4]
- A low macular pigment density (see below).[2,4,5]

A review of the prevalence and potential risk factors for AMD in three racially similar populations in North America, Europe and Australia suggests there may be a threshold effect for sunlight exposure; exposure throughout life might influence the likelihood of developing AMD. Another environmental factor strongly associated with AMD is exposure to tobacco smoke.[5] At present, the main nutraceuticals for eye health are lutein and its stereoisomer zeaxanthin.

Lutein and zeaxanthin

There is interest in the possible roles of lutein and zeaxanthin in preventing onset or progression of AMD, improving vision and benefiting some types of cataracts and other eye conditions.

Lutein and zeaxanthin are usually derived from the diet, particularly dark green leafy vegetables such as kale and spinach.[6] Foods that are yellow, such as egg yolk, corn, orange juice, honeydew melon and orange pepper, are also good sources.[7,8] Lutein and zeaxanthin are naturally found together, with lutein usually in much higher concentrations.[3]

Lutein and zeaxanthin are unique compared with other dietary carotenoids because they selectively accumulate in the retina of mammals.[4] They give the area of the retina that serves central vision, the macula lutea, its yellow colour[9] by making up a screening pigment referred to as the macular pigment. This pigment may have both acute and chronic effects on visual performance.[5] Lutein and zeaxanthin are carried in human serum, mainly by high-density lipoproteins. In contrast, the carotenes are preferentially carried by low-density lipoprotein.[3]

Possible roles of lutein and zeaxanthin include antioxidant activity and their ability to filter blue light.

Antioxidant activity

Lutein and zeaxanthin are able to quench singlet oxygen, a highly reactive free radical that can damage deoxyribonucleic acid (DNA).[10]

There is evidence that lutein and zeaxanthin are even more effective at preventing lipid peroxidation, and are themselves better protected against secondary oxidative breakdown when melatonin, glutathione, alpha-tocopherol and ascorbate are also present, interacting in a cascade.[7] Direct oxidation products of both DNA and lipids have been found in the human retina.[11] Lutein and zeaxanthin are better antioxidants than hydrocarbon carotenoids, such as beta-carotene. They undergo a 2e-oxidation of hydroxyl groups as opposed to the 1e-oxidation of hydrocarbon carotenoids.[10]

Ability to filter blue light

Ultraviolet light is filtered by the cornea and lens in the anterior aspect of the eye but visible light reaches the retina. Visible light in the blue spectrum is the most damaging – short wavelength light (400–500 nm) has been shown to be 30 times more damaging than long wavelength light (510–749 nm).[7] Macular pigment absorbs blue light as it enters the inner retinal layers, reducing the amount reaching the fovea. This reduces the potential for photo-oxidation of reactive saturated lipids of photoreceptors.[10,11]

In people with normal amounts of macular pigment, 20–40% of light at 460 nm is absorbed. However, up to 90% can be absorbed in those with higher than normal amounts of macular pigment.[10] There is a high degree of individual variability in concentration of lutein and zeaxanthin in the fovea.[12]

Increasing numbers of people taking lutein and zeaxanthin supplements for their proposed prophylactic benefits also report improvements in vision, such as higher contrast sensitivity, less glare, and improved colour perception.[5] Within cells, lutein and zeaxanthin may selectively bind to tubulin, a structural protein necessary in the formation of the cytoskeleton within axons. This could improve structural integrity and function of the cytoskeleton,[5] thus helping maintain eye health and quality of vision.

Epidemiological evidence

There is evidence that a diet high in carotenoids is associated with a lower risk of AMD. One case–control study, after adjusting for other risk factors, found a 43% lower risk of AMD in individuals consuming the highest levels of carotenoids (especially lutein and zeaxanthin) compared with those consuming the least. The study also evaluated individual foods and found a strong inverse association for spinach.[13] This is supported by a further study, which found that for patients with low lutein and antioxidant intake the prevalence of AMD was about twice as high as patients with a high intake.[14] However, not all studies agree with this association. The Beaver Dam Eye Study reports only slightly (and not significantly) lower lutein and zeaxanthin serum concentrations in subjects with AMD compared with controls. This may be because of a relatively low intake of these carotenoids by these subjects.[15]

In the normal Western diet, there is a great deal of variation in the dietary intakes of these carotenoids. A study of Canadian dietary intake found the combined lutein and zeaxanthin intake to be 1.3–3 mg/day, with a standard deviation of 2.45 mg/day.[10] In 2001, the Institute of Medicine in the USA reported the mean dietary intake of combined lutein and zeaxanthin in Americans to be 1.71 mg/day. After further study, consumption by the general population was considered to be 2 mg/day less than a sensible intake based on recommended dietary guidelines.[12]

Macular pigment optical density and serum levels

Due to the invasive nature of the methods available to measure levels of compounds in the lens there are, as yet, no studies relating dietary lutein intakes to levels in the lens.[6] Although the amount of lutein and zeaxanthin in the retina cannot be measured directly in living subjects, it is relative to the optical density of the macular pigment.[16] A number of studies have shown that serum levels can be influenced by dietary supplementation or modification of the diet, as can the optical density of macular pigment.[7]

The serum half-life of lutein and zeaxanthin is around one to two weeks, so fasting before taking blood samples will not greatly affect the results.[9] A blood test will only reflect recent dietary intake and may not represent an average intake. The normal range of concentrations of lutein and zeaxanthin in serum is between 0.08 and 0.35 mg/mL. Associated food frequency questionnaires allow the relationship between diet and serum concentration to be assessed through calculating average daily consumption of these carotenoids.

Macular pigment optical density responds slowly to changes in serum concentration. Studies show that it can take several weeks from when a significant serum response is seen, before a change in macular pigment optical density is observed. In addition, macular pigment optical density falls slowly after stopping supplementation with lutein and zeaxanthin.[9,11] The authors of one study comparing the effects of supplementing with different doses of lutein (between 2.4 and 30 mg/day) and high-dose zeaxanthin (30 mg/day) suggest that continued high-dose supplementation of lutein and zeaxanthin may not be necessary to maintain a high macular pigment density, and that a high dose may only be needed initially to increase density followed by a lower maintenance dose.[15]

Nutraceuticals

There are two forms of lutein available for use in supplements and functional foods – purified crystalline lutein and lutein esters. The latter are less prevalent in the diet. Both types have been shown to increase serum levels and macular pigment optical density in intervention trials.[6]

The flower of *Tagetes erecta* (marigold) provides one possible source of crystalline lutein, the extract containing 86% by weight of the macular carotenoids.[12] GRAS status has been established for crystalline lutein from this source (confirmed by the US Food and Drug Administration (FDA) in June 2003),[17] allowing addition of lutein and zeaxanthin to some foods and making it possible to supplement a deficient diet through modified dietary intake.[12] Many supplements are already commercially available and lutein supplements have shown substantial sales growth in the past 2–3 years.[17]

The largest prospective, randomised, placebo-controlled study looking at the effect of taking supplements on eye disease is the Age-Related Eye Disease Study (AREDS). Over 6 years, nearly 4000 patients were given either a placebo or combination oral supplements. Lutein was not included as it was not commercially available, but the study showed that a high-dose antioxidant supplement slowed the progression of AMD significantly.[6] The Lutein Antioxidant Supplementation Trial (LAST) was carried out as a follow-up. It was a double-blind, placebo-controlled trial involving 90 patients with AMD who were given 10 mg lutein, 10 mg lutein and a mixed antioxidant, or placebo daily for 12 months. Significant improvements were seen in several objective measurements of visual function, such as glare recovery, contrast sensitivity and visual acuity, as well as a 50% increase in macular pigment optical density in the lutein-supplemented group compared with placebo. In the group taking the combined supplement slightly better results were seen.[6]

There are individual differences in absorption and metabolism of lutein and zeaxanthin.[11] Other components in the diet (particularly fat) influence carotenoid uptake into the blood.[9,15] The bioavailability of lutein esters, when consumed as part of a low fat meal (~3 g fat) has been shown to be significantly lower compared with consumption as part of a high fat meal (~36 g fat). Purified or synthetic beta-carotene has been shown to diminish serum lutein concentrations,[3] and this could be important in combined supplements or recommendations regarding dosage of supplements to maintain carotenoid balance in the body.

After reviewing toxicological and other data on the safe use of lutein or zeaxanthin derived from *Tagetes erecta*, the Food and Agriculture Organization of the United Nations (FAO) and the World Health Organization (WHO) set an acceptable intake of 2 mg/kg per day. This equates to about 145 mg lutein or zeaxanthin a day for a 72.6 kg person.[18] As regards the optimum dosage or combination of antioxidant vitamin and mineral supplements, there are few published data.[3]

High dietary intake of lutein and zeaxanthin from green leafy vegetables and coloured fruits will also be combined with a high intake of other phytochemicals. Lutein and zeaxanthin might work synergistically with other nutrients. If this is so, supplementation with lutein and zeaxanthin alone would not be as beneficial as dietary changes. Higher macular pigment levels might be a biomarker of better nutritional status.[5]

Current supplements containing the macular carotenoids might not contain them in sufficient quantities. For example, the manufacturer of Centrum, a widely used multivitamin and multimineral supplement, has started to add 250 mg lutein to its supplements. However, many studies showing lutein to have benefits in the prevention of onset or progression of AMD use 3–6 mg lutein per day.

Combination of acetyl-L-carnitine, n-3 fatty acids and coenzyme Q10

One clinical trial involving 106 patients with diagnosis of early AMD evaluated the benefits of supplementation with a proprietary formulation containing 100 mg acetyl-L-carnitine, 530 mg of *n*-3 fatty acids and 10 mg of coenzyme Q10 (Co Q10). Two capsules daily were taken by the test group over 12 months, and changes recorded in visual field mean effect, visual acuity, foveal sensitivity and fundus alterations. The treated group of patients showed improvement in all four parameters tested.[19]

Other eye conditions

Although research has focused on the links between the macular carotenoids and AMD, lutein and zeaxanthin have also been shown to have beneficial effects in other eye diseases.

Retinitis pigmentosa

Retinitis pigmentosa has been described as 'a genetically and clinically heterogeneous group of incurable retinal degenerative diseases'.[20] It has no cure and symptom alleviation is limited. Retinitis pigmentosa is characterised by progressive loss of rod photoreceptors, leading to night blindness, followed by atrophy of the receptors, resulting in tunnel vision and blindness. Macular pigment has been suggested to have a protective role for central vision through antioxidant and filtering effects. Short-term improvement in visual acuity and central field diameter has been seen following supplementation with lutein 20 mg/day for four months.[7] Another study looking at macular pigment and lutein supplementation in retinitis pigmentosa found central vision in patients to be unchanged after taking 20 mg/day of purified lutein for six months. However, macular pigment optical density increased in approximately half of the patients.[6] The researchers also noted that macular pigment optical density in their patient group did not differ from the normal range, although disease expression tended to be more severe in those with lower macular pigment levels.

Cataracts

Age-related cataract is the world's leading cause of blindness. In the USA it is prevalent in 40% of adults aged over 75 years and cataract extraction is one of the most common types of surgery in the elderly.[6] Development occurs when oxidatively damaged protein deposits form on or in the lens, clouding vision.[6]

Lutein and zeaxanthin are the only carotenoids that have been found in the human crystalline lens[21] but concentrations here are much lower than in the macular pigment and not high enough to absorb visible light. They may have a role protecting against oxidative damage from UV light and helping to prevent oxidation of epithelial lipids.[8,15]

Studies have indicated that people who eat more fruit and vegetables are less likely to develop a cataract. A prospective study has shown specifically that spinach consumption was inversely related to cataract development. This was followed by three prospective studies showing intake of lutein and zeaxanthin to be inversely associated with cataract development, with a 20–50% risk reduction.[6] Two large epidemiological studies looking at dietary intake of these carotenoids and cataract development found people in the highest quintile of dietary intake to have less chance of developing cataracts by 20% compared with people in the lowest quintile of dietary intake.[5]

There are a number of other nutraceuticals that might have beneficial effects regarding vision and the eye.

Astaxanthin

Astaxanthin is another carotenoid associated with eye health. It is found in many types of seafood, including lobster, shrimp and salmon, and is responsible for their pink colour when cooked. Microalgae, specifically *Haematococcus pluvialis*, is the main source, however, for companies producing astaxanthin for human consumption.[22] Astaxanthin is a powerful antioxidant and is able to cross the blood–brain barrier. Animal studies have shown it to accumulate in the retina and reduce photobleaching of the retina from exposure to high-intensity light.[23]

Pycnogenol

The results from five clinical trials carried out since 1960 support the use of the pine bark extract Pycnogenol in the treatment and prevention of diabetic retinopathy.[24]

It is estimated that about 5% of adults in developed countries have diabetes (about 1.4 million people in the UK) and diabetic retinopathy will be present in 10–50% of adults with diabetes.[25] This is characterised by vascular lesions, exudate deposits and haemorrhages, leading to loss of vision. Early treatment can prevent 98% of vision loss but there are no symptoms or warning signs during onset so the condition is often not diagnosed until it is advanced. Regular screening of people with diabetes is, therefore, needed, especially if blood glucose levels are not well controlled.

Pycnogenol is a highly potent antioxidant with a high affinity for collagen. Larger procyanidins, which are oligomers and polymers composed of catechin or epicatechin subunits, bind to proteins of damaged blood vessels to lower capillary permeability and reduce basement membrane leakage. Pycnogenol increases production of nitric oxide, which may be impaired in diabetes, by stimulating endothelial nitric oxide synthetase. Nitric oxide relaxes constricted blood vessels. Pycnogenol has anti-inflammatory action, reducing leukocyte-mediated degeneration of retinal capillaries, and has also been shown to prevent increased platelet activity without increasing bleeding time.[24]

Pycnogenol has been shown to be well tolerated at doses of up to 150 mg a day in trials lasting up to eight months. Its mode of action also suggests possible use in the prevention and treatment of a number of venous disorders and in the prevention of complications after cataract removal in people with diabetes.[24]

Docosahexaenoic acid

Fatty acids have been shown to influence function of the retina and to play a role in many pathological eye conditions. The bilayer membranes of the outer segments of the light-sensitive rod and cone photoreceptors in the retina contain membrane phospholipids. These are primarily esterified with high concentrations of docosahexaenoic acid (DHA), a long-chain n-3 polyunsaturated fatty acid (PUFA).[26] The essential n-3 fatty acid α-linolenic acid can be converted to DHA in the liver or retinal epithelium.

Evidence for the role of DHA in the development of visual function has been found from the study of premature babies.[26] Accumulation of DHA in retinal tissue is highest during the last three months of pregnancy (when retinal membranes develop) and until six months after birth. It has been shown that premature babies fed formula milk lacking DHA have compromised visual acuity compared with those fed formula milk enriched with fish oil containing DHA at levels approximating those found in breast milk. This poor visual acuity was related to an immaturity in rod cell function. For breastfed babies DHA intake will depend on the mother's diet.

The best dietary sources of DHA are coldwater fish, such as mackerel and tuna. Supplementation of DHA may be suitable for pregnant or breastfeeding women whose diets may be low in DHA, but more research is needed.

The role of fatty acids in retinitis pigmentosa has also been researched. Patients with this condition are consistently found to have abnormal blood levels of fatty acids. In particular, DHA is reduced and this might be due to an impairment in the final steps of DHA synthesis.[26] There may be a role for DHA in maintaining optimal visual function, and supplementation with DHA may be of value. People with high intakes of DHA have also been shown to be less likely to suffer from dry eye syndrome (when not enough tears are produced), which can lead to corneal scarring and vision loss.[27]

A further application of the *n*-3 PUFAs DHA and eicosapentaenoic acid (EPA) is in the common eye condition called dry eye syndrome.[28] Dry eye syndrome leads to lower visual acuity and difficulty in reading/writing and night vision. Inflammation or blockage of the lacrimal duct is frequently responsible, and artificial tears provide incomplete symptomatic relief. A sample (1546 patients) out of 39 876 female health professionals who were affected by the syndrome had their dietary fat intakes investigated using a food frequency questionnaire. A high ratio of *n*-6 to *n*-3 fatty acid consumption was associated with an increased risk of the syndrome, and tuna consumption was inversely associated with risk.[28]

α-Lipoic acid

α-Lipoic acid has antioxidant properties. It is both water- and fat-soluble and can cross cell membranes, helping to reduce free radical damage inside and outside cells. α-Lipoic acid also helps to recycle other antioxidants such as vitamins C and E, and glutathione, returning them to their oxidative states.[29] Dietary sources of α-lipoic acid include spinach, beef, kidney and heart. Humans can also produce α-lipoic acid in small amounts.

Doses of α-lipoic acid between 50 and 400 mg a day have been suggested for general antioxidant purposes but they are far in excess of normal physiological levels. Recently, pure *R*-lipoic acid has become available as a supplement.

α-Lipoic acid can lower glucose and insulin levels in people with diabetes, so care should be taken to monitor glucose levels in patients taking these supplements. Prevention of the damaging effects of hyperglycaemia is the main therapeutic indication for α-lipoic acid.[29]

Conclusions

Lutein and zeaxanthin have not been proven conclusively to improve eye health but there is compelling evidence to suggest this may be the case, particularly in AMD. If controlled clinical trials show that lutein and zeaxanthin reduce the progression and onset of AMD, retinitis pigmentosa and other retinal degenerations they may fulfil criteria to be considered essential nutrients.[7]

There is a need to educate consumers about eye health and how dietary habits and supplementation can help. As well as improving the natural antioxidant and protective defences of the eye (such as through increasing macular pigment optical density), reducing retinal oxidative stress may also help. Preventive strategies include stopping smoking, reducing the amount of blue light that reaches the eye through use of narrow-band yellow filters in glasses or contact lenses, and reducing intake of saturated fatty acids.[6,13]

Probably the best advice is to follow dietary guidelines and increase consumption of fruit and vegetables, specifically those rich in these carotenoids. In those who find it difficult to achieve the suggested fruit and vegetable intake, addition of lutein and zeaxanthin in supplement form might be of benefit. Advice could be to take supplements with food containing some fat to increase absorption. However, there is a need to carry out further research into the effectiveness and safety of such supplements in disease prevention. Trials would have to be long-term because diseases such as AMD are thought to be the result of many years of oxidative stress and exposure to other contributory factors. Studies are also needed to look at interactions of lutein and zeaxanthin with other antioxidants (e.g. alpha-tocopherol, ascorbate and glutathione) and deprivation studies looking at the effect of a lack of lutein and zeaxanthin in the diet and the effects of high light exposure.[7]

Future supplements containing synergistic combinations of in- gredients need established efficacious doses. Future research could also be carried out to identify possible candidate genes that might predispose people to AMD and allow them to take extra precautions that may involve supplementation with lutein and zeaxanthin.

References

1. Evans J R, Fletcher A E, Wormald R P L. Causes of visual impairment in people aged 75 and older in Britain: an add-on study to the MRC trial of assessment and management of older people in the community. *Br J Ophthalmol* 2004; 88: 365–371.
2. Smith W, Assink J, Klein R *et al*. Risk factors for age-related macular degener- ation, pooled findings from three continents. *Am J Ophthalmol* 2001; 108: 697–704.
3. Landrum J T, Bone R A. Lutein, zeaxanthin and the macular pigment. *Arch Biochem Biophys* 2001; 385: 28–40.
4. Bone R A, Landrum J T, Dixon Z *et al*. Lutein and zeaxanthin in the eyes, serum and diet of human subjects. *Exp Eye Res* 2000; 71: 239–245.
5. Mozaffariieh M, Sacu S, Wedrich A. The role of the carotenoids, lutein and

zeaxanthin, in protecting against age-related macular degeneration: a review based on controversial evidence. *Nutrition J* 2003; 2: 20.

6. Alves-Rodrigues A, Shao A. The science behind lutein. *Toxicol Lett* 2004; 150: 57–83.
7. Semba, R, Dagnelie, G. Are lutein and zeaxanthin conditionally essential nutrients for eye health? *Med Hypotheses* 2003; 61: 465–472.
8. Mayer J. The role of carotenoids in human health. *Nutr Clin Care* 2002; 5: 56–65.
9. Hammond B Jr, Wooten B, Curran-Celentano J. Carotenoids in the retina and lens: possible acute and chronic effects an human visual performance. *Arch Biochem Biophys* 2001; 385: 41–46.
10. Kruger C L, Murphy M, DeFreitas Z *et al.* An innovative approach to the determination of safety for a dietary ingredient derived from a new source: case study using a crystalline lutein product. *Food Chem Toxicol* 2002; 40: 1535–1549.
11. Beatty S, Koh H, Henson D, Boulton M. The role of oxidative stress in the pathogenesis of age-related macular degeneration. *Surv Ophthalmol* 2002; 45: 115–134.
12. Ahmed A. Lutein receives GRAS status. www.chiro.org/nutrition/FULL/Lutein_Receives_GRAS_Status.html (accessed 18 May 2006).
13. Seddon J M, Anji U A, Sperduto R D *et al.* Dietary carotenoids, vitamins A, C, and E, and advanced age-related macular degeneration. *JAMA* 1994; 272: 1413–1420.
14. Snellen E L M, Verbeek A L M, Van den Hoogen G W P *et al.* Neovascular age-related mascular degeneration and its relationship to antioxidant intake. *Acta Ophthalmol Scand* 2002; 80: 368–371.
15. Wright, T. Eye health ingredients have taken centre stage. http://www.nutraceuticalsworld.com/articles/2002/05/eye-health.php (accessed 18 May 2006).
16. Johnson E J, Hammond B R, Yeum K J *et al.* Relation among serum and tissue concentrations of lutein and zeaxanthin and macular pigment density. *Am J Clin Nutr* 2000; 71: 1555–1562.
17. Bartlett H, Eperjesi F. A randomised controlled trial investigating the effect of nutritional supplementation on visual function in normal, and age-related macular disease affected eyes: design and methodology. *Nutr J* 2003; 2: 12.
18. Bone R A, Landrum J T, Guerra L H, Ruiz C A. Lutein and zeaxanthin dietary supplements raise macular pigment density and serum concentrations of these carotenoids in humans. *J Nutr* 2003; 133: 992–998.
19. Feher J, Kovacs B, Kovacs I *et al.* Improvement of visual functions and fundus alterations in early age-related macular degeneration treated with a combination of acetyl-L-carnitine, *n*-3 fatty acids, and coenzyme Q10. *Ophthalmologica* 2005; 219: 154–166.
20. US Food and Drug Administration. International Food Ingredient Safety Panel take action to affirm safety of free lutein and zeaxanthin for human consumption. http://foodingredientsfirst.com/newsmaker_article.asp?idNewsMaker=6451&fSite=AO545&next=pr (accessed 18 May 2006).
21. Aleman T S, Duncan J L, Bieber M L *et al.* Macular pigment and lutein

supplementation in retinitis pigmentosa and Usher syndrome. *Invest Ophthalmol Vis Sci* 2001; 42: 1873–1881.

22. Gale C R, Hall N F, Phillips D I W, Martyn C N. Plasma antioxidant vitamins and carotenoids and age-related cataract. *Ophthalmology* 2001; 108: 1992–1998.

23. Madley RH (ed.). Seeing is believing. www.nutraceuticalsworld.com/mayjune001.htm (accessed 29 March 2004).

24. Schonlau F, Rohdewald P. Pycnogenol for diabetic retinopathy, a review. *Int Ophthalmol* 2002; 24: 161–171.

25. Walker R, Edwards C. *Clinical Pharmacy and Therapeutics*, 3rd edn. London: Churchill Livingstone, 2003.

26. Hoffman D R. Fatty acids and visual dysfunction. In: Chow C K, ed. *Fatty Acids in Foods and their Health Implications*, 2nd edn. New York: Food Science and Technology, 2000: 817–841.

27. Denoon D. Fish oil benefits your eyes. http://my.webmd.com/content/article/64/72431.htm (accessed 18 May 2006).

28. Miljanovic B, Trivedi K A, Dana M R *et al.* Relation between dietary *n*-3 and *n*-6 fatty acids and clinically diagnosed dry eye syndrome in women. *Am J Clin Nutr* 2005; 82: 887–893.

29. The Linus Pauling Institute. Alpha-lipoic acid. http://lpi.oregonstate.edu/infocenter/othernuts/la/ (accessed 18 May 2006).

8

Mental health

Two of the most important mental ailments are cognitive decline and depression. The most commonly available nutraceuticals claimed to be effective in age-related cognitive decline include acetyl-L-carnitine, phosphatidylserine, n-3 fatty acids, particularly docosahexaenoic acid (DHA), soy isoflavones, citicoline (cytidine diphosphate choline), reduced form of nicotinamide adenine dinucleotide (NADH), green tea and carnosine. Depression has been treated with n-3 fatty acids and S-adenosyl methionine (SAMe).

Many people believe that their memory declines with age. Many changes do occur in the ageing brain, including loss of myelin, accumulation of lipofuscin and a reduction in the branching of dendrites,[1] consequently the brain makes fewer new connections. Other changes that may occur during ageing are reduced availability of acetylcholine and reduced cerebral blood flow. The central nervous system does not generally divide or regenerate cells; it relies on a regular supply of glucose to continuously repair the neurons. Memory loss is probably related to the death of neurons. Increased glutamate and intracellular calcium levels will lead to necrosis, which can cause inflammation of the brain. Hydroxyl radicals and hydrogen peroxide can be produced as by-products of respiration under given conditions, and these are extremely reactive species and will attack DNA, enzymes and lipid membranes. The body's natural defences against these radicals are antioxidants: superoxide dismutase, vitamin C and alpha-tocopherol (vitamin E).[2] Normal memory loss is believed to be caused by a combination of these factors taking place over many years in the brain.

Alzheimer's disease is a form of dementia that has no specific precipitating factors. It is diagnosed by patients scoring 27 or less on the Mini-Mental State Examination (MMSE). The brain tissue shrinks and there is a loss of neurons, particularly in the hippocampus. Other specific aspects of the disease are the formation of amyloid plaques and neurofibrillary tangles. These cause damage and are thought to subject the brain to more oxidative stress and ischaemia.[2] Another major feature of Alzheimer's disease is the loss of cholinergic neurons; all the drugs used in the UK to treat mild to moderate Alzheimer's are acetylcholinesterase inhibitors. Donepezil, rivastigmine and galantamine have a success rate of up to 50% in slowing the disease process.[3] These products are not without side-effects and there is great interest in developing dietary and supplementary regimens to help the memory.

Another form of memory loss is that associated with cardiovascular disease. Arteriosclerosis in the cerebral arteries can lead to transient ischaemic attacks, in which not enough blood reaches one part of the brain for a short period of time, or in the worst case scenario, stroke occurs.

Small memory lapses may be early symptoms of ischaemia, and the degree of ischaemia and subsequent loss of respiration in the brain have been linked to the severity of certain dementias.[4]

The current pharmacological treatments for dementia are only partially effective. There is a great deal of interest in whether diet and/or supplementation could slow down or reverse the ageing process in the brain. The following nutraceuticals are marketed as enhancing 'brain power'.

Acetyl-L-carnitine

Acetyl-L-carnitine is a common nutraceutical sold to combat cognitive decline or to enhance memory. The acetyl form of carnitine can easily cross the blood–brain barrier and it appears to be well tolerated and safe in humans.[5] Acetyl-L-carnitine is a very promising agent for the treatment of patients with mild Alzheimer's disease. It is thought to have many actions on brain cells and to increase the availability of acetylcholine to neurons, possibly by providing acetyl groups to conjugate with choline. It is also believed to be a partial cholinergic agonist, working in a similar way to the current pharmacological treatments for Alzheimer's disease.[6] In addition, acetyl-L-carnitine assists the movement of fatty acids from the cytoplasm into mitochondria, where they are converted to ATP, and helps with the removal of toxic long-chain fatty acids.[6] This could lead to a synergism with long-chain fatty acids such as the n-3 group; acetyl-L-carnitine is sometimes combined with α-linolenic acid in supplements.

Acetyl-L-carnitine has also been shown to increase the levels of nerve growth factor (NGF),[7] one of a group of substances known as neurotrophins. NGF is involved in the formation of neurons in the developing brain, and has been recently discovered to be implicated in the repair and maintenance of neurons and the formation of new connections between them.[1] The branching of dendrites and formation of new connections is critical in the memory storage process. Acetyl-L-carnitine may also boost the levels of phosphomonoesters, which are phospholipid components that are reduced in Alzheimer's disease patients.[7,8] This means that acetyl-L-carnitine might synergise with another nutraceutical called phosphatidylserine, which has beneficial effects on the neuron membrane.[9] Other reports state that it could increase protein kinase C (PKC) activity and reverse an age-related decline in glutamate N-methyl D-aspartate receptors,[1] possibly reducing the risk of excitotoxicity (the death of neurons stimulated by glutamate).

Acetyl-L-carnitine has been shown to cause a slowdown in the decline of cognitive measures in a number of studies conducted on subjects with mild Alzheimer's disease or mild cognitive impairment. However, one of the double-blind trials conducted on its use in Alzheimer's disease showed very little difference between acetyl-L-carnitine and placebo.[10] This trial used the Alzheimer's Disease Assessment Scale, cognitive section (ADAS-Cog) as the main endpoint for analysis. The trial was then reanalysed by another group of researchers[11] who stated that the younger patients with Alzheimer's disease, who fully complied with the treatment, benefited significantly more from acetyl-L-carnitine treatment than older patients. Trends observed by the group included a slowdown of decline on the Clinical Global Impression (CGI) scale, and concluded that acetyl-L-carnitine benefits patients less than 61 years old. This conclusion was somewhat contradicted by a study published in 2000,[12] in which patients with early-onset (age 45–65 years) Alzheimer's disease were specifically chosen for the trial. The results showed that there was no significant difference between ADAS-Cog scores for the placebo and acetyl-L-carnitine treatment groups after one year's treatment.[1] However, there was a significantly reduced deterioration on one aspect of the MMSE test in these patients, and the placebo group did not display a rapid deterioration during the year as had been predicted earlier.

Both of the studies discussed above have been included in a recent meta-analysis of all the double-blind, controlled clinical trials of acetyl-L-carnitine.[6] The study concentrated on patients treated with acetyl-L-carnitine who had mild cognitive impairment or mild Alzheimer's disease, and found that of 21 studies conducted, 17 showed that acetyl-L-carnitine had a positive effect on patients; this included some unpublished trials. The meta-analysis used two endpoints for its results: the CGI used in most studies and the Integrated Summary of Clinical Tests referred to as the $ES_{all\ scales}$. The $ES_{all\ scales}$ was a statistical method used to combine the results of the many different tests (e.g. ADAS-Cog, MMSE, and word-list recall) that were used in the clinical trials into one factor. This enabled the authors to compare all the trials and come to their conclusion. It was believed that this was relevant, on the basis that the psychometric tests all essentially measure the same thing. As many different factors affect and cause Alzheimer's disease, the CGI is a good way of measuring overall and general change (e.g. it takes into account memory, behaviour and the ability to look after oneself).

The $ES_{all\ scales}$ result was 0.201 when all 21 studies were combined, with a positive score showing advantage for acetyl-L-carnitine over placebo. A funnel plot was used to test the results for bias and only one result fell outside this plot, suggesting that it could be biased in a positive manner, as was later claimed.[7] This was a small study including seven patients with Alzheimer's disease. Only patients who could cope with magnetic resonance imaging (MRI) scanning were selected for treatment, and because of this the trial could have been biased towards favourable results with acetyl-L-carnitine.[6] When this study was excluded, a significant benefit on clinical and psychometric tests was still found with acetyl-L-carnitine ($ES_{all\ scales}$ = 0.191). The integrated summary for CGI (ES_{CGI-CH}) was 0.32, which also suggested that acetyl-L-carnitine treatment benefits overall performance and behaviour. A subsidiary examination showed that acetyl-L-carnitine provided most benefit on intellectual and memory functions, which are more prevalent in mild cognitive impairment.

Acetyl-L-carnitine appears to have been well tolerated at doses of 1.5–3 g/day in all studies. Side-effect profiles appear to have been similar to placebo, with body odour, increased appetite, rash and restlessness reported.[5,6]

Overall, acetyl-L-carnitine has great potential as a treatment for people with early-stage Alzheimer's disease or those with mild cognitive impairment. Future large-scale trials may be required on patients with these conditions to conclusively prove its value. Studies have shown that younger people with these conditions may benefit more, and any future trials should pay specific attention to the age of patients that seem to experience the most benefit. Future trials could also attempt to determine whether acetyl-L-carnitine has any effect on the memory of 'normally ageing' subjects.

Phosphatidylserine

Phosphatidylserine is a membrane phospholipid found in every cell in the body and is part of a normal diet. It is particularly concentrated in the central nervous system, and is usually found on the inside of the neuron plasma membrane.[9] It was originally derived from bovine brain but with fears about Creutzfeldt–Jakob disease in recent years the production source has been switched to soy.[9] Like other nutraceuticals, phosphatidylserine has many proposed mechanisms of action. Levels are thought to decline with age, which has consequences for the communication and transmission between neurons. Phosphatidylserine supplementation is thought to maintain the ability of the neurons to transmit electrical potentials, which aids the communication between neurons necessary for the formation of memory. It also activates PKC, a substance that helps the release of neurotransmitters such as dopamine, serotonin and acetylcholine, from synaptic vesicles. PKC also upregulates genes that are believed to produce the long-term changes needed to form memory. In addition to this it has been postulated that it could reduce the age-related loss in the number of dendritic spines formed by neurons.[13]

Clinical trials have shown that phosphatidylserine produces minimally significant benefits in a number of clinical and psychometric tests. However the trial with the best results for phosphatidylserine appears to have used subjects who were significantly less mentally impaired than in the rest of the clinical studies.[14] Phosphatidylserine has generally been tested in patients with mild to moderate dementia, or those with mild cognitive impairment. A double-blind crossover study later[13] reported that the CGI of patients treated with phosphatidylserine was significantly increased compared with the placebo group, and these effects continued for weeks after phosphatidylserine had stopped being administered. However, amongst a battery of psychometric tests administered to the subjects, only reaction times were significantly reduced (no improvements were measured in tests such as logical memory and mental arithmetic). CGI is the most sensitive of tests and only a modest improvement was observed in this work.

Use of phosphatidylserine has been shown to result in a consistent improvement in verbal memory tests[13] (e.g. immediate word-list recall) and was found to be better than placebo for face recognition in a trial conducted on normally ageing adults.[15] This trial found benefits for a specific group of patients who had no diagnosis of dementia, but poor memories compared with other people of a similar age. Significant benefits were observed in these patients for 'primary memory measures' such as name–face recognition and recall, and phone number recall.

Phosphatidylserine has also been reported to improve the cooperation and friendliness of patients with advanced dementia.[9] The latest study conducted in this area states that soy phosphatidylserine at 300 mg/day or 600 mg/day had no effect on learning and memory tests. This trial was carried out on 120 patients with age-associated memory impairment, but no CGI scores were available.[16]

Overall, PS appears to provide very few benefits for patients with mild cognitive impairment or Alzheimer's disease. There is some debate as to whether soy phosphatidylserine has the same effects as bovine phosphatidylserine; the latest study with soy phosphatidylserine shows no positive outcomes.[16] The only promise appears to be in a specific group of elderly people with no dementia or cognitive decline but poor memory for their age.

Docosahexaenoic acid

Docosahexaenoic acid (DHA) is widely available from fish oils, and the prevalence of Alzheimer's disease correlates negatively with fish consumption.[17] There are high levels of DHA in the brain, and DHA deficiency has been reported to cause a reduction in learning ability in rats.[18] A diet containing a high ratio of n-6 to n-3 fatty acids was shown to have a negative effect on the maintenance of the cognitive functions of the brain, whereas a low ratio was beneficial, using the MMSE evaluation in men aged 69–89 years.[17] A 4:1 ratio of n-6 to n-3 fatty acids was shown to give the best results in learning tasks in rats, and was later tested in 100 patients with Alzheimer's disease. Overall improvement was reported in 49 out of the 60 patients receiving the preparation of fatty acids.[19]

A further study produced similar results, in which participants who consumed fish once weekly or more had a 60% lower risk of Alzheimer's disease compared with those who rarely or never ate fish. Total n-3 polyunsaturated fatty acids (PUFAs) and DHA were associated with reduced risk, but eicosapentaenoic acid (EPA) had no association with Alzheimer's disease.[20]

Lack of sufficient quantities of n-3 and n-6 fatty acids is known to be a limiting factor in brain development,[21] and an inverse association between cognitive decline and the ratio of n-3 to n-6 fatty acids in erythrocyte membranes has been revealed. This latter marker is also implicated in an association with low DHA levels in depressive patients.[22]

The increased interest of the public in *n*-3 fatty acids has recently fuelled research into the effects on IQ, which has resulted in publication of an article in the *Economist* magazine.[23] It was shown that children of mothers who ate food containing low levels of *n*-3 fatty acids during pregnancy had a lower IQ, found social relations more demanding and were less physically coordinated than those with higher maternal consumption.

Soy isoflavones

Research into feeding a high soy isoflavone diet (0.6 mg/g isoflavones) to rats investigated the neurobehavioural effects. It was found that soy consumption resulted in very high plasma isoflavone levels, which significantly altered dimorphic brain regions, anxiety, learning and memory.[24] Few trials have been carried out in humans, and most of these concentrated on the effects in menopausal women. Evidence that post-menopausal women suffer cognitive decline is possibly due to decreased oestrogen levels, and soy has been considered to be an alternative to hormone replacement therapy (HRT), after controversy over evidence suggesting this leads to increase risk in breast cancer, and additionally that the cognitive benefits of HRT may actually be reversed over long-term usage.[25] There is limited evidence to substantiate the benefits of soy isoflavones, one trial on 53 postmenopausal women over six months showed a significant improvement in one of five cognitive tests, insignificant improvement in two tests and no improvement in the rest.[26] Other work using low levels of isoflavone (60 mg) over short time periods (12 weeks) has been reported to increase memory, pattern recognition and mental flexibility.[25] Another trial carried out with young subjects over a ten-week period found that a dose of 100 mg per day of total isoflavones caused significant cognitive improvements in both young males and females, in both short- and long-term memory, but also in mental flexibility.[27] Soy phytoestrogens have been subjected to a number of investigations in the area of cognitive function in both menopausal and postmenopausal women (see Chapter 13).

Other nutraceuticals

Choline compounds, such as phosphatidylcholine, found in lecithin, have been postulated as having beneficial effects on dementia by increasing the brain levels of acetylcholine. They work in a similar way to the current pharmaceutical treatments, cholinesterase inhibitors, and it is thought that increased acetylcholine levels help any remaining neurons in a diseased brain to work more efficiently. Other forms of choline include citicoline and choline alphoscerate. Citicoline is a combination of choline and cytidine, which may work synergistically to promote dopamine levels, as well as acetylcholine levels.[28]

Only two out of 29 studies have reported a benefit for phosphatidylcholine over placebo in the treatment of Alzheimer's disease, suggesting that it is unlikely to be effective.[1] The use of lecithin for the treatment of dementia and cognitive impairment has been investigated in a Cochrane Systematic Review of 12 clinical trials.[29] The conclusions were not positive, and evidence did not support its use. Citicoline is used in Europe for cerebrovascular dementia, and the doses used in clinical trials have been varied, and as a result inconsistencies have been found. Trials suggest that it has a moderate benefit for patients with cerebrovascular disease, but that choline alphoscerate may be more safe and efficacious.[30] Citicoline appears to improve memory and learning capabilities but has no effect on attention. CGI scores have been strongly improved on treatment. It appears to be most beneficial in cerebrovascular disease and it also seems to improve recall in people with poor memories but no dementia.[31,32] The most effective dose of citicoline is subject to some question: a recent double-blind trial on 30 subjects revealed no beneficial effect of 1000 mg/day citicoline when compared with placebo,[33] but at 2000 mg/day citicoline produced many benefits for normal patients with poor memory.[32] Side-effects included stomach upset, insomnia, headache and rash. Further studies are required to identify a specific daily dose and to determine if choline compounds can have a long-term benefit in mild cognitive impairment or dementia.

NADH has been proposed as a possible treatment for Alzheimer's disease, possibly because it stimulates dopamine release. Good results were reported in an open label trial on 17 patients, whose average improvement on the MMSE was 8.35 points,[34] which was far more than the average increase caused by currently available drugs. However a similar trial was carried out and found no significant effects of NADH supplementation; it was believed that exogenous NADH would not be able to penetrate the blood–brain barrier.[35] A double-blind placebo-controlled trial is needed before any conclusions can be drawn about the possible efficacy of NADH treatment.

The polyphenols from teas, particularly green tea, may possess neuroprotective activity that may help to ameliorate diseases such as cognitive decline. Epidemiological research in Japan has found that a higher consumption of green tea is associated with lower prevalence of cognitive impairment in >70 year olds. Green tea was found to be superior to either black or oolong, and consumption of up to two cups daily was the highest effective level of consumption tested. A dose–response relationship was evident.[36]

Carnosine, a naturally occurring dipeptide, has been postulated as a future anti-ageing product. It is believed to act in three ways: as an antioxidant, a metal binder and as an antiglycating agent. It disrupts the binding of protein to advanced glycosylation end product receptors, which can reduce the toxicity of amyloid plaques. It binds to carbonyl groups present on glycated proteins,[37] which inhibits the cross-linking of proteins to other proteins (amyloid plaque aggregation) and the formation of protein–DNA cross-linking, which will lead to cell death. The presence of carbonyl groups on proteins is often used as a signal of ageing, and these are especially abundant in diabetics. Carnosine has been shown *in vitro* to increase the lifespan of human fibroblasts beyond the normal length,[7,38] and could theoretically be used as a future treatment for Alzheimer's disease.

The evidence for the application of a number of other plant-derived constituents, including vinpocetine, in treating cognitive decline has recently been reviewed.[39]

Treatments for depression

Mental depression is thought to affect 8–10% of people in Europe, associated with psychological, environmental and hereditary factors. Epidemiological research has shown that populations with low intakes of seafood have a higher prevalence of severe depression.[40] As with risk factors associated with cognitive impairment, red blood cell DHA and EPA levels are significantly lower in people with depression.[41] Two studies investigating the effect of supplementation with *n*-3 fatty acids have shown significant improvements in depressive symptoms in patients. Supplementation with 6.2 g EPA and 3.4 g DHA daily for four months,[42] and 2 g EPA for four weeks[43] showed positive results, but supplementation with 2 g DHA daily for six weeks was found to produce no significant effect.[44]

S-Adenosyl methionine (SAMe) is the most widely investigated nutraceutical for treatment of depression, and has been the subject of clinical trials since 1973.[45] SAMe is a methyl donor and is involved in the synthesis of neurotransmitters in the brain. It is believed that it is as effective as tricyclic antedepressants in alleviating depression, and may even potentiate their activity.[46] Most investigations involved either parenteral dosing at 45–400 mg per day or 200–1600 mg orally daily, and meta-analyses appear to confirm the efficacy of SAMe. Two analyses report significant improvement when compared with placebo,[47,48] and a third agrees a definite role for its use.[49]

Conclusions

Acetyl-L-carnitine and citicoline may be useful supplements for age-related decline of varying causes. Further research, specifically large-scale, placebo controlled, double-blind trials should be carried out into their use before their efficacy is firmly established. Phosphatidylserine appears to have a minimal effect, but it may be beneficial when used in combination with other products.

The mechanisms that cause dementia and mild cognitive impairment are not clearly understood. Loss of memory could be caused by a number of factors including ischaemia, amyloid plaques, a decrease in cholinergic neurons, loss of phospholipid components and oxidative stress. It is likely that combinations of these pathologies are present in any patient with memory loss. Diagnostic tests should improve in the future and scans may be able to show what is really happening in the brain to cause memory loss. Physicians may then be able to prescribe a specific treatment(s) for a specific patient.

References

1. McDaniel M A, Maier S F, Einstein G O. 'Brain-specific' nutrients: a memory cure? *Nutrition* 2003; 19: 957–975.
2. Rang H P, Dale M M, Ritter J M. *Pharmacology*, 4th edn. London: Churchill Livingstone, 1999.
3. British Medical Association and Royal Pharmaceutical Society of Great Britain. *British National Formulary 51*, March 2006.
4. Branconnier R. The efficacy of the cerebral metabolic enhancers in the treatment of senile dementia. *Psychopharmacol Bull* 1983; 19: 212–219,
5. Rapport L, Lockwood B. *Nutraceuticals*. London: Pharmaceutical Press, 2002.
6. Montgomery S A, Thal L J, Amiren R. Meta-analysis of double-blind randomized controlled clinical trials of acetyl L-carnitine versus placebo in the treatment of mild cognitive impairment and mild Alzheimer's disease. *Int Clin Psychopharmacol* 2003; 18: 61–71.
7. Pettegrew J W, Klunk W E, Panchalingam K *et al.* Clinical and neurochemical effects of acetyl-L-carnitine in Alzheimer's disease. *Neurobiol Aging* 1995; 16: 1–4.
8. Pettegrew J W, McClure R J. Acetyl L-carnitine as a possible therapy for Alzheimer's disease. *Exp Rev Neurother* 2002; 2: 647–654.

9. Kidd P M. A review of nutrients and botanicals in the integrative management of cognitive dysfunction. *Altern Med Rev* 1999; 4: 144–161.

10. Thal L J, Carta A, Clark W R *et al.* A 1-year multicenter placebo-controlled study of acetyl-L-carnitine in patients with Alzheimer's disease. *Neurology* 1996; 47: 705–711.

11. Brooks J O III, Yesavage J A, Carta A, Bravi D. Acetyl L-carnitine slows decline in younger patients with Alzheimer's disease: a reanalysis of a double-blind, placebo controlled study using the trilinear approach. *Int Psychogeriatrics* 1998; 10: 193–203.

12. Thal L J, Calvani M, Amato A, Carta A. A 1-year controlled trial of acetyl-L-carnitine in early-onset AD. *Neurology* 2000; 55: 805–810.

13. Engel R R, Satzger W, Gunther W *et al.* Double-blind cross-over study of phosphatidylserine vs. placebo in patients with early dementia of the Alzheimer type. *Eur Neuropsychopharmacol* 1992; 2: 149–155.

14. Amaducci L, Crook T H, Lippi A *et al.* Use of phosphatidylserine in Alzheimer's disease. *Ann N Y Acad Sci* 1991; 640: 245–249.

15. Crook T H, Tinklenburg J, Yesavage J *et al.* Effects of phosphatidylserine in age associated memory impairment. *Neurology* 1991; 41: 644–649.

16. Jorissen B L, Brouns F, Van Boxtel M P *et al.* The influence of soy-derived phosphatidylserine on cognition in age-associated memory impairment. *Nutr Neurosci* 2001; 4: 121–134.

17. Horrocks L A, Yeo Y K. Health benefits of docosahexaenoic acid (DHA). *Pharmacol Res* 1999; 40: 211–224.

18. Linko Y, Hayakawa K. Docosahexaenoic acid: a valuable nutraceutical? *Trends Food Sci Technol* 1996; 7: 59–63.

19. Yehuda S, Rabinowitz S, Carasso R L, Mostofsky D I. Essential fatty acids preparation (SR-3) improves Alzheimer's patients quality of life. *Int J Neurosci* 1996; 87: 141–149.

20. Morris M C, Evans D A, Bienias J L *et al.* Consumption of fish and *n*-3 fatty acids and risk of incident Alzheimer disease. *Arch Neurol* 2003; 60: 940–946.

21. Heude B, Ducimetiere P, Berr C. Cognitive decline and fatty acid composition of erythrocyte membranes – The EVA Study. *Am J Clin Nutr* 2003; 77: 803–808.

22. Peet M, Laugharne J D, Mellor J, Ramchand C N. Essential fatty acid deficiency in erythrocyte membranes from chronic schizophrenic patients, and the clinical effects of dietary supplementation. *Prostaglandins Leukot Essent Fatty Acids* 1996; 55: 71–75.

23. Anon. Food for thought; nutrition (omega 3 fatty acids' effect on health). *Economist* 2006; 378: 1.

24. Lephart E D, West T W, Weber K S *et al.* Neurobehavioral effects of dietary soy phytoestrogens. *Neurotoxicol Teratol* 2002; 24: 5–16.

25. Hill C E, Dye L. Phytoestrogens and cognitive performance: a review of the evidence. *Curr Top Nutr Res* 2003; 1: 203–212.

26. Kritz-Silverstein D, Von Muhlen D, Barrett-Connor E, Bressel M A B. Isoflavones and cognitive function in older women: the SOy and Postmenopausal Health In Aging (SOPHIA) Study. *Menopause* 2003; 10: 196–202.

27. File S E, Jarrett N, Fluck E *et al.* Eating soya improves human memory. *Psychopharmacology* 2001; 157: 430–436.

28. Fonlupt P, Martinet M, Pacheco H. Effect of CDP-choline on dopamine metabolism in central nervous system. In: Zappia V, Kennedy E P, Nilsson B I, Galletti P. *Novel Biochemical, Pharmacological and Clinical Aspects of CDP-choline*. New York: Elsevier Science, 1985: 169–177.

29. Higgins J P T, Flicker L. Lecithin for dementia and cognitive impairment. *Cochrane Database Syst Rev* 2003; 3: CD001015.

30. Amenta F, Di Tullio M A, Tomassoni D. The cholinergic approach for the treatment of vascular dementia: evidence form pre-clinical and clinical studies. *Clin Exp Hypertens* 2002; 24: 697–713.

31. Fioravanti M, Yanagi M. Cytidinediphosphocholine (CDP choline) for cognitive and behavioural disturbances associated with chronic cerebral disorders in the elderly. *Cochrane Database Syst Rev* 2000; 4: CD000269.

32. Abad-Santos F, Novalbos-Reina J, Gallego-Sandin S, Garcia A G. Treatment of mild cognitive impairment: value of citicoline. *Rev Neurologia* 2002; 35; 675–682.

33. Cohen R A, Browndyke J N, Moser D J *et al.* Long-term citicoline (cytidine diphosphate choline) use in patients with vascular dementia: neuroimaging and neuropsychological outcomes. *Cerebrovasc Dis* 2003; 16: 199–204.

34. Birkmayer J G D. Coenzyme nicotinamide dinucleotide. New therapeutic approach for improving dementia of the Alzheimer type. *Ann Clin Lab Sci* 1996; 26: 1–9.

35. Rainer M, Kraxberger E, Haushofer M *et al.* No evidence for improvement from oral nicotinamide adenine dinucleotide (NADH) in dementia. *J Neural Transmission* 2000; 107: 1475–1481.

36. Kuriyama S, Hozawa A, Ohmori K *et al.* Green tea consumption and cognitive function: a cross-sectional study from the Tsurugaya Project. *Am J Clin Nutr* 2006; 83: 355–361.

37. Hipkiss A R, Brownson C, Carrier M J. Carnosine, the anti-ageing, anti-oxidant dipeptide, may react with protein carbonyl groups. *Mech Ageing Dev* 2001; 122: 1431–1445.

38. Hipkiss A R. Carnosine, a protective, anti-ageing peptide? *Int J Biochem Cell Biol* 1998; 20: 863–868.

39. Berry J, Lockwood B. Can nutraceuticals offer hope for future treatments for cognitive decline? *Pharm J* 2004; 273: 610–614.

40. Hibbeln J R. Seafood consumption, the DHA content of mothers' milk and prevalence rates of postpartum depression: a cross-national, ecological analysis. *J Affect Disord* 2002; 69: 15–29.

41. Maes M, Smith R, Christophe A *et al.* Fatty acid composition in major depression: decreased omega 3 fractions in cholesteryl esters and increased C20:4 omega 6/C20:5 omega 3 ratio in cholesteryl esters and phospholipids. *J Affect Disord* 1996; 38: 35–46.

42. Stoll A L, Locke C A, Marangell L B, Severus W E. Omega-3 fatty acids and bipolar disorder : a review. *Prostaglandins Leukot Essent Fatty Acids* 1999; 60: 329–337.

43. Nemets B, Stahl Z, Belmaker R H. Addition of omega-3 fatty acid to

maintenance medication treatment for recurrent unipolar depressive disorder. *Am J Psychiatry* 2002; 159: 477–479.

44. Marangell L B, Martinez J M, Zboyan H A, *et al*. A double-blind, placebo-controlled study of the omega-3 fatty acid docosahexaenoic acid in the treatment of major depression. *Am J Psychiatry* 2003; 160: 996–998.

45. Fetrow C W, Avila J R. Efficacy of the dietary supplement S-adenosyl-L-methionine. *Ann Pharmacother* 2001; 35: 1414–1425.

46. Mischoulon D, Fava M. Role of S-adenosyl-L-methionine in the treatment of depression: a review of the evidence. *Am J Clin Nutr* 2002; 76: 1158S–1161S.

47. Bressa G M. S-Adenosyl-L-methionine (SAMe) as antidepressant: meta-analysis of clinical studies. *Acta Neurol Scand Suppl* 1994; 154: 7–14.

48. Anon. Agency for Healthcare Research and Quality, 2002. S-Adenosyl-L-methionine for treatment of depression, osteoarthritis, and liver disease. http://www.ahrq.gov/clinic/epcsums/samesum.pdf (accessed 23 May 2006).

49. Williams A-L, Girard C, Jui D, Sabina A, Katz D L. S-Adenosylmethionine (SAMe) as treatment for depression: a systematic review. *Clin Invest Med* 2005; 28: 132–139.

9

Sleep enhancement

Melatonin is the most important nutraceutical used for the enhancement of sleep, but limited use may also be made of carnitine.

Melatonin

Melatonin has been investigated for many different applications, based on its physiological roles. As it has a role in the control of circadian rhythms, it has been widely researched as an aid to shiftwork adaptation, jet lag and for problems of insomnia. Endogenous levels occur as a result of production by the pineal gland, normally starting as darkness falls, with maximal production between 2 and 4 am. The 'melatonin replacement' hypothesis states that age-related decline in melatonin production contributes to insomnia, and replacement with physiological doses improves sleep.[1] Melatonin has also been found to be a powerful free-radical scavenger and its use as an antioxidant in ageing and related problems has been studied.

Shiftwork adaptation

An increasing proportion of the world's workers are involved in shiftwork; it is believed, for example, that 20% of the US workforce, approximately 15 million workers, are required to work in shifts. A range of symptoms are often experienced by these workers, including sleep disturbance, increased risk of accidents and major chronic disease states. The main causes of these problems are disruption and desynchronisation of circadian rhythms. Because melatonin is known to be a factor in the circadian organisation of both sleep and other biological rhythms its effects in relation to sleep patterns have been studied. One study investigated urinary 6-hydroxymelatonin sulfate (6-OHMS) levels and variability in work–sleep patterns in shift workers. It was found that melatonin levels are usually 5–10 times greater during sleep, than during daytime or non-sleep periods, and workers sleeping during daytime showed up to 45% lower 6-OHMS levels. In addition, workers with sleep–work ratios of <1 were found to be 3.5–8 times more liable to experience symptoms than those with ratios >1.[2]

Jet lag

Jet lag can be an unfortunate consequence of air travel, and is particularly evident when moving through a number of time zones, specifically in an easterly direction. When the internal body clock (or circadian rhythm) is not synchronised with the external 'local' time (light–dark cycle) jet lag is experienced. The symptoms, which vary between individuals, include tiredness, inability to sleep at the new bedtime, inability to concentrate and disturbed sleep for several days after a long flight, as well as headache and gastrointestinal problems. A study involving 39 subjects travelling from the UK to either Sydney or Brisbane questioned whether subjective symptoms could predict perception of jet lag. It was concluded that the amount of perceived jet lag was predicted by the level of fatigue at that time.[3] It may also cause considerable problems for training and performance in sports competitions and should be taken into account when planning journey times. Symptoms are also more marked in older travellers, and as more time zones are crossed.[4,5]

Both endogenous and supplemented melatonin is chronobiotic and can alter circadian rhythms. An early double-blind trial was carried out in 1986, using 17 volunteers, between the ages of 29 and 68, who flew from London to San Francisco (eight time zones west). After 14 days, once the subjects had adapted to the local time, they were flown back to London. For 3 days before the return flight, a dose of 5 mg melatonin or placebo was taken at 6 pm local time and on return to the UK the dose was continued for a further 4 days, between 10 pm and midnight local time. On day 7 after arriving home, the subjects were asked to assess the jet lag that they had experienced. None of the melatonin group had suffered appreciable jet lag, but six out of nine placebo subjects had.[6] This small study reported the first results using melatonin for prophylaxis of jet lag.

In a later similar double-blind study,[7] 20 volunteers (aged 28–68 years) flew eastwards from Auckland, New Zealand to London, through 12 time zones, and returned after three weeks. Subjects took either placebo or 5 mg melatonin for the first journey and the other for the second journey, in a double-blind test. Less jet lag was experienced in the travellers taking melatonin than in the placebo group. The dose of

5 mg melatonin was well tolerated with few side-effects reported (a mild sedative effect in two subjects and a relaxed feeling in another). As in the former study the results were favourable, but more research was necessary to determine the optimum dose and dosing schedule. Also, the symptoms of jet lag were not standardised in either study and were subjective, making comparisons difficult. Baseline symptoms, such as previous fatigue, stress due to travel preparations and the flight itself, or inability to sleep in a new environment or due to other activities, were not taken into account.

In a more recent study,[4] these problems were addressed. The number of passengers was large ($n = 257$) and a scale was used to assess the severity of the jet lag experienced, including daytime symptoms, when travelling from New York to Oslo (six time zones eastwards). A randomised, double-blind procedure was used in which subjects received either placebo or 5 mg melatonin at bedtime, 0.5 mg melatonin at bedtime or 0.5 mg melatonin taken on a shifting schedule, starting at bedtime and taken 1 hour earlier each day. The results were somewhat surprising, with melatonin not showing significant improvement over placebo. Symptoms of sleep disturbance, which are associated with jet lag, were not investigated, but rather daytime disturbance and times of sleep onset at night, and awakening in the morning. Also the subjects stayed for only 4 days at their destination before flying back and may not have fully adjusted to the local time. There may also have been a large placebo effect, as the subjects knew that they had three out of four chances of receiving melatonin, which could make the actual melatonin effect even smaller. The authors concluded that more work was needed to assess the use of melatonin in jet lag.

The latest study in 2004 compared the effects of controlled-release caffeine (300 mg daily) and melatonin (5 mg daily) on symptoms of jet lag when travelling from Texas to France. Melatonin and caffeine were administered daily to the different groups on days 1–5, and the 27 participants had their activities controlled, including their sleeping time. Sleep architecture was assessed by polysomnographic recordings such as encephalography. It was concluded that both treatments had some benefits for jet lag symptoms, however melatonin treatment showed significant rebound of slow wave sleep on night 1, and sleepiness was reported to be objectively increased.[8]

A Cochrane review of trials of melatonin use in jet lag was carried out in 2002, and included ten trials. Eight of the ten trials showed that daily doses of melatonin from 0.5 to 5.0 mg had similar effects when taken close to the target bedtime at the destination, when traversing five or more time zones. Doses of 5 mg seemed to be no more effective. A controlled-release 2 mg formulation was relatively ineffective, possibly because a short-lived higher peak concentration works better. The benefit is also likely to be greater with more time zones crossed, but less for travel in a westerly direction. Not surprisingly, dosing at times different to the optimum time (10–12 pm) is liable to be detrimental to good sleep and to cause sleepiness at the wrong time![9]

Sleep disorders

Sleep disturbances are very common, especially in the elderly. These can be primary, such as age-related disorders, or side-effects of medicines such as beta-blockers, illness, anxiety or stress. Side-effects of medication may include increased urination, gastrointestinal effects and nausea which can also interfere with sleep.[10] As it is involved in the circadian rhythm and the sleep–wake cycle, it is logical that melatonin might be used in the treatment of primary sleeping problems. It is important to try to eliminate secondary causes of sleep disorders when recruiting volunteers for melatonin studies, to ensure that only the primary cause is being studied.

Six healthy young men were used in a study to investigate the effect of melatonin given at night.[11] None of the subjects suffered from any sleep disorders or took any medication, and they refrained from alcohol and caffeine for 24 hours before each session. It was found that doses of 0.3 mg and 1 mg melatonin given at 8 pm or 9 pm produced acute hypnotic effects. These effects were assessed both subjectively and using polysomnographs. The authors suggested that a critical plasma melatonin level may be necessary for sleep induction. There was no residual hypnotic effect in the morning following melatonin administration, determined from mood and performance tests carried out by the volunteers. This outcome may be helpful in insomniac patients.

In another study[12] involving 20 subjects who met the criteria for primary insomnia, plasma samples were taken every half-hour between 6.00 pm and 11.00 pm. It was found that between 6.00 pm and 11.00 pm there were significantly lower concentrations of melatonin in the plasma of insomniacs than in 20 controls matched for sex and age. This small study suggests that the lower plasma melatonin levels could have affected sleep in these subjects.

Melatonin has a half-life of only 40–50 minutes, with serum concentrations after oral dosing reaching peak levels after 20 minutes.

To ensure high serum levels throughout the night, administration of a controlled-release formulation of melatonin is needed. A 2 mg melatonin controlled-release tablet was administered to 12 elderly insomniacs who were taking various medications for chronic illnesses (six had hypertension, five had ischaemic heart disease, four had spondyloarthrosis, three had Parkinson's disease and two had diabetes mellitus).[10] These elderly subjects were taking between one and six drugs, nitrates, calcium-channel blockers, diuretics, aspirin, beta-blockers and analgesics, for a range of illnesses, and also used sleep medication. Before starting the study, subjects were woken every 3 hours during one night, to measure urinary 6-OHMS. This was compared with values from an earlier study by the authors using elderly people without insomnia. In all subjects, the peak excretion of 6-OHMS was between 3 and 6 am, rather than beginning at midnight as in young adults and elderly people without insomnia. This indicated that the sleep disorders might well be due to a shift in plasma melatonin secretion.

Actigraphy recording wrist movements to assess sleep patterns was then carried out for three nights. Subjects were given 2 mg controlled-release melatonin, or placebo, 2 hours before bedtime, for three weeks. Actigraphy was used again for three nights, at the end of the study. Results showed an overall improvement in sleep quality in the test subjects, despite chronic disease states and concomitant medication. It was concluded that it is necessary to establish melatonin deficiency in the trial subjects, and the controlled-release of melatonin may have prevented desensitisation to large doses required for the same plasma concentration. A minimum of three weeks treatment is also important, as it has been shown in animal studies that melatonin receptors can be reduced in the elderly and need to be resensitised by long-term exposure. A further reason given is that the internal clock in the elderly is sometimes not synchronised with the light–dark cycle and exogenous melatonin will correct this over a few weeks.[10]

A systematic review of six double-blind trials of melatonin for insomnia in the elderly has been published. Doses of melatonin ranged from 0.5 to 6 mg, 30–120 minutes before bedtime, and the study concluded that 'melatonin was most effective in elderly people with insomnia who chronically used benzodiazepines and/or with documented low melatonin levels during sleep'.[1] Measures of sleep quality were variable and found to improve; no early-morning sleepiness occurred, but subjective sleep quality did not improve.

Meta-analysis

A recent meta-analysis on evidence for the use of melatonin in managing secondary sleep disorders and sleep disorders accompanying sleep restriction such as shiftwork and jet lag has been published. Evidence from six trials on secondary sleep disorders revealed there to have been no effect on sleep onset latency, and evidence from a further nine trials showed no effect on shiftwork and jet lag symptoms.[13] The editorial from the same issue of the *British Medical Journal* argued that meta-analysis of trials concerning these two latter cases of sleep restriction – shiftwork and jet lag – should not have been linked in the same analysis, due to their inherent differences.[14]

Miscellaneous

Twenty-one female patients with Rett syndrome were given 100 mg/kg carnitine daily in two divided doses for six months in an investigation into its possible benefits on sleep patters. It was found that in patients with less than 90% baseline sleep efficiency, the carnitine treatment led to significant improvements in sleep pattern, as well as energy levels and communication skills.[15]

References

1.   Olde Rikkert M G, Rigaud A S. Melatonin in elderly patients with insomnia. A systematic review. *Z Gerontol Geriatr* 2001; 34: 491–497.
2.   Burch J B, Yost M G, Johnson W, Allen E. Melatonin, sleep, and shift work adaptation. *J Occup Environ Med* 2005; 47: 893–901.
3.   Waterhouse J, Edwards B, Nevill A *et al*. Do subjective symptoms predict our perception of jet-lag? *Ergonomics* 2000; 43: 1514–1527.
4.   Spitzer R L, Terman M, Williams J B W *et al*. Jet lag: clinical features, validation of a new syndrome-specific scale, and lack of response to melatonin in a randomised, double-blind trial. *Am J Psychiatry* 1999; 156: 1392–1396.
5.   Waterhouse J, Reilly T, Atkinson G. Jet lag. *Lancet* 1997; 350: 1611–1615.
6.   Arendt J, Aldhous M, Marks V. Alleviation of jet lag by melatonin: preliminary results of controlled double blind trial. *BMJ* 1986; 292: 1170.
7.   Petrie K, Conaglen J V, Thompson L, Chamberlain K. Effect of melatonin on jet lag after long haul flights. *BMJ* 1989; 298: 705–707.
8.   Beaumont M, Batejat D, Pierard C *et al*. Caffeine or melatonin effects on sleep and sleepiness after rapid eastward transmeridian travel. *J Appl Physiol* 2004; 96: 50–58.
9.   Herxheimer A, Petrie K J. Melatonin for the prevention and treatment of jet lag. *Cochrane Database Syst Rev* 2002; 2: CD001520.

10. Garfinkle D, Laudon M, Nof D, Zisapel N. Improvement of sleep quality in elderly people by controlled-release melatonin. *Lancet* 1995; 346: 541–544.

11. Zhdanova I V, Wurtman R J, Lynch H J *et al.* Sleep inducing effects of low doses of melatonin ingested in the evening. *Clin Pharmacol Ther* 1995; 57: 552–558.

12. Attenburrow M E J, Dowling B A, Sharpley A L, Cowen P J. Case-control study of evening melatonin concentration in primary insomnia. *BMJ* 1996; 312: 1263–1264.

13. Buscemi N, Vandermeer B, Hooton N *et al.* Efficacy and safety of exogenous melatonin for secondary sleep disorders and sleep disorders accompanying sleep restriction: meta-analysis. *BMJ* 2006; 332: 385–393.

14. Herxheimer A. Does melatonin help people sleep? *BMJ* 2006; 332: 373–374.

15. Ellaway C J, Peat J, Williams K *et al.* Medium-term open label trial of L-carnitine in Rett syndrome. *Brain Dev* 2001; 23: S85–S89.

10

Cancer prevention

Approximately 10 million people worldwide are diagnosed with cancer each year, and more than 6 million people a year die from the disease. The most common cancers (excluding skin cancers other than melanoma) are lung (12.3% of all cancers), breast (10.4%) and colorectal cancer (9.4%). The chances of developing cancer of the lung, large bowel, breast, prostate and bladder are greatest in developed countries, and the rates of these cancers in northern Europe are about three times greater than in sub-Saharan Africa, where large bowel, breast and lung cancer are virtually unknown. Overall, there are major variations in the incidence of certain cancers in different geographical areas. For example, colon cancer is 20 times more prevalent in the USA than in India. There is evidence that this variation is mainly due to environmental factors and lifestyle, rather than genetic factors, as immigrants from low-incidence countries to high-incidence areas acquire the cancer pattern of the host country within a relatively short period of time, for example within in a single generation, and genetic changes would take longer than one generation to show an effect.

It has been estimated that 32–35% of cancers can be attributed to nutrition, although the contribution of diet to specific types of cancer varies from as little as 10% for lung cancer, to 80% for cancer of the large bowel.[1] Interestingly, data from countries with seemingly comparable socio-economic status, such as Mediterranean and non-Mediterranean European states, show very different cancer rates for specific forms of cancer. It has been suggested that this association is strongly influenced by the traditional diet of such countries.

Cancer is the cause of 26% of all deaths in the UK (155 180 deaths in 2002), which far outnumbers the deaths from heart disease. The major cause of mortality is lung cancer, which is responsible for 22% of deaths; large bowel, breast and prostate cancers account for 24% collectively.[2] The numbers of cancer cases are increasing annually and cancer prevention has become a major international health issue. In an attempt to address this problem many screening programmes were introduced in the UK and other countries in the late 1980s. However, although screening was shown to identify cancer cases at an earlier stage of the disease, it failed to reduce the total incidence of cancer. In addition, concerns over the safety and efficacy of conventional cancer therapies have stimulated the search for new alternatives.[3] It is now widely accepted that the best way to limit the incidence of cancer is by prevention.

The complexity and diversity surrounding each type of cancer, and the resulting morbidity and often mortality, has led researchers to explore the use of a number of nutraceuticals. Soy, green tea, lycopene, flaxseed, polyunsaturated fatty acids (PUFAs), coenzyme Q10 (Co Q10), melatonin and conjugated linoleic acid (CLA) have all been proposed as preventive treatment for a range of cancers, including leukaemia, lymphoma, prostate, breast, lung and colon.

A wide range of research studies have demonstrated that soy or soy phytoestrogens have the ability to inhibit the growth of various cancer cell lines, including prostate, breast and lung cancer cells. They have been shown to exert actions on a number of biochemical pathways and molecular mechanisms essential to cell growth and survival. This may be useful in delaying or even preventing the development of clinically significant cancer.

Epidemiological evidence for soy

It has been estimated that more than two-thirds of human cancers could be prevented through changes in lifestyle, and it has been reported that 10–70% of cancers are attributable to diet.[4] Dietary constituents are implicated in both cancer development and prevention, and epidemiological studies have revealed great differences between cancer incidence data taken from different countries.

Asian countries where soy products are regularly consumed, such as Japan, China, Korea and Indonesia, have some of the lowest incidences of breast, prostate, and colon cancer. However, the incidence of such cancers is now rising in these countries due to changes in diet and lifestyle. Soy may be a contributory factor in cancer prevention, but a number of other dietary factors such as low saturated fat intake have also been linked to low cancer risk.[5]

The death rate from prostate cancer in the Japan is about 25% the level found in the USA,[6] and in the Japanese men with prostate cancer, many tumours are much smaller on average, suggesting that soy may slow the growth of tumours and delay the onset of cancer. If this is the case then soy may not only prevent cancer developing, but also lessen its impact on the individual where cancer is already present.

Epidemiological studies have shown an inverse relationship between soy consumption and cancer risk and, in particular, the mortality from clinically diagnosed prostate cancer has been shown to be lower in countries with high soy consumption.[7]

Asian emigrants who move to the USA and change their dietary habits show a marked increase in the risk of developing prostate or breast cancer, reaching levels comparable to those found in indigenous inhabitants.[8] This is likely to be a result of the higher fat and much lower soy isoflavone content of the diet, suggesting that the protective effect found in inhabitants of Asian stock is not genetically determined. It has been shown that women who had consumed tofu during adolescence were less likely to develop both premenopausal and postmenopoausal breast cancer as adults. This contrasts with inconclusive results found in Western patients who did not consume soy before diagnosis.[9]

Genistein and daidzein have similar stereochemical structures to the endogenous oestrogens such as oestradiol (see Chapter 2). Due to their similar spatial conformation, they have the ability to bind weakly to oestrogen receptors in mammalian tissue and to influence oestrogen-regulated gene products.[10,11] It was initially suggested that the anticancer properties demonstrated by soy were due to this oestrogen receptor binding. It should be noted, however, that this activity could either be oestrogenic, if the binding stimulates a response, or anti-oestrogenic if the isoflavones compete with endogenous hormones for the receptors.[12]

The oestrogen antagonist tamoxifen is widely used as treatment for breast cancer. This activity may also be related to its structural similarity to oestrogen.

Biological activities of soy phytoestrogens

Early studies on the biological activity of the isoflavones centred on their oestrogenic activity, but recently, wide-ranging activities have been investigated.

The *in vivo* antioxidant activity of soy isoflavones has been studied in humans. Healthy 18- to 35-year-old women were given either low or high soy isoflavone diets over a 13-week period, and antioxidant status was assessed by measurement of endogenous lipophilic urinary metabolites. Decreased levels of these metabolites appear in the urine as products of lipid peroxidation *in vivo*, and indicate *in vivo* antioxidant protection. The levels of individual isoflavones in commercial soy protein powders were 55% genistein, 37% daidzein and 8% glycetin, and subjects were fed 0.15 (control), 1.01, and 2.01 mg total isoflavones/kg body weight daily. Levels of the six urinary metabolites, C-4 to C-7 alkanals and alkanones, were significantly reduced with both the low and high isoflavone supplementation.[13]

Antioxidant effects of have been studied and it is believed that activity is related to structure. However, these studies investigated effects at supraphysiological levels.[14] Other reported activities include inhibition of enzymes such as topoisomerase II, protein kinase, aromatase, thyroid peroxidase, as well as antiangiogenesis properties, induction of cell differentiation, and weak oestrogenic and anti-oestrogenic activities.[15] It has been suggested that the action of genistein and daidzein may be tissue-selective, which could have great benefits if specific cells such as cancerous tissue can be targeted without adverse effects on other tissues.[16]

Oestrogenic activity

Cancers can be described as oestrogen-dependent or androgen-dependent. Cancer of the breast and prostate are influenced by the levels of circulating androgens in the body.[8] The development and growth of these types of cancers are strongly influenced by the sex hormones, and it is known that postmenopausal women are at much higher risk of developing breast cancer due to lower levels of circulating oestrogen.

Isoflavones have a range of binding affinities to the two oestrogen receptors, ERα and ERβ, as shown in Table 10.1. Genistein and daidzein bind to the receptors to a lesser extent than to oestrogen itself, and it has been postulated that their anticancer properties are associated with this ability. They exert a weak oestrogen-like activity, comparable to that of tamoxifen.[17] Competition takes place between the isoflavones and oestrogen for the oestrogen receptors. Genistein and daidzein compete with androgens at their target site, thus affecting the clearance rates and availability of the hormones. This difference suggests that genistein and daidzein may have different biological activities in cancer cells, not simply related to their binding affinities. Further complications in activity may occur due to the metabolism of the isoflavones, and these metabolites having further differing affinities for the receptors.[18] This mechanism has the potential to slow the growth of certain oestrogen-dependent cancers and also possibly to prevent their development.

Table 10.1 Comparative binding affinities of phytoestrogens to oestrogen receptors[19]

Compound	ERα	ERβ
17β-Oestradiol	100	100
Genistein	4	87
Daidzein	0.1	0.5
Formononetin	<0.01	<0.01
Biochanin A	<0.01	<0.01
Ipriflavone	<0.01	<0.01

Non-oestrogenic activity

Although the oestrogenic and antioxidant properties of genistein may contribute to the anticancer effect demonstrated by soy, it is unlikely that these are the only mechanisms by which the isoflavones act. Although daidzein has exhibited anticancer effects both *in vitro* and animal models, most research has concentrated on genistein. In human stomach cancer cell lines genistein caused inhibition of growth apparently by stimulation of a signal transduction pathway leading to DNA fragmentation, indicating apoptosis. This effect was dose-dependent.[20] Genistein arrests cell cycle progression at the G_2–M phase in cells derived from human gastric cancer, oestrogen receptor positive and negative human breast carcinoma, leukaemic cells and melanoma cells.[21] It has also been shown to inhibit the growth of cancer cells by modulating genes related to homeostatic cell cycle controls and apoptosis. It may do this by inhibiting the activation of the nuclear transcription factor (NFκB) and Akt signalling pathways, both of which maintain a balance between cell survival and apoptosis. It is also an angiogenesis inhibitor, and also inhibits metastasis.[22]

Interestingly, genistein is able to interfere with cell processes by inhibiting DNA topoisomerase and protein tyrosine kinase (PTK).[23] Genistein is thought to target specific PTKs, particularly the epidermal growth factor receptor, and blocks the EGF-mediated pathway by preventing phosphorylation of tyrosine receptors, thereby causing cell death.[24] This may result in apoptosis of cancerous cells. Genistein also interacts with metalloproteinase (ras-MAP) kinases and DNA topoisomerase II and S6 kinase.[15,25,26] Genistein causes increased levels of transforming growth factor beta (TGF-β), which has a major role in the inhibition of growth of cancer cells by causing DNA strand breakage, leading to cell death.[27]

Genistein has also been shown to stimulate the ATPase activity of membranes from GLC4/ADR cells, thus affecting multidrug resistance protein (MRP) transport of anticancer drugs via direct interaction with the MRP.[28] MRPs are frequently expressed in human tumours, causing cellular resistance to cytotoxic drugs.[29,30] This means that genistein may prevent the development of this cellular resistance by inhibiting the efflux of drug molecules, thus enhancing the effectiveness of cancer drug therapy.

In another study genistein was shown to inhibit angiogenesis,[21] which could significantly restrict the growth of cancer by inhibiting the tumour-stimulated growth of new blood vessels within the tumour. This could be applied to all cancers, possibly enabling control of their development and progression.

Unlike genistein, daidzein has not been shown to inhibit PTK activity, but it does possess other actions similar to those of genistein. Isoflavones, including daidzein, have demonstrated inhibitory effects on aromatase enzymes,[31,32] which are involved in the conversion of androgen precursors to oestrogens. They can therefore have a direct effect on the amount of circulating oestrogens. As oestrogens can positively stimulate the growth of hormone-dependent cancers such as breast and prostate cancer, a reduction in oestrogen could limit the growth of cancer.

Pharmacokinetics and bioavailability

In order to demonstrate anticancer activity, genistein and daidzein have to be bioavailable. Their bioavailability depends on the relative uptake rates of the conjugated and free forms of genistein and daidzein, hydrolysis of glycosides in the gut, further metabolism in the liver, and their excretion rates. Bioavailability, absorption, plasma levels, metabolism and excretion, and distribution is dealt with in Chapter 2.

Breast cancer

Genistein may induce early mammary gland differentiation, thus suppressing the development of breast cancer.[33] Evidence from many studies has shown that early consumption of soy phytoestrogens is vital for protection against breast cancer. Early genistein exposure promotes cell differentiation in breast tissue, which suppresses the development of mammary cancer in adulthood by decreasing the activity of the epidermal growth signal pathway.[34] Pregnancy early in a woman's life is a predisposing factor that has been shown to protect against cancer. Early exposure to oestrogen causes differentiation of mammary tissue, thereby reducing susceptibility to chemically induced breast cancer.[35] Genistein appears to stimulate cell proliferation and to enhance the maturation of mammary glands. This has the effect of reducing the number of terminal end buds, the least differentiated structures in mammary tissue and the most susceptible to carcinogens.[35] Less differentiated terminal ducts of mammary tissue are more susceptible to chemical carcinogens, therefore genistein may act by enhancing differentiation in a mechanism similar to that of oestrogens during pregnancy. This increase in cell proliferation during early life has been associated with a less active EGF-signalling pathway in adulthood that in turn suppresses the development of breast cancer [35]. This may also suggest a possible reason for the lower incidence of breast cancer where average consumption of soy is high.

Sustained soy intake throughout life may have beneficial effects.[5] One large case–control study in Shanghai showed that independent of adult soy intake, women who consumed approximately 11 g soya protein/day during adolescence (13–15 years), were almost 50% less likely to develop breast cancer as adults than women who consumed ≤2 g soy protein/day during this period.[34]

Apart from the role of soy phytoestrogens in prevention of breast cancer, there is also need for an oestrogen-replacement treatment for women who have survived cancer. As they act as weak oestrogens, particularly in a low-oestrogen environment, it has been suggested that they show anti-oestrogenic activity in a high-oestrogen environment; prior to menopause there is a high-oestrogen environment and phytoestrogens may protect against breast cancer, but after menopause the reverse may occur, with consequent stimulation of breast cancer.[36]

Prostate cancer

Nearly 200 000 cases are diagnosed annually in the USA, and 1 in 32 die of the disease.[37] One meta-analysis of relevant clinical trials showed that high concentrations of oestrogen have been shown to affect the growth of prostate cancer and benign prostatic hyperplasia, so it is possible that the isoflavones will also show a similar effect. It has been observed that the soy isoflavone genistein induces apoptosis and inhibits growth of both androgen-sensitive and androgen-independent prostate cancer cells *in vitro*.[7] Genistein and daidzein have been shown to bind to receptors for endogenous androgens and stimulate the hepatic synthesis of sex hormone-binding globulin (SHBG).[38] Regular soy consumption causes increasing serum SHBG levels which result in decreased bioavailability of testosterone.[39] Soy isoflavones have been reported to inhibit the steroid-metabolising enzymes 5α-reductase and 17β-hydroxysteroid dehydrogenase, which lowers the levels of free androgens in the body.[40] Men around the age of 50 show a decline in testicular activity and an increase in SHBG and associated testosterone levels, which is thought to be a predominant factor in the subsequent development of prostate cancer.

One study using steroid hormone levels and total prostate-specific antigen levels as surrogate markers of disease progression concluded that the prolonged and consistent consumption of soy (60 mg/day for 12 weeks) might reduce the risk of developing prostate cancer and delay its onset.[37] The plasma concentration of isoflavonoids in Japanese men is high, and higher still in prostatic fluid, and there appears to be a relationship with prostate cancer incidence. Treatment of prostate cancer with oestrogens results in inhibition of cancer growth, but these hormones are also associated with development of benign prostatic hyperplasia and prostate cancer, therefore dietary phytoestrogens may be both benificial and detrimental to prostate disease.[5]

Colon cancer

There are no useful epidemiological data for the effects of soy consumption on colon cancer incidence due to conflicting conclusions, and few significant data from case–control studies. A few recent studies in rats have shown that soy has either no effect on colon cancer or even mildly procarcinogenic effects.[5] Limited research on the effects of isoflavones on colonic cancer cells has yielded results consistent with those for other cancer cell lines.

Although not typically associated with endogenous hormones, colon cancer can be hormonally influenced. It has been suggested that genistein at normal physiological isoflavone concentrations in humans may reduce colonic cancer risk by slowing the growth of normal cells rather than by inhibiting their growth.[3]

Other cancer types

Genistein has been shown to inhibit cell growth in cancer of the stomach, lung and blood. An *in vitro* study of human stomach cancer cells found that genistein stimulates apoptosis via a signal transduction pathway.[41]

Genistein has also been shown to inhibit growth of leukaemia cells.[24] From studies both *in vitro* and *in vivo* there seems to be evidence to suggest that growth of bladder cancer cells are also inhibited by soy isoflavones,[42] although one study reported a high intake of soy foods to cause elevated risk of bladder cancer.[43] Soy isoflavones have been linked to effects on endometrial cancer. Levels of isoflavones around 1.5 mg/day are typical of a US diet, and have been shown to be inversely related to the risk of endometrial cancer.[44]

Colorectal cancer is one of the most common forms of cancer in the UK, with 17 000 new cases being reported each year, but incidence in other countries, such as Japan, is much lower. Conflicting results have been shown from epidemiological data, but none of these studies have studied the role of the phytoestrogens. Lung cancer is also one of the most common cancer forms in the UK. In addition to evidence from *in vivo* studies showing inhibition of experimentally induced tumours, one study has reported a protective effect between non-smokers and high intake of soy isoflavone.[14]

Conclusions

Available epidemiological data suggest that consumption of soy isoflavones in a quantity equivalent to that found in a typical Chinese or Japanese diet should potentially reduce the risk of developing cancer. It would appear that a consumption of 30 mg (aglycone) per day appears reasonable, based upon one study reporting the isoflavone intake of over 3000 Japanese adults to be around 30–40 mg daily.[45] The quantity of soy products that would need to be consumed to reach these levels of intake varies considerably, depending on the dietary form of the soy. Whole soybean contains many constituents, as well as protein and isoflavonoids, so there is the possibility for synergistic effects to be seen.

It has also been proposed that as the half-life of genistein is relatively short, around 6–9 hours, and that repeat exposure is required to maintain claimed therapeutic levels.[21] However, long-term regular consumption of soy may not confer adequate protection against cancer, because soy isoflavones are able to induce their own metabolism.[8] This explains why there is a relatively low plasma concentration of genistein and daidzein in Japanese men who regularly consume soy as part of their normal diet.

As genistein has a very large therapeutic index, concentrations in the body would need to be much higher than typical therapeutic doses before toxicity is experienced.

It is evident from the body of research material published to date that soy isoflavones may act as dietary or nutraceutical cancer prevention agents. The wide range of activities shown is very promising. However, not all studies on soy ingestion showed positive activity. One study, for example, found that dietary genistein may stimulate the growth of oestrogen-dependent tumours in humans with low estrogen levels.[46] In another study, women with breast tumours who were treated with 45 mg isoflavones for two weeks prior to breast surgery showed higher rates of breast cancer cell proliferation.[47] There is a need for much more research to identify and elucidate the specific action of soy, as much of the research has been concentrated on the isoflavones.

Interest has recently been shown in a novel peptide called lunasin, found at concentrations of 0.10–1.3% in soy flour.[48] The anticancer activity of this may be independent to that of the isoflavones, or there may be complex interactions. From the body of published epidemiological data, it is most likely that soy and the isoflavones have positive health benefits when consumed as part of a healthy diet.

Tea

A number of chemical constituents are thought to be responsible for the anticancer activity associated with tea, but the overall activity is probably due to a combined or synergistic effect of all or some of the components.[49] (—)-Epigallocatechin gallate (EGCG) has been claimed to be the most important active constituent. One study investigated the activity of the four major tea catechins in inhibiting the growth of human lung cancer cell lines. (—)-Epicatechin gallate (ECG) was found to be most active, followed by EGCG, then (—)-epigallocatechin (EGC), but (—)-epicatechin (EC) was innactive. The major catechin, EGCG, is thought to be the major active constituent,[50] although it is known to have low bioavailability.[51] It is possible that synergistic activity is demonstrated as cancer growth inhibition by EGCG was increased when EC was also present.[50] Theaflavin-3,3′-digallate appears to have similar activity to that of EGCG and therefore the inhibitory activity of black tea against the development of cancer may be due to the combination of catechins and theaflavins.[51]

The pharmacokinetics of tea polyphenols has been reviewed in great detail,[49] and is discussed in Chapter 2.

Mode of action

Tea polyphenols have been proposed to act via a number of different mechanisms to exert their cancer chemopreventive effects. Studies have shown that EGCG acts specifically on certain cancer cells through induction of apoptosis, cell cycle arrest and inhibition of cell growth, but does not cause these effects in normal cells.[52,53] The inhibition of cell growth is thought to be caused by the involvement of tea polyphenols in the activation of genes, via signalling mechanisms.[54]

Inhibition of growth factor signalling, for example, by blocking the binding of epidermal growth factor (EGF) to its receptor, can inhibit cell growth and promote apoptosis. EGCG has been shown to inhibit the activities of the EGF receptor and prevent binding of EGF to the receptor,[53] thereby preventing cell proliferation.

Tea polyphenols such as EGCG and theaflavins are known to be antioxidant.[51,56,57] Their antioxidant activities include scavenging of free radicals[57] and inhibition of reactive oxygen species (ROS).[54] Tea polyphenols may also prevent the formation of ROS by inhibiting activity of the enzyme xanthine oxidase, which is involved in their formation.[58]

Other studies have suggested that tea polyphenols act through their pro-oxidant activity in the induction of apoptosis. One investigation using human lung cancer H661 cells demonstrated that EGCG induced apoptosis and was inhibited by the enzyme catalase, but found that catalase did not inhibit the growth inhibition activity of EGCG.[51,55]

Tea polyphenols may cause induced apoptosis, cell growth inhibition and antioxidant activity through increasing levels of p53, which regulates cell cycle arrest and apoptosis and therefore has a fundamental role in protecting cells from tumorigenesis. Antioxidants increase levels of p53 by promoting biosynthesis and also alter the redox potential, which results in the activation of p53.[53]

The activities of transcription factors such as AP-1 are induced by tumour promoters.[57] AP-1 is involved in the regulation of transforming growth factors, apoptosis and also in direct repression of p53.[53] EGCG and theaflavins have been shown to inhibit the activation of AP-1.[57] This inhibition may be caused by decreased activation of mitogen-activated protein kinase pathways, in particular jun N-terminal kinase, which thus prevents successful AP-1 binding.[51] Tea polyphenols have been shown to prevent cell transformation and cell growth by inhibiting the activity of AP-1.[56]

Administration of both green and black tea to rats was shown to induce the phase II enzymes cytochrome P450 1A1, 1A2 and 2B1.[54,58]

Levels of UDP-glucuronosyl transferase, a phase II enzyme, were increased significantly after drinking tea. This enzyme system detoxifies environmental chemicals such as heterocyclic amines, which are known to be mutagenic. Animals consuming tea produced detoxified metabolites of heterocyclic amines together with increased UDP-glucuronosyl transferase enzymes.[54]

Urokinase is a u-plasminogen activator involved in metastasis that is regularly expressed in human cancers. EGCG has been proposed to inhibit urokinase and hence to have a chemopreventive effect.[50,52,57] Using molecular modelling, EGCG was shown to block various amino acids needed for the catalytic activity of urokinase.[57]

EGCG has also been found to inhibit the activity of the enzyme topoisomerase I, which is involved in the relaxation of DNA, but not topoisomerase II in colon cancer. The concentration of EGCG needed to inhibit the activity of topoisomerase I was less than that required to inhibit cell growth.[55]

Inhibition of tumour necrosis factor alpha (TNF-α) could be the mechanism of action of tea polyphenols.[50,51,55] One investigation has supported this mechanism and shown the importance of TNF-α in cancer. It also indicated that ECG, EGCG and EGC all inhibited TNF-α release from human stomach cancer cells in the cell line KATO-III.[50]

Angiogenesis involves the formation of new blood vessels; these provide oxygen and nutrients to a tumour, which are essential for tumour growth and mestastasis. Polyphenols in green tea have been shown through *in vivo* and *in vitro* studies to be antiangiogenic. Tea polyphenols have been shown to inhibit the expression of vascular endothelial growth factor and matrix metalloproteinase-2, which are both important proangiogenic factors. Tea polyphenols have also been shown to inhibit the growth of endothelial cells, which are required for angiogenesis to occur.[59]

The therapeutic effects of tea

Early research into the chemopreventive effects of tea reported that application of EGCG to mouse skin inhibited tumour promotion.[60,61] Later studies have involved both green and black tea, decaffeinated tea and also fractionated tea, specifically individual components such as EGCG.

Epidemiological studies

Apparently contradictory results from Japan have been published. In an epidemiological study 8552 individuals over 40 years of age were surveyed over a period of 11 years. The age of cancer onset in women was increased from 65.7 years in those who drank fewer than three cups of green tea a day, to 74.4 years in those consuming over ten cups a day. The age of cancer onset in men was shown to increase from 63.3 years to 68.3 years. The smaller delay in age seen in men was thought to be attributable to the higher number of male smokers.[65] However, the incidence of cancer increased in individuals consuming over ten cups of tea a day, once the age of 80 years was reached. The increase in incidence was higher than in those who drank fewer cups of green tea.[61]

One case–control study in Shanghai showed a negative correlation between tea consumption and the risk of gastric cancer,[62] but contra-dictory evidence from Japan found no correlation between gastric cancer and tea consumption.[63]

Further studies have been reviewed. One in the USA studying post-menopausal women showed a lower risk of digestive tract and urinary tract cancers in tea drinkers. Most subjects in this study drank black tea, however, in another study observing the effects of black tea ingestion, no reduction in risk was observed. A cohort study in the Netherlands showed that drinking black tea had no effect on stomach, colorectal, lung or breast cancers.[56]

Studies in China using green tea and in the UK using black tea have shown a negative correlation between tea consumption and the risk of colon cancer,[64,65] but a study in Finland has shown a positive correla-tion between black tea consumption and the risk of colon cancer in males.[66]

One epidemiological study in Taiwan examined the effects primarily of oolong tea consumption on incidence of bladder cancer, and revealed that oolong tea was associated with an increased risk of bladder cancer. Drinking tea before the age of 40 and continuous consumption of tea for over 30 years showed an increased risk of cancer.[67]

Combination therapy with chemotherapeutic anticancer medication

Concomitant treatment of cancer with a chemotherapeutic agent plus tea has been proposed. The combination of EGCG with the non-steroidal anti-inflammatory drug sulindac has been evaluated *in vivo*, and apoptosis was induced 20 times more strongly than when either of the agents were given alone. This combination was also shown to inhibit tumour formation in multiple intestinal neoplasia in mice to a greater extent than the individual components. This synergistic effect is thought to be caused by new modulation of gene expression.[68]

Activity against cancers caused by smoking

Lung, oral and oesophageal cancers in particular are caused by cigarette smoking. Cigarette smoke contains compounds that can generate ROS, which can cause damage to DNA and lead to development of cancer.[69] The incidence of lung cancer in men in the USA is twice that in Japan, even though the prevalence of smokers in Japan is nearly twice that of the USA. This could be due to a number of other factors, including genetic and environmental factors. Green tea is consumed far more in Japan than in the USA,[53] which suggests possible chemopreventive effects of tea against smoking-induced cancers.

The effects of both green and black tea on lung cancer in mice and rats have been observed. The mice and rats were both treated with the carcinogen 4-(methylnitrosamine)-1-(3-pyridyl)-1-butanone (NNK), which is present in cigarette smoke.[53,58] Green and black teas were shown to inhibit the NNK-induced tumours in mice by 45% and 28% respectively compared with controls. Animals treated with black tea had a 19% incidence of tumours compared with 47% in the control.[53]

It has been reported that drinking ten Japanese-size cups (10 × 120 mL) of green tea a day, providing approximately 3000–4000 mg of EGCG, produces a chemopreventive effect.[68] Another study concluded that 6–10 cups of tea a day would result in chemopreventive effects, but there was insufficient evidence to show that drinking fewer than four cups a day provided any chemopreventive effect.[58] This, however, contradicts the findings of a separate study that showed a dose–response relationship between consumption of tea and cancer prevention.[69] In general, data suggest that a large daily consumption of tea (e.g. ten cups) is more beneficial than having just one cup a day.

One clinical trial used a biomarker of oxidative DNA damage, 8-hydroxydeoxyguanosine (8-OHdG), to investigate the effects of tea. The study showed that the levels of urinary 8-OHdG were significantly reduced by 31% after drinking four cups of decaffeinated green tea per day for four months, but decaffeinated black tea was shown to have no effect on urinary 8-OHdG in smokers. Higher levels of 8-OHdG are present in cancerous tissues and smokers are also associated with higher levels of this compound.[70] This reduction in biomarker levels supports the antioxidant mechanism of action, but does not necessarily translate into a definitive reduction in the level of cancer. Another trial involving smokers has observed enhanced apoptosis of oral cells and induced p53 expression following green tea consumption.[53]

Effect of the caffeine content

Caffeine has been shown to inhibit tumour growth and to strengthen the effect of tea in a trial involving NNK-induced lung tumours in mice. Whole tea had an even greater inhibitory action than ECGC and caffeine used alone.[53] Further studies comparing tea with and without caffeine have shown an increased inhibitory effect for regular tea against a carcinogen, compared with decaffeinated tea.[58]

Synergistic effects of caffeine and tea polyphenols are supported by the fact that these effects are not seen with coffee, which contains more caffeine than tea. Caffeine may exert its effects through the induction of specific cytochromes and inhibition of cell growth.[58]

Adverse effects

In a survey of 100 people, drinking ten Japanese-size cups of tea a day was tolerated by 90% of the participants and no biochemical abnormalities were observed. The side-effects experienced at this dose included: abdominal bloating, heartburn, nausea and insomnia; which were largely attributable to the caffeine content.[68]

The first clinical phase I trials, in humans in the USA, were started in 1997 to determine the maximum tolerated dose and to observe any side-effects of tea. These trials were conducted using green tea extract containing both catechins and caffeine formulated in a tablet, in cancer patients. The maximum tolerated dose was found to be 1.6–2.2 g of green tea extract, three times a day. This is equivalent to 7–8 Japanese size cups of green tea, three times a day. Drinking tea three times a day was better tolerated than once a day, and the side-effects were similar to those observed following ten cups of tea a day, and were dose-limited. Again the caffeine content was thought to be the cause of the side-effects.[71]

Conclusions

It is difficult to conclude whether tea has chemopreventive effects, partially because of the variety of tea products used in tests, and the inconsistency in results.[69] The mechanism of action is still unclear and results surrounding bioavailability are inconclusive.

Cancer is a complex disease with many factors, including age, sex, diet, lifestyle and environment, contributing to its development. Hereditary cancer incidence, socio-economic status and body mass index may all contribute to development. Unfortunately, the use of a range of tea varieties and variability in the constituents and their levels make overall conclusions from published clinical trials difficult. In addition, there is no clear correlation with the measurement of biological markers of cancer (e.g. 8-OHdG) as these are not directly related to cancer development.

New trends in tea drinking, such as the consumption of iced black tea, have not been investigated in detail. One report has suggested that the chemopreventive effects of tea are lost when the beverage is cold! Therefore, the number of consumers of the active constituents of tea may be an overestimation. It has also been suggested that the beneficial effects of tea may actually be due to the effects of not drinking coffee! Few studies conducted have considered coffee consumption as a cause of cancer.[69] Little research has been carried out on the effect of adding milk to tea. Green tea is always consumed without milk, but an investigation into the effects of adding milk to black tea showed no effect on the inhibitory effects of tea or on the absorption of tea polyphenols.[54] The effect of temperature of tea has rarely been considered. One study found that drinking tea at a high temperature increased the risk of bladder cancer.[67] This highlights the difficulty in assessing studies that are affected by a large number of variables.

In conclusion it can be said that tea consumption has few side-effects. Animal and *in vivo* studies look promising with a negative correlation between tea consumption and the risk of cancer. However, the effects of tea in humans, and the mechanism of action, are not yet clear.

Lycopene

Tomatoes and tomato-based products, which are the major source of many of the dietary carotenoids, especially lycopene, have shown promise for the prevention of some cancers.[72]

The ability of lycopene to act as an antioxidant and free radical scavenger is considered by the majority of researchers to be the most likely mechanism that could account for its beneficial effects in cancers.[73] ROS are the main source of oxidative damage that can generate structural alterations in DNA and decrease DNA repair by damaging essential proteins, and ultimately cause cancer.[74]

Animal studies have shown that a large proportion of ingested lycopene is excreted in the faeces and that 1000-fold more lycopene is absorbed and stored in the liver than accumulates in other target organs.[75] However, physiologically significant levels of lycopene have also been measured in other key organs such as breast, prostate, lung and colon, and there is an approximate dose–response relationship between lycopene intake and blood levels.[76] Research has also revealed that the general diet of the individual can affect the uptake and distribution of lycopene, and has provided evidence that lycopene in tomatoes is absorbed more efficiently than lycopene alone, making the raw material the more effective form.[75]

Lycopene and cancers of the digestive tract

A series of clinical experiments have shown a consistent inverse relationship between tomato consumption and the risk of cancers of the digestive tract. Preliminary case–control studies carried out in Italy during the early 1990s found that a high frequency of tomato intake reduced the risk of developing cancers of the oral cavity, pharynx and oesophagus, and also of the stomach and colon. A later, much larger study, also carried out in Italy, used patients below the age of 80 with incident, histologically confirmed cancer of the oral cavity and pharynx, oesophagus, colorectum, breast and ovary who had been admitted into hospital. The comparison group, in total, included approximately 5000 patients, also below the age of 80, with acute, non-neoplastic, non-hormone-related diseases, unrelated to long-term diet modifications. Information regarding each patient's diet was collected. The trials provided supportive evidence that tomato consumption is inversely related to the risk of upper digestive neoplasms. Levels of cancer of the oral cavity, pharynx and oesophagus decreased with increasing levels of lycopene intake. A similar relationship was also found in colorectal cancers. The association with lycopene, however, was less consistent in cancers of the ovary and breast.[77]

Researchers have also attempted to assess whether elevated levels of lycopene and other carotenoids in the lung provide a greater degree of protection against oxidative and ozone-induced damage.

Lung cancer

A randomized clinical trial looked at the effects of supplementation of carotenoid-rich vegetable juice (V-8) on lung macrophage levels of carotenoids and in moderating ozone-induced lung damage. Lycopene was the predominant carotenoid in the vegetable juice, representing 88% of total carotenoids. The dose of lycopene that the subjects received was 23 mg/day. Healthy young adults were exposed to 0.4 ppm ozone for 2 hours after either two weeks of antioxidant supplementation (one can of V-8 juice daily) or placebo. Mean lung concentrations of lycopene increased by 12% in supplemented subjects. The decreases in forced expiratory volume in 1 second (FEV_1) and forced vital capacity (FVC) were 30% and 24% smaller respectively, in the supplemented subjects compared with the placebo subjects. However, there was no difference in markers of inflammation in the lung between both sets of subjects. This may be because antioxidants only have a role in protecting the lung from damaging ozone and maintaining lung function, and play no part in mediating the inflammatory response. Although the study showed no significant change in peripheral blood lymphocyte DNA damage in either supplemented or placebo subjects, the lung epithelial cell DNA damage as measured by the Comet Assay was 20% lower in supplemented subjects. This provided evidence that these carotenoids protect the lung from DNA damage caused by oxidative stresses, in particular that associated with ozone exposure.[78]

This study demonstrated the presence of lycopene in the human lung following supplementation, and provided preliminary evidence that an increased intake of lycopene might provide an additional level of protection against oxidative damage. It is supported by epidemiological literature showing that diets rich in tomatoes are associated with low lung cancer rates.[75,77,78]

Prostate cancer

Prostate cancer is the most common of all male cancers,[4] yet preventable measures for this malignancy are not well established.[3] Recent epidemiological studies have shown that a high intake of lycopene in the diet lowers the risk of developing prostate cancer.[79] Three mechanisms have been put forward to explain how lycopene may help to prevent prostate cancer: inhibition of growth and induction of differentiation in prostate cancer cells; upregulation of the tumour suppressor protein Cx43 alongside improved intercellular communication; and prevention of oxidative DNA damage.[80]

One of the studies providing the strongest evidence concerning tomatoes and prostate cancer prevention was published in 1995. The dietary habits of over 47 000 men enrolled in the Health Professionals Follow-Up Study were examined. This is the only dietary study that showed estimated concurrent plasma lycopene levels in a sample of participants.[81] During the follow-up period 773 of the participants were diagnosed with prostate cancer. The only fruits or vegetables or products containing them found to be associated with a reduced risk of prostate cancer were: raw tomatoes, tomato sauce and pizza. In men who had more advanced prostate cancer, consuming ten servings of tomato products per week compared with less than 1.5 servings per week, lycopene was found to be significantly protective. The study identified a correlation between plasma and dietary lycopene. In addition, a high intake of tomatoes and tomato products, which accounted for 82% of lycopene, was associated with a 35% lower risk of total prostate cancer, and a 53% lowered risk of advanced prostate cancer. Tomato sauce had the strongest inverse association with prostate cancer; a slightly weaker inverse association was found with tomatoes and pizzas. This decline in protective effect from tomato sauce to tomatoes and pizza corresponded with a mirrored decline in plasma lycopene levels.[73] This study showed an association between intake of tomato products and a lower risk of prostate cancer.

A pilot study was conducted to investigate the biological and clinical effects of lycopene supplementation in patients with localised prostate cancer. Newly diagnosed prostate cancer patients were given either tomato extract containing 30 mg of lycopene, or no supplementation, for three weeks before radical prostatectomy. Prostatic tissue lycopene levels were 47% higher in the intervention group; however, plasma lycopene levels were not significantly different between the groups nor did they change significantly within each group. Mean plasma prostate-specific antigen (PSA) levels (a clinical parameter of prostate cancer burden) decreased by 18% in the supplemented patients and increased by 14% in the control group. Seventy-three per cent of patients in the intervention group had involvement of surgical margins and/or extraprostatic tissues with cancer, compared to 18% of patients in the control group. In addition, the intervention group was found to have smaller tumours. Eighty per cent in the lycopene group had tumours that measured 4 mL or less compared with only 45% in the control group.[80]

Intake of tomato products, equating to 30 mg lycopene/day, over a three-week period was shown to cause a decrease in lipid peroxides, a reduction in DNA strand breaks in circulating lymphocyte DNA, and a decline in nucleoside damage in the form of 8-hydroxydeoxyguanosine/deoxyguanosine (8-OHdG/dG) in circulating leukocytes, indicating antioxidant activity.[82] It is probable that the prostate, because of greater chronic inflammation of prostate epithelial cells and faster cell turnover together with reduced levels of DNA repair enzymes compared with other tissues, may be more susceptible to oxidative damage. After the three-week intervention, the patients' serum and prostate lycopene concentrations had increased 1.97- and 2.92-fold respectively. There was a positive correlation between leukocyte and prostate 8-OHdG/dG, which may allow leukocyte 8-OHdG/dG measurement to be used as a prognostic biomarker of oxidative stress in clinical practice. However, there was no inverse linear correlation between plasma or prostate lycopene concentrations and 8OHdG/dG in leukocytes or prostate tissue.[82]

Staining of the biopsy and resected tissue samples showed that there had been a decrease in DNA damage in cancer cells after tomato sauce consumption; mean cancer cell nuclear density had decreased by 40% and by 36% in mean area. Mean serum PSA concentrations decreased by 17.5% and apoptotic index was higher in hyperplastic and neoplastic cells in the resected tissue following supplementation. It is probable that the decreased DNA damage in these neoplastic cells leads to the induction of apoptosis (and therefore fewer viable cancer cells), thus producing an elevated apoptotic index.[82]

Meta-analysis

A meta-analysis of observational studies on the role of tomato products and lycopene in the prevention of prostate cancer also supported the protective effect of lycopene. Again data suggested that the protective effect of lycopene is somewhat better when tomatoes are consumed rather than lycopene alone.[79] This combination may comprise an efficient system that keeps lycopene in an antioxidant state in cell membranes.[82] In addition, the protective effect is slightly stronger for high intakes of cooked tomato products than for high intakes of raw tomatoes. This may be due to either higher concentrations of lycopene in tomato-based products or differences in lycopene bioavailability in processed tomato products compared with raw tomatoes.[79]

Conclusions

These preliminary studies have provided us with evidence to suggest that tomato consumption, lycopene intake and serum lycopene levels are associated with a reduced risk of developing cancer, most notably prostate and lung cancer. The beneficial effects of lycopene, owing to its ability to act as an antioxidant, may allow it to be used as an adjunct therapy in the treatment of some cancers. Due to the lack of information we have on its mechanism of action and safety in homogeneous patient populations, larger clinical trials are needed to warrant the use of lycopene in the prevention of cancer. A problem arises in ascertaining the most suitable tomato-based product, as lycopene content varies immensely between formulations and brands. The lycopene content of the tomatoes themselves can vary significantly with variety and ripening stage of tomatoes.[73] Lycopene concentrations in the red strains approach 50 mg/kg, compared with only 5 mg/kg in yellow varieties. High-quality supplements are one alternative. Also the form in which lycopene should be delivered to patients poses the greatest subject for deliberation, since this appears to have a profound impact on its effectiveness.[79,82]

Flaxseed

Flaxseed contains two possibly beneficial substances: the lignans and α-linolenic acid (ALA). Flaxseed has several plant lignans, including matairesinol, pinoresinol, isolariciresinol and the major lignan secoisolariciresinol diglucoside (SDG).

Anticancer activity

Studies have shown that flaxseed has anticancer properties. These have largely been attributed to the lignan component, but a recent study has demonstrated the contribution of both the lignans and the flaxseed oil to activity against metastasis.[83] In this experiment, different groups of mice with oestrogen receptor (ER)-negative breast cancer were given either flaxseed, flaxseed oil, or both SDG and flaxseed oil; tumour growth and metastasis was reduced in all cases but the groups did not differ in their effects, suggesting that both the SDG and flaxseed oil contribute to the anticancer activity. Furthermore, the lung and total metastasis incidences were significantly lowest in the group given SDG and flaxseed oil, indicating that SDG and flaxseed oil complement each other against metastasis.[83]

In a study from eastern Finland in humans it was found that there was a significant inverse relationship between the metabolite enterolactone serum level and breast cancer incidence.[84]

Mode of action

The lignan metabolites enterodiol and enterolactone are structurally very similar to the natural oestrogen, 17β-oestradiol, and are thought to be weakly oestrogenic and/or anti-oestrogenic.[85] This suggests that they may be of use against hormone-dependent cancers.

There is some evidence that lignans may stimulate liver production of SHBG and thus reduce the free sex hormone concentration and prolong the menstrual cycle, leading to reduced breast cancer risk; this evidence is controversial though, as SHBG only appears to be increased by lignans in women who have low SHBG in the first place.[5]

In general, therefore, lignans may reduce oestrogen exposure by being anti-oestrogenic, by decreasing 17β-oestradiol in cancer cells or by provoking the production of less oestrogenic metabolites; in effect the bioavailability of 17β-oestradiol to cancer cells is reduced. Further-more, lignans have been shown to inhibit tumour growth of ER-positive MCF-7 cells with already low oestrogen concentration and also to inhibit growth of ER-negative tumour cells, showing that flaxseed has non-hormonal anticancer roles too.[86]

There are many more sites of action that also appear to be targets, including reduction in growth factors, inhibition of membrane ATPase, ornithine decarboxylase, tyrosine protein kinase and DNA topoiso-merases, leading to inhibition of growth and proliferation. Lignans may inhibit the enzyme that produces primary bile acids from cholesterol; this means there are fewer primary bile acids to be converted in the colon to secondary bile acids, which correlate with colon cancer. Antioxidant properties have also been linked to lignans.[87]

Conclusions

The experimentally observed anticancer effects of flaxseed are mainly due to the lignan fraction.[88] Flaxseed oil is less likely to be the major active anticancer agent although it probably has some contribution.

Lignans have so far been well tolerated in animal studies but safety data are still lacking. Enterodiol and enterolactone have not been found to be mutagenic in bacteria, animals or humans,[89] but more rigorous long-term studies are required.

n-3 Polyunsaturated fatty acids

The amount and type of fat that we consume in our daily diet may affect our risk of developing cancer. Several influential organisations, such as the World Cancer Research Fund, have advised that we limit our intake of fat, particularly animal fat, in an attempt to decrease the incidence of cancer. Dietary fat is known to be able to affect changes in genetic structure and genetic expression, both of which have been linked to the causes of cancer.

High dietary fat intake has been identified as a causative factor in the development of colon, breast, prostate and pancreatic cancer, particularly when there is evidence of a high intake of meat and mono-unsaturated fat in the diet. Saturated fat has been found to be a risk factor for ovarian cancer, and polyunsaturated fats for hepatic cancer. A meta-analysis of experimental animal studies found *n*-6 fatty acids to significantly enhance carcinogenesis, saturated fatty acids to slightly enhance carcinogenesis, monosaturated fatty acids to have no effect, and *n*-3 fatty acids to inhibit carcinogenesis.[90]

Nutritionists have long accepted the association between a high dietary intake of very long-chain *n*-3 fatty acids found in fish and a reduced risk of death from coronary heart disease. However, it has only more recently come to light that consumption of ALA, the parent compound of all *n*-3 fatty acids may be linked to an increased risk of prostate cancer. The highest proportion of our daily ALA intake is from plants and vegetable oils; its intake in wealthy countries is 5–10 times higher than that of *n*-3 fatty acids from fish.[91]

Clinical evidence

A meta-analysis was carried out to quantitatively estimate the association between ALA intake, mortality from heart disease, and occurrence of prostate cancer in observational studies. Data from nine observational studies investigating the relationship between prostate cancer incidence and intake or blood levels of ALA were identified and reviewed. These studies all suggested that a high intake or blood level of ALA increased the incidence of prostate cancer.[91]

The question is, should we consume high levels of ALA for its protective effect on coronary heart disease or avoid it because of its association with an increased risk of prostate cancer? For men with a predisposed, increased risk of developing heart disease the benefits of ALA probably outweigh the risks.

The *n*-3 PUFAs found mainly in fish oils are promising molecules in both cancer prevention and possibly cancer treatment.[92]

It has been reported that certain types of fish (oil) might protect against colorectal cancer because *n*-3 PUFA is able to inhibit some steps in colon carcinogenesis. In addition, diets containing *n*-3 PUFA as fish oil have been found to reduce both mammary and lung tumour metastasis.[92]

A number of clinical trials have reported effects of *n*-3 fatty acids in many types of cancers, with varying success. One large meta-analysis of clinical trials investigating the incidence of cancers after supplementation with *n*-3 fatty acids has been published. Overall, 20 cohorts from seven countries have been studied for incidence of 11 different types of cancers. No significant benefits were detected for supplementation for aerodigestive, bladder, ovarian, pancreatic or stomach cancer, or lymphomas. Statistically significant associations were found with four studies on breast cancer, one study on colorectal cancer, two for lung cancer, and two for prostate cancer. Unfortunately there were found to be both increased and decreased risks for breast, lung and prostate cancers, and there was an increased risk with skin cancer.[93]

Coenzyme Q10

The reduced form of Co Q10 is a powerful antioxidant and, as oxidative damage to DNA, proteins and lipids is associated with carcinogenesis,[94] there is great interest in Co Q10 as a potential chemopreventive or chemotherapeutic agent in cancer. In addition, deficiency in Co Q10 has been shown to be significantly higher in cancer patients than in healthy people.[95]

Antioxidant activity

The relationship between Co Q10 and cancer can be shown by measuring Co Q10 levels in cancer tissue. Normal blood levels of Co Q10 are 0.9 ± 0.2 µg/mL. Two studies in the USA and Sweden showed that about 20% of breast cancer patients in those studies had Co Q10 levels of 0.5 µg/mL or lower.[96]

A clinical trial of 200 breast cancer patients showed that plasma Co Q10 levels were reduced both in cancer and non-malignant lesions compared with the control. Large-volume tumours and patients with poor prognosis exhibited more dramatic reduction in Co Q10 levels.[97] Breast cancer may, in part, be attributed to the lack of Co Q10 antioxidant defence activity.

In another study, a patient with high-risk breast cancer who showed partial tumour regression on treatment with antioxidants, fatty acids and 90 mg of Co Q10 daily, was stepped up from 90 mg to 390 mg of Co Q10 and within two months mammography showed no signs of tumour. The investigators were so encouraged by this that they treated another patient who had residual tumour post surgery with 300 mg of Co Q10 daily; after three month no tumour tissue remained.[96] Unfortunately clinical trials are lacking in the area.

Melatonin

The lifestyles of people in industrialised countries tend not to follow the day/night cycle as closely as in the past; shiftwork results in exposure to light at night, thus suppressing melatonin secretion, and this has been blamed for a contribution to increased cancer risk. Melatonin has been shown to be anti-oestrogenic *in vitro* and *in vivo* and many studies have linked a lack of melatonin to increased cancer risk/growth. To further the link between melatonin and oestrogen levels, another study has shown that oestrogen receptor (ER)-positive tumours have much lower melatonin peaks at night than ER-negative tumours. The higher the tumour ER concentration, the lower the melatonin peak is, indicating that a low/no nocturnal melatonin peak may predict increased risk of hormone-dependent cancer.[98]

Observational studies have shown that light pollution at night increases the risk of breast cancer; the longer women work night shifts, the greater the breast cancer risk.[99] A meta-analysis looking at the relationship between shiftwork and breast cancer concluded that night shiftwork, including the work of flight attendants, increased breast cancer risk by 48%. This figure is strikingly significant and attenuates the idea that female flight attendants are at increased risk of breast cancer because of increased exposure to radiation, however melatonin deficiency may well be involved in tumour development.[100] The reduced risk of breast cancer in blind women, who cannot perceive light and therefore do not have reduced melatonin levels, also strengthens the argument for the anticancer effects of melatonin.[99]

The increased cancer risk associated with reduced melatonin levels may be explained by associated increased oestrogen levels, but melatonin does not appear to act entirely by that mechanism since light at night seems to increase the risk of other non-hormonally dependent cancers too. For example, women doing night shiftwork for more than 15 years have been shown to be at increased risk of colorectal cancer.[99]

In 2005, the first meta-analysis looking at the impact of melatonin therapy on various cancers, either on its own or along with conventional chemotherapy, was published. It considered ten randomised controlled trials between 1992 and 2003 and entailed 643 patients. Taking melatonin was found to reduce the death risk at 1 year, with similar effects in different cancers. No severe side-effects were reported, and this, combined with melatonin's apparent anticancer efficacy and low cost, indicates that melatonin may have good potential as a cancer treatment.[101]

Melatonin is a potent antioxidant and acts as a direct free radical scavenger. It is also involved in oxidative defence by stimulating enzymes that metabolise and inactivate free radicals.[102]

Melatonin is both proapoptotic and appears to inhibit apoptosis in immune cells and neurons. Therefore, while melatonin may be considered for cancer therapy, its activity in relation to apoptosis may depend on both the type of the cell and the functional state of the cell.[103]

Melatonin and the immune system

An *in vivo* study has shown that optimal immune function in mammals relies on an evening 'dose' of melatonin. Melatonin helps to develop haematopoietic and lymphoid cells in the bone marrow, thymus, spleen and lymph node and also enhances lymphocyte- and phagocyte-mediated immunity.[104]

Not only can melatonin reverse metabolic changes and enhance lymphocyte and macrophage response to tumours, but also, by acting at G protein-coupled membrane receptors, it can stimulate cytokine release and thus help to mount an immune response. For example, melatonin administered with the cytokine interleukin 2 might act synergistically to prolong survival of a cancer patient.[105]

Melatonin as an adjunct in chemotherapy

It has been shown that melatonin exhibits anticancer properties but, in clinical practice, it is more realistic that it will be used as an adjunct to conventional chemotherapy.

Various studies have shown that melatonin may enhance chemotherapy efficacy and reduce the toxic side-effects experienced by cancer patients. One such study looked at 1-year survival status in advanced cancer patients with poor clinical status. When chemotherapy was combined with 20 mg/day of melatonin the number of patients surviving at 1 year was significantly increased (63/124 compared with 29/126 for chemotherapy without melatonin). Also, the tumour regression rate was significantly increased. This is probably both because of the powerful antioxidant properties of melatonin, which had been shown to enhance the cytotoxicity of chemotherapeutic agents, and because of its proapoptotic nature. The increased survival rate may also be due to the ability of melatonin to reduce the immunosuppression induced by chemotherapy. Melatonin reduced the incidence of thrombocytopenia, cardiotoxicity, neurotoxicity and other adverse effects induced by chemotherapy. Chemotherapy often entails generating free radicals, and melatonin, being the most active natural antioxidant, can help counteract the toxicity from such therapy. No side-effects from melatonin itself were noticed. It appears that in patients with advanced cancer, the efficacy and toxicity of chemotherapy may be increased and decreased respectively by melatonin.[106]

To further these findings, another longer term study was carried out that investigated the 5-year survival in 100 patients with metastatic non-small cell lung cancer. The results here further the evidence that melatonin should be used in cancer treatment. Chemotherapy alone (cisplatin and etoposide) left no patients alive after 2 years, whereas the same chemotherapy combined with 20 mg/day melatonin resulted in 6% of patients living after 5 years. Not only does melatonin prolong survival but it increases the quality of the patient life during that extended survival period,[107] probably due to the anticachetic effects.

Cachexia is a wasting away of the human body with noticeable weight loss. This is not just due to malnutrition, but also partly due to increased release of TNF-α, which has antitumour effects but also metabolic side-effects causing cachexia. Melatonin and TNF-α secretion are possibly related by a feedback mechanism and a study has shown that when given along with supportive care melatonin significantly decreases TNF-α levels compared with supportive care alone. Corresponding to this, weight loss in the group of patients receiving melatonin was 10% less than in the group receiving only supportive care. The study thus provides evidence that melatonin may treat neoplastic cachexia by its effect on TNF-α levels. Furthermore, possibly by virtue of this inhibition of TNF-α secretion, respiratory problems due to cancer appear to be attenuated in this study.[108]

Conclusions

The characteristic melatonin peak at night in healthy people is widely seen to be disrupted in cancer patients.[109] What is not known is information about the time of day that melatonin might have its greatest benefit. The circadian nature of melatonin means it may have different effects at different times of the day, and this has been demonstrated in mice.[104] Linoleic acid, an *n*-6 PUFA, is known to stimulate tumour growth, particularly at night, when melatonin levels are lowest, and melatonin supplementation has been shown to cause a dose-dependent reduction in linoleic acid uptake and tumour growth. Melatonin may also have an optimum time of day at which it inhibits fatty acid uptake, which itself exhibits circadian rhythm.[110] It is known that cancers coordinate their cell cycles and vary in their susceptibility to chemotherapy throughout the day.[109]

The clinical evidence for melatonin has shown increased survival times and amelioration of the toxicities of conventional chemotherapy.[109] The safety of melatonin has been largely confirmed, with doses of 1–300 mg or 1 g melatonin daily for 30 days exhibiting no side-effects, although bone marrow toxicity has been shown to be worsened with melatonin use.[105] Also, the chief melatonin metabolite 6-hydroxy-melatonin has been found to be carcinogenic.[111] Not only has melatonin exhibited anticancer activity, an ability to reduce the side-effects of conventional anticancer drugs and an antioxidant ability to minimise radiation therapy damage, but it has also been shown to reduce levels of anxiety in patients and improved their overall quality of life.[112]

Conjugated linoleic acid

The anticancer activity of this mixture of linoleic acid isomers has been widely investigated at the molecular level. In addition, a study of women from Finland showed that CLA levels were significantly lower in breast cancer cases than in control healthy people.[55]

Mode of action

There is a 40–50% reduction in colorectal cancer relative risk in those who use non-steroidal anti-inflammatory drugs (NSAIDs) continuously; this has led to the suggestion that inhibition of eicosanoid synthesis (NSAIDs block production of prostaglandins (PG) – eicosanoids) may have anticancer effects.[113] Arachidonic acid leads to eicosanoid production; it has been shown that eicosanoid products such as prostaglandin E_2 (PGE$_2$) are involved in carcinogenesis and that they can influence cell proliferation and tissue differentiation.[114] Enzymes involved in eicosanoid manufacture include cyclooxygenase (COX) and lipoxygenase (LOX).[115]

It is known that CLA is incorporated into phospholipids and competes with arachidonic acid, possibly thus displacing it from cell membranes. This would alter subsequent eicosanoid production.[116] For example, CLA has been shown to reduce arachidonic acid-derived PGE_2, and this correlates with a reduction in tumorigenesis.[57] Colon cancer is associated with increased expression of COX-2 enzyme and enhanced synthesis of eicosanoids, especially prostaglandins. In a colon cancer study in rats, 1% CLA reduced arachidonic acid levels in phospholipids and led to a significant reduction in PGE_2 and thromboxane, eicosanoid products of arachidonic acid. The researchers concluded that eicosanoid levels were reduced by modulation of arachidonic acid availability rather than involvement with COX-2 expression, as levels of this enzyme were unchanged throughout the experiment. The reduced eicosanoid levels could contribute to increased apoptosis and reduced cell proliferation.[113]

CLA may oppose the tumour-inducing effects of linoleic acid because of their structural similarity.[117] CLA is metabolised by desaturation and elongation and it has been proposed that the enzymes involved may also be used by linoleic acid. Addition of 1% CLA significantly reduced levels of arichidonic acid and other linoleic acid metabolites in rat mammary tissue, indicating that there is competition for enzymes between CLA and linoleic acid and that this can lead to reduced eicosanoid synthesis from arachidonic acid.[118]

CLA may also interfere with the LOX pathway, thus modulating cell proliferation and apoptosis. A study looking at this pathway found that the *trans*10, *cis*12 CLA isomer significantly reduced 5-HETE (5-hydroxyeicosatetraenoic acid) levels (the normal 5-LOX metabolite) and tumour cell growth. This occurred by CLA competing with arachidonic acid (5-LOX substrate) and by altering expression of a protein that enables 5-LOX to form 5-HETE. As malignant tissue shows increased expression of 5-LOX, treatment with *trans*10, *cis*12 CLA may be useful in anticancer therapy.[115]

CLA may modulate eicosanoid production and therefore have anticancer activity by competing with the normal substrates in the pathway, by altering expression of enzymes and also by inhibiting COX and LOX enzymes.[119]

Conclusions

The CLA isomers differ in their mechanism of action and they may also differ in their benefit against different tissues. For example, the *trans*10, *cis*12 isomer works better against colorectal cancer proliferation.[120] *trans*10, *cis*12 CLA appears to be the best isomer for use in androgen-dependent prostate cancer[121] and is better than *cis*9, *trans*11 CLA in

ER+ breast cancer cell inhibition.[122] Another isomer, *cis*-9, *cis*-11 CLA has proven to be the best radiosensitiser and this could justify its use in radiotherapy for breast cancer.[123] CLA should now be investigated more closely in its constituent isomers rather than as a mixture.

CLA has established anticancer properties and they manifest themselves at levels as low as 0.1% by weight in the diet.[119] However, most studies have been carried out *in vitro* or on animals; data on humans are rare.[116]

Overall conclusions

Cancer patients are increasingly turning to the use of preventive medication or nutraceuticals alongside their conventional chemotherapeutic drugs, either to enhance the anticancer effects, ameliorate the negative effects of conventional drugs or to improve their quality of life. Over the years, research has been devoted to unravelling the relationship between nutraceuticals and cancer, but there is still much work to be carried out before we may see compounds such as these nutraceuticals used regularly in therapy and side-by-side with cancer drugs.

Much of the available evidence for nutraceuticals is based on *in vitro* and *in vivo* studies in animals. To date there are few epidemiological and clinical data for these nutraceuticals, but it is becoming evident that we can decrease the incidence of cancer through dietary selection.

Encouraging information from these nutraceuticals indicates that they have good safety profiles and are generally well-tolerated; however, conflicting data on the anticancer efficacy of these nutraceuticals are available.

References

1. Bingham S, Riboli E. Diet and cancer – the European Prospective Investigation into Cancer and Nutrition. *Nat Rev Cancer* 2004; 4: 206–215.
2. Cancer Research UK Statistics (2006) http://info.cancerresearchuk.org/cancerstats/reports/#rep (accessed 29 June 2006).
3. Senior H, Lockwood B. Soy isoflavones: Their role in cancer prevention. *Nutrafoods* 2005; 4: 5–17.
4. Surh Y-J. Cancer chemoprevention with dietary phytochemicals. *Nat Rev Cancer* 2003; 3: 768–780.
5. Adlercreutz H. Phyto-oestrogens and cancer. *Lancet Oncol* 2002; 3: 364–373.
6. American Cancer Society (1998) http://www.cancer.org/STT Facts and Figures (accessed 29 June 2004).

7. Hussain M, Banerjee M, Sarkar FH *et al.* Soy isoflavones in the treatment of prostate cancer. *Nutr Cancer* 2003; 47: 111–117.

8. Adlercreutz H, Honjo H, Higashi A *et al.* Urinary excretion of lignans and isoflavenoid phytoestrogens in Japanese men and women consuming a traditional Japanese diet. *Am J Clin Nutr* 2001; 54: 1093–1100.

9. Messina M J, Loprinzi C L. Soy for breast cancer survivors: a critical review of the literature. *J Nutr* 2001; 131: 3095S–3108S.

10. Makiewicz L, Garey J, Aldercreutz H, Gurpide E. In vitro bioassays of non-steroidal phytoestrogens. *J Steroid Biochem Mol Biol* 1993; 45: 399–405.

11. Mayr U, Butsch A, Schneider S. Validation of two in vitro test systems for estrogenic activities with zearalenone, phytoestrogens and cereal extracts. *Toxicology* 1992: 74: 135–149.

12. Dixon R A, Ferreira D. Molecules of Interest: Genistein. *Phytochemistry* 2002; 60: 205–211.

13. Fritz K L, Seppanen C M, Kurzer M S, Saari Csallany A. The in vivo antioxidant activity of soybean isoflavones in human subjects. *Nutr Res* 2003 23: 479–487.

14. Boyle C, Moizer K, Barlow T *et al.* Phytoestrogens and health. In: Johnson I, Williamson G, eds. *Phytochemical Functional Foods.* Boca Raton, FL: CRC Press, 2003: 65–87.

15. Constantinou A, Kiguchi K, Huberman E. Induction of differentiation and DNA strand breakage in human HL-60 and K-562 leukaemia cells by genistein. *Cancer Res* 1990; 50: 2618–2624.

16. Peterson G. Evaluation of the biochemical targets of genistein in tumour cells. *J Nutr* 1990; 125: 7845S–7895S.

17. Endogenous Hormones and Breast Cancer Collaboration Group. Endogenous sex hormones and breast cancer in post-menopausal women: reanalysis of nine prospective studies. *J Natl Cancer Inst* 2002; 94: 606–616.

18. Barnes S, Kim H, DarelyUsmar V *et al.* Beyond ER alpha and ER beta: estrogen receptor binding is only part of the isoflavone story. *J Nutr* 2000; 130: 656S–657S.

19. Kuiper G G, Lemmen J G, Carlsson B *et al.* Interaction of estrogenic chemicals and phytoestrogens with estrogen receptor beta. *Endocrinology* 1998; 139: 4252–4263.

20. Yanagihara K, Ito A, Toge T, Numoto M. Anti-proliferative effects of isoflavones on human cancer cell lines established from the gastro-intestinal tract. *Cancer Res* 1993; 53: 5815–5821.

21. Messina M, Bennick M. Soyfoods, isoflavones and risk of colonic cancer: a review of the in vitro and in vivo data. *Bailliere's Clin Endocrinol Metab* 1998; 12: 707–725.

22. Sarkar F H, Yiwei Li. Mechanisms of cancer chemoprevention by soy isoflavone genistein. *Cancer Metastasis Rev* 2002; 21: 265–280.

23. Akiyama T, Ishida J, Nakagawa S *et al.* Genistein, a specific inhibitor of tyrosine-specific protein kinases. *J Biol Chem* 1987; 262: 5592–5595.

24. Uckun F M, Evans W E, Forsyth C J *et al.* Biotherapy of B-cell precursor leukaemia by targeting genistein to CD19-associated tyrosine kinases. *Science* 1995; 267: 886–891.

25. Thorburn J, Thorburn A. The tyrosine kinase inhibitor, genistein, prevents

α-adrenergic-induced cardiac muscle cell hypertrophy by inhibiting activation of the Ras-MAP kinase signalling pathway. *Biochem Biophys Res Commun* 1994; 202: 1586–1591.

26. Linassier C, Pierre M, Le Peco J-B, Pierre J. Mechanism of action in NIH-3T3 cells of genistein, an inhibitor of EGF receptor tyrosine kinase activity. *Biochem Pharmacol* 1990; 39: 187–193.

27. Peterson T G, Barnes S. Genistein potentially inhibits the growth of human primary breast epithelial cells: correlation with a lack of genistein metabolism. *Mol Biol Cell* 1994; 5: 384a.

28. Hooijberg J H, Broxterman H J, Heijn M *et al*. Modulation by (iso)flavonoids of the ATPase activity of the multidrug resistance protein. *FEBS Lett* 1997; 413: 344–348.

29. Critchfield J W, Welsh C J, Phang J M, Yeh G C. Modulation of adriamycin® accumulation and efflux by flavonoids in HCT-15 colon cells: activation of P-glycoprotein as a putative mechanism. *Biochem Pharmacol* 1994; 48: 1437–1445.

30. Versantvoort C H M, Schuurhuis G J, Pinedo H M *et al*. Genistein modulates the decreased drug accumulation in non-P-glycoprotein mediated multidrug resistant tumor cells. *Br J Cancer* 1993; 68: 939–947.

31. Kao Y C, Zhou C, Sherman M *et al*. Molecular basis of the inhibition of human aromatase (estrogen synthetase) by flavone and isoflavone phyto-estrogens: a site-directed mutagenesis study. *Environ Health Prospect* 1998; 106: 85–92.

32. Naik H R, Lehr J E, Pienta K J. An in vitro and in vivo study of anti-tumour effects of genistein on hormone refractory prostate cancer. *Anticancer Res* 1994; 14: 2617–2620.

33. Lamartiniere C A. Protection against breast cancer with genistein: a component of soy. *Am J Clin Nutr* 2000; 71: 1705S–1707S.

34. Shu X O, Jin F, Dai Q *et al*. Soyfood intake during adolescence and subsequent risk of breast cancer among Chinese women. *Cancer Epidemiol Biomark Prev* 2001; 10: 483–488.

35. Russo J, Wilgus G, Russo I H. Susceptibility of the mammary gland to carcinogenesis: differentiation of the mammary gland as a determinant of tumour incidence and type of lesion. *Am J Pathol* 1979; 96: 721–736.

36. Ososki A L, Kennelly E J. Phytoestrogens: a review of the present state of research. *Phytother Res* 2003; 17: 845–869.

37. Kumar N B, Cantor A, Allen K *et al*. The specific role of isoflavones in reducing the prostate cancer risk. *Prostate* 2004; 59: 141–147.

38. Aldercruetz H, Hockerstedt K, Bannwart C *et al*. Effects of dietary components, including lignans and phytoestrogens on enterohepatic circulation and liver metabolism of estrogens and on sex hormone-binding globulin. *J Steroid Biochem* 1987; 27: 1135–1144.

39. Adlercreutz H, Markkanen H, Watanabe S. Plasma concentrations of phyto-estrogens in Japanese men. *Lancet* 1993; 342: 1209–1210.

40. Evans B A J, Griffiths K, Morton M. Inhibition of 5α-reductase and 17β-hydroxysteroid dehydrogenase in genital skin fibroblasts by dietary lignans and isoflavonoids. *J Endocrinol* 1995; 147: 295–302.

41. Yanagihara K, Ito A, Toge T, Numato M. Anti-proliferative effects of

isoflavones on human cancer cell lines established from the gastro-intestinal tract. *Cancer Res* 1993; 53: 5815–5821.

42. Su S J, Yeh T M, Lei H Y, Chow N H. The potential of soybean foods as a chemoprevention approach for human urinary tract cancer. *Clin Res* 2000; 6: 230–236.

43. Anderson J W, Johnston B M, Cook-Newell M E. Meta-analysis of the effects of soy protein intake on serum lipids. *N Engl J Med* 1995; 333: 276–282.

44. Horn-Ross P L, John E M, Canchola Al J *et al*. Phytoestrogen intake and endometrial cancer risk. *J Nat Cancer Inst* 2003; 95: 1158–1164.

45. Wakai K, Egami I, Kato K *et al*. Dietary intake and sources of isoflavones among Japanese. *Nutr Cancer* 1999; 33: 139–145.

46. Hsieh C Y, Santell R C, Haslam S Z, Helferich W G. Estrogenic effects of genistein on the growth of estrogen receptor-positive human breast cancer (MCF-7) cells in vitro and in vivo. *Cancer Res* 1998; 58: 3833–3838.

47. McMichael-Phillips D F, Harding C, Morton M *et al*. Effects of soy-protein supplementation on epithelial proliferation in the histologically normal human breast. *Am J Clin Nutr* 1998; 68: 1431S–1436S.

48. de Mejia E G, Vasconez M, de Lumen B O, Nelson R. Lunasin Concentration in different soybean genotypes, commercial soy protein, and isoflavone products. *J Agric Food Chem* 2004; 52: 5882–5887.

49. Hartley C, Lockwood B. Tea polyphenols: Their role in cancer prevention. *Nutrafoods* 2005; 4: 5–14.

50. Fujiki H. Two stages of cancer prevention with green tea. *J Cancer Res Clin Oncol* 1999; 125: 589–597.

51. Chhabra S K, Chung J Y, Lee M-J *et al*. Tea and tea polyphenols in cancer prevention. *J Nutr* 2000; 130: 472S–478S.

52. Yang C S, Landau J M. Effects of tea consumption on nutrition and health. *J Nutr* 2000; 130: 2409–2412.

53. Lambert J D, Yang C S. Mechanisms of cancer prevention by tea constituents. *J Nutr* 2003; 133: 3262S–3267S.

54. Adhami V M, Afaq F, Ahmad N *et al*. Antioxidants of the beverage tea in promotion of human health. *Antiox Redox Signal* 2004; 6: 571–582.

55. Chung F, Herzog C R, Schwatz J, Yang Y. Tea and cancer prevention: studies in animals and humans. *J Nutr* 2003; 133: 3268S–3274S.

56. Weisburger J H. Prevention of coronary heart disease and cancer by tea, a review. *Environ Health Prevent Med* 2003; 7: 283–288.

57. Ahmad N, Mukhtar H. Tea polyphenols: prevention of cancer and optimizing health. *Am J Clin Nutr* 2000; 71: 1698S–1702S.

58. Chung F, Weisburger J H. Mechanisms of chronic disease causation by nutritional factors and tobacco products and their prevention by tea polyphenols. *Food Chem Toxicol* 2002; 40: 1145–1154.

59. Bedoui J E, Oak M-H, Schini-Kerth V B. Antiangiogenic properties of natural polyphenols from red wine and green tea. *J Nutr Biochem* 2005; 16: 1–8.

60. Imai K, Suga K, Nakachi K. Cancer-preventive effects of drinking green tea among a Japanese population. *Prevent Med* 1997; 26: 769–775.

61. Imai K, Matsuyama S, Miyake S *et al*. Preventive effects of drinking green tea

on cancer and cardiovascular disease: epidemiological evidence for multiple targeting prevention. *BioFactors* 2000; 13: 49–54.

62. Gao Y, Lee M, Ross R *et al.* Urinary tea polyphenols in relation to gastric and esophageal cancers: a prospective study of men in Shangai, China. *Carcinogenesis* 2002; 23: 1497–1503.

63. Fukao A, Hisamichi S, Hsieh C *et al.* Green tea and the risk of gastric cancer in Japan. *N Engl J Med* 2001; 344: 632–636.

64. Blot W, Chow W, Dai Q *et al.* Green tea consumption and the risk of pancreatic and colorectal cancers. *Int J Cancer* 1997; 70: 255–258.

65. Goldblatt P, Kinlen L, Willows A, Yudkin J. Tea consumption and cancer. *Br J Cancer* 1988; 58: 397–401.

66. Albanes D, Hartman T, Malila N *et al.* Tea and coffee consumption and risk of colon cancer and rectal cancer in middle-aged Finnish men. *Nutr Cancer* 1998; 31: 41–48.

67. Huang C-H, Huang J-K, Hsieh C-C *et al.* Tea consumption: fluid intake and bladder cancer risk in southern Taiwan. *Urology* 1999; 54: 823–828.

68. Fujiki H, Imai K, Nakachi K, Suganuma M. Green tea: cancer preventive beverage and/or drug. *Cancer Lett* 2002; 188: 9–13.

69. Arab L, Il'yasova D. The epidemiology of tea consumption and colorectal cancer incidence. *J Nutr* 2003; 133: 3310S–3318S.

70. Agarwal S, Brown S, Chow H *et al.* Effects of increased tea consumption on oxidative DNA damage among smokers: a randomised controlled study. *J Nutr* 2003; 133: 3303S–3309S.

71. Pisters K M, Newman R A, Coldman B *et al.* Phase I trial of oral green tea extract in adult patients with solid tumours. *J Clin Oncol* 2001; 19: 1830–1838.

72. Giovannucci E. A review of epidemiologic studies of tomatoes, lycopene, and prostate cancer. *Exp Biol Med* 2002; 227: 852–859.

73. Hadley C, Miller E, Schwartz S, Clitons S. Tomatoes, lycopene, and prostate cancer: progress and promise. *Exp Biol Med* 2002; 227: 869–880.

74. King R J B. What is cancer? In: *Cancer Biology*, 2nd edn. Harlow, UK: Pearson Education Limited, 2000: 1–7.

75. Cohen L. A review of animal model studies of tomato carotenoids, lycopene, and cancer chemoprevention. *Exp Biol Med* 2002; 227: 864–868.

76. Nishino H, Murakoshi M, Ii T, Takemura M *et al.* Carotenoids in cancer chemoprevention. *Cancer Metastasis Rev* 2002; 21: 257–264.

77. Vecchia C. Tomatoes, lycopene intake, and digestive tract and female hormone-related neoplasams. *Exp Biol Med* 2002; 227: 860–863.

78. Arab L, Steck-Scott S, Fleishauer A. Lycopene and the lung. *Exp Biol Med* 2002; 227: 894–899.

79. Etminan M, Takkouche B, Caamano-Isorna F. The role of tomato products and lycopene in the prevention of prostate cancer: A meta-analysis of observational studies. *Cancer Epidemiol Biomarker Prev* 2004; 13: 340–345.

80. Kucuk O, Sarkar F, Djouric Z *et al.* Effects of lycopene supplementation in patients with localized prostate cancer. *Exp Biol Med* 2002; 227: 881–885.

81. Giovannucci E, Ascherio A, Rimm E B *et al.* Intake of carotenoids and retinol in relation to risk of prostate cancer. *J Natl Cancer Inst* 1995; 87: 1767–1776.

82. Bowen P, Chen L, Stacewicz-Sapuntzakis M *et al.* Tomato sauce supplementation and prostate cancer: Lycopene accumulation and modulation of biomarkers of carcinogenesis. *Exp Biol Med* 2002; 227: 886–893.

83. Wang L, Chen J, Thompson L U. The inhibitory effect of flaxseed on the growth and metastasis of estrogen receptor negative human breast cancer xenografts is attributed to both its lignan and oil components. *Int J Cancer* 2005; 116: 793–798.

84. Pietinen P, Stumpf K, Mannisto S *et al.* Serum enterolactone and risk of breast cancer: a case-control study in eastern Finland. *Cancer Epidemiol Biomarker Prev* 2001; 10: 339–344.

85. Saarinen N, Makela S, Santti R. Mechanism of anticancer effects of lignans with a special emphasis on breast cancer. In: Thompson L U, Cunnane S C., eds. *Flaxseed in Human Nutrition*, 2nd edn. Champaign, IL: AOCS Press, 2003: 223–231.

86. Chen J, Hui E, Ip T, Thompson L U. Dietary flaxseed enhances the inhibitory effect of tamoxifen on the growth of estrogen-dependent human breast cancer (MCF-7) in nude mice. *Clin Cancer Res* 2004; 10: 7703–7711.

87. Thompson, L U. Flaxseed, lignans and cancer. In: Thompson L U, Cunnane S C, eds. *Flaxseed in Human Nutrition*. Champaign, IL: AOCS Press, 1995: 219–236.

88. Donaldson M S. Nutrition and cancer: A review of the evidence for an anticancer diet. *Nutr J* 2004; 3 pp. (e-journal).

89. van de Poll L. Phytoestrogens: health benefits, bioavailability and safety. *Agro Food Ind Hi-Tech* 2004; 15: 9–11.

90. Glauert H. Dietary fatty acids and cancer. In: Chow C, ed. *Fatty Acids in Foods and their Health Implications*, 2nd edn. New York: Marcel Dekker, 2000: 865–881.

91. Brouwer I, Katan M, Zock P. Dietary α-linolenic acid is associated with reduced risk of fatal coronary heart disease, but increased prostate cancer risk: a meta-analysis. *J Nutr* 2004; 134: 919–922.

92. Bougnoux P. *n*-3 Polyunsaturated fatty acids and cancer. *Curr Opin Clin Nutr Care* 1999; 2: 121–125.

93. MacLean C H, Newberry S J, Mojica W A *et al.* Effects of omega-3 fatty acids on cancer risk: a systematic review. *JAMA* 2006; 295: 403–415.

94. Portakal O, Ozkaya O, Inal M E *et al.* Coenzyme Q10 concentrations and antioxidant status in tissues of breast cancer patients. *Clin Biochem* 2000; 33: 279–284.

95. Roffe L, Schmidt K, Ernst E. Efficacy of coenzyme Q10 for improved tolerability of cancer treatments: a systematic review. *J Clin Oncol* 2004; 22: 4418–4424.

96. Lockwood K, Moesgaard S, Folkers K. Partial and complete regression of breast cancer in patients in relation to dosage of coenzyme Q10. *Biochem Biophys Res Commun* 1994; 199: 1504–1508.

97. Jolliet P, Simon N, Barre J *et al.* Plasma coenzyme Q10 concentrations in breast cancer. Prognosis and therapeutic consequences. *Int J Clin Pharmacol Ther* 1998; 36: 506–509.

98. Tamarkin L, Danforth D, Lichter A *et al.* Decreased nocturnal plasma

melatonin peak in patients with estrogen receptor positive breast cancer. *Science* 1982; 216: 1003–1005.

99. Schernhammer E S, Schulmeister K. Melatonin and cancer risk: does light at night compromise physiologic cancer protection by lowering serum melatonin levels? *Br J Cancer* 2004; 90: 941–943.

100. Megdal S P, Kroenke C H, Laden F *et al*. Night work and breast cancer risk: a systematic review and meta-analysis. *Eur J Cancer* 2005; 41: 2023–2032.

101. Mills E, Wu P, Seely D, Guyatt G. Melatonin in the treatment of cancer: a systematic review of randomized controlled trials and meta-analysis. *J Pineal Res* 2005; 39: 360–366.

102. Tomas-Zapico C, Coto-Montes A. A proposed mechanism to explain the stimulatory effect of melatonin on antioxidative enzymes. *J Pineal Res* 2005; 39: 99–104.

103. Trubiani O, Recchioni R, Moroni F *et al*. Melatonin provokes cell death in human B-lymphoma cells by mitochondrial-dependent apoptotic pathway activation. *J Pineal Res* 2005; 39: 425–431.

104. Haldar, C. Apoptosis, cancer, immunity and melatonin. In: Haldar C, Singaravel M, Maitra S K, eds. *Treatise on Pineal Gland and Melatonin*. Enfield, NH: Science Publishers, 2002: 535–542.

105. Maestroni G J M. The photoperiod transducer melatonin and the immune-hematopoietic system. *J Photochem Photobiol B: Biol* 1998; 43: 186–192.

106. Lissoni P, Barni S, Mandala M *et al*. Decreased toxicity and increased efficacy of cancer chemotherapy using the pineal hormone melatonin in metastatic solid tumor patients with poor clinical status. *Eur J Cancer* 1999; 35: 1688–1692.

107. Lissoni P, Chilelli M, Villa S *et al*. Five years survival in metastatic non-small cell lung cancer patients treated with chemotherapy alone or chemotherapy and melatonin: a randomized trial. *J Pineal Res* 2003; 35: 12–15.

108. Lissoni P, Paolorossi, F, Tancini G *et al*. Is there a role for melatonin in the treatment of neoplastic cachexia? *Eur J Cancer A* 1996; 32A: 1340–1343.

109. Hrushesky W J M. Melatonin cancer therapy. *Pineal Gland Cancer* 2001; 476–508.

110. Sauer L A, Dauchy R T, Blask D E. Polyunsaturated fatty acids, melatonin, and cancer prevention. *Biochem Pharmacol* 2001; 61: 1455–1462.

111. Sakano K, Oikawa S, Hiraku Y, Kawanishi S. Oxidative DNA damage induced by a melatonin metabolite, 6-hydroxymelatonin, via a unique non-*o*-quinone type of redox cycle. *Biochem Pharmacol* 2004; 68: 1869–1878.

112. Vijayalaxmi, Reiter R J, Tan D-X *et al*. Melatonin as a radioprotective agent: a review. *Int J Radiation Oncol Biol Physic* 2004; 59: 639–653.

113. Park H S, Cho H Y, Ha Y L, Park J H Y. Dietary conjugated linoleic acid increases the mRNA ratio of Bax/Bcl-2 in the colonic mucosa of rats. *J Nutr Biochem* 2004; 15: 229–235.

114. Belury M A. Inhibition of carcinogenesis by conjugated linoleic acid: potential mechanisms of action. *J Nutr* 2002; 132: 2995–2998.

115. Kim J-H, Hubbard N E, Ziboh V, Erickson K L. Attenuation of breast tumor cell growth by conjugated linoleic acid via inhibition of 5-lipoxygenase activating protein. *Biochim Biophys Acta, Mol Cell Biol Lipid* 2005; 1736: 244–250.

116. Kritchevsky D, Pariza M W. Conjugated linoleic acid as a tumor preventive agent. In: Kelloff G J, Hawk E T, Sigman C C, eds. *Cancer Chemoprevention*, Vol 1: *Promising Cancer Chemoprevention Agents*. Totowa, NJ: Humana Press, 2004: 583–589.

117. Pariza M W, Park Y, Cook M E. Conjugated linoleic acid and the control of cancer and obesity. *Toxicol Sci* 1999; 52: 107–110.

118. Banni S, Angioni E, Casu V *et al*. Decrease in linoleic acid metabolites as a potential mechanism in cancer risk reduction by conjugated linoleic acid. *Carcinogenesis* 1999; 20: 1019–1024.

119. Lee K W, Lee H J, Cho H Y, Kim Y J. Role of the conjugated linoleic acid in the prevention of cancer. *Crit Rev Food Sci Nutr* 2005; 45: 135–144.

120. Palombo J D, Ganguly A, Bistrian B R, Menard M P. The antiproliferative effects of biologically active isomers of conjugated linoleic acid on human colorectal and prostatic cancer cells. *Cancer Lett* 2002; 177: 163–172.

121. Ochoa J J, Farquharson A J, Grant I *et al*. Conjugated linoleic acids (CLAs) decrease prostate cancer cell proliferation: different molecular mechanisms for cis-9, trans-11 and trans-10, cis-12 isomers. *Carcinogenesis* 2004; 25: 1185–1191.

122. Tanmahasamut P, Liu J, Hendry L B, Sidell N. Conjugated linoleic acid blocks estrogen signaling in human breast cancer cells. *J Nutr* 2004; 134: 674–680.

123. Drouin G, Douillette A, Lacasse P P B. Radiosensitizing effect of conjugated linoleic acid against breast cancer cells MCF-7 and MDA-MB-231. *Can J Physiol Pharmacol* 2004; 82: 94–102.

11

Nutraceuticals and bone health

Our skeletons provide us with a strong yet light protective framework, due to a unique structure comparable to reinforced concrete. It is not merely an inert material, however, but a highly dynamic metabolic reservoir of calcium ions containing 99% of the total body calcium content.[1]

There are two main types of bone in the skeleton based on their microscopic architecture. Cortical bone is hard and dense, and forms the shafts of the long bones which bear most of the body's weight. Cancellous or trabecular bone is found at the ends of the long bones and in the vertebrae and pelvis. This has a honeycomb-like structure, with plates known as trabeculae arranged in such a way as to provide resistance to forces. There is also a larger internal surface area and more blood supply than for cortical bone, which means it has a greater involvement in calcium homeostasis.

Bone consists of an organic phase (matrix) and an inorganic mineral phase together with a highly diverse population of cells responsible for its development and maintenance. The matrix is composed of structural proteins, collagen and mucopolysaccharides, which provide resistance and flexibility. The main mineral present is hydroxyapatite (crystalline calcium phosphate) which is responsible for the rigidity and compressibility of bone.

Bone growth (modelling) begins in fetal development and continues to the age of 25–40 years when peak bone mass is said to be attained.[2] During puberty there is an accelerated period of growth where most of this mass is laid down. The timing and nature of this process is initially dictated by genetic factors, followed by environmental factors in adulthood which are described below.

After modelling there follows a process of consolidation known as remodelling, which is necessary to allow the skeleton to respond to external forces and maintain body mineral levels. There is continued restructuring at up to 10% of existing bone per year[3] at sites known as bone multicellular units (BMUs). BMUs consist of teams of osteoblasts and osteoclasts acting in a coordinated fashion under the influence of numerous cellular factors. The resorption process follows a clear series of stages lasting approximately 100 days.[2] First, osteoclasts initiate remodelling through specific activation of their membrane receptors. They attach to internal bone surfaces and secrete protons and enzymes which degrade and release minerals from the tissue. Second, osteoblasts replace the resorbed material with immature matrix protein (osteoid) which later becomes mineralised.

The factors necessary to coordinate the activities of osteoblasts and osteoclasts include calcium availability, mechanical forces experienced by the skeleton, and autocrine, paracrine and endocrine factors. The last category is of particular significance once peak bone mass is attained.

Endocrine factors are released into the systemic circulation and have a generalised effect on the skeleton. Parathyroid hormone (PTH) is a peptide hormone secreted in response to low concentrations of serum calcium and directly enhances osteoclast activation via interaction with a membrane receptor. This stimulates resorption and release of free calcium ions to restore the imbalance. Vitamin D is obtained from the diet and is synthesised in the skin by the action of ultraviolet light; it acts by increasing intestinal calcium absorption and promoting osteoclast resorption. Calcitonin is a peptide hormone that inhibits the action of osteoclasts in response to elevated serum calcium levels. Growth hormone (GH) promotes the synthesis of collagen and other bone proteins by osteoblasts. Oestrogens such as oestradiol are thought to be important in maintaining bone mass in women, and are thought to act by inhibiting paracrine factors that promote bone resorption (see below). Androgens such as testosterone have a similar role to oestrogens in men, and also contribute to the sudden growth spurt at puberty.[1]

Autocrine and paracrine factors are secreted by cells present within bone tissue and have more localised targets of action. Prostaglandins derive from membrane lipid precursors and are thought to be the main local mediators of bone metabolism. Prostaglandins E_1 and E_2 (PGE_1, PGE_2) both act through their binding to various membrane receptors, and their effects are also mediated through cytokines known as insulin-like growth factors (IGF). PGE_1 is made constitutively through the action of the enzyme cyclooxygenase-1 (COX-1) in many tissues and is thought to increase bone formation, inhibit osteoclasts and promote calcium uptake.

PGE_2 is synthesised by the COX-2 isoenzyme in response to factors released during inflammation, and can inhibit bone formation and promote osteoclast activity. This may be through promoting expression of IGF. Cytokines and growth factors are peptides secreted by osteoblasts and other cells, and have both inhibitory and stimulatory effects on bone remodelling. Examples of these cytokines include inter-leukin-1 (IL-1) and tumour necrosis factor alpha (TNF-α).[4]

The effects of both local and systemic molecules are ultimately mediated by transcription factors. Osteoblasts are thought to initially secrete an osteoclast-differentiation factor following stimulation by vitamin D or PTH. This factor (known as 'receptor activator of nuclear factor-kappa' or the RANK ligand) is a transmembrane protein which specifically binds to a RANK receptor on the immature osteoclast membrane and promotes its maturation. Opposing this action is a second protein known as osteoprotegerin (OPG), also secreted by the osteoblast, which inhibits the differentiation of osteoclasts through binding and blocking of the RANK ligand.

In addition to the RANK/OPG system, another potential transcription factor mechanism has been identified, known as core binding factor alpha-1 which promotes expression of genes in osteoblasts necessary for their development from marrow precursor cells. This factor is thought to be more active during fetal and childhood development.[5]

BMUs are thus tightly regulated to prevent overall changes in bone mass, but this can be lost with ageing or disease. Up to peak mass formation 100% of the BMUs are active, followed by a gradual decline in bone strength and increasing porosity due to reduced activity at each BMU, resulting in reduction with age by 30% in men and 50% in women.[3] This can lead to the most prevalent disease affecting bone, osteoporosis.

Osteoporosis

Osteoporosis literally means 'porous bones' and is defined as a progressive, systemic skeletal disease that leads to loss of bone and its microscopic structure.[1] The consequences of this are reduced strength and an increased risk of low-impact fracture. This can lead to associated complications of mortality, morbidity and reduced quality of life. The three most common sites of fracture are due to their having the greatest proportion of cancellous bone, namely the hip (femoral neck), lumbar vertebrae and the forearm/wrist. Hip fractures are clinically the most serious and require very long stays in hospital.[3] Osteoporosis is a clinically silent condition whose prevalence increases with age (seen in up to 70% of people over 80[3]), and which often evades diagnosis until a fracture occurs.

With increasing life expectancy in the West, osteoporosis looks set to become increasingly prevalent. The World Health Organization (WHO) has estimated that over 75 million osteoporotic fractures will occur per year by 2025 in Europe, Japan and the USA.[3] The disease therefore represents a significant financial burden to healthcare systems in terms of secondary care for fractures and long-term primary and social care, with current estimated costs to the National Health Service in the UK estimated at £5 million per day.[6]

Aetiology

Besides advancing age, with a corresponding decline in osteoblast activity and reduced calcium absorption and retention, there are a number of other risk factors for osteoporosis. Women have a lower peak bone mass than men and generally live longer, and so have a longer period of bone loss. Combined with the effects of the menopause described below, this results in primary osteoporosis being three times more common in women than in men.[3] During the menopause, which occurs in women between the ages of 45 and 55, there is a period of accelerated bone loss (2–3% per year) before it returns to the same rate as men (0.25–1% per year).[2] This is due to a decline in oestrogen levels, favouring bone resorption over formation. There can be a difference in bone mass of up to 5% between men and women over the age of 60.[1]

Diets low in calcium, vitamin D or high in animal protein can increase the risk of osteoporosis. Though protein is necessary in the diet, a large intake of animal-derived protein containing large quantities of acidic/sulfurous amino acids will interfere with renal calcium reabsorption. Smoking is also a significant risk factor for osteoporosis. Toxic free radicals in cigarette smoke interfere with the blood supply to bone and directly damage osteoblasts. In women, smoking can reduce active oestrogen levels and promote an earlier onset of menopause.

Alcohol has both direct and indirect toxic effects on bone formation by directly inhibiting osteoblast activity and interfering with the balance of cytokine activity. Excessive alcohol consumption is becoming an increasingly prevalent problem in the form of binge drinking, particularly in young women, and increases the risk of osteoporosis later in life.

There are a number of drug-related risk factors for osteoporosis: corticosteroids are strongly associated with osteoporosis and increased fracture risk, particularly at vertebrae.[6] They mediate their effects via osteoblast receptors, and can reduce their activity and bone mineral content within months of their initiation.[3] They can also cause adrenal suppression which reduces oestrogen and androgen synthesis, and consequently exacerbate the situation.

Prevention and treatment

Due to its slow onset over many years, much of the focus on osteoporosis therapy is concerned with prevention from a young age rather than active treatment. Prevention aims to promote a larger peak bone mass in youth and slow the rate of bone loss with age, unlike treatment to prevent fractures or further fracture after diagnosis. These measures ideally need to be adopted from childhood and include a balanced diet and adequate exercise. A balanced diet, including adequate levels of calcium, vitamin D and protein is essential. A diet generally lacking in any essential requirements can lead to malnutrition, oestrogen deficiencies in women and direct loss of bone mass in both sexes. Adequate exercise is required, including regular weight-bearing exercise at least three times a week from a young age. Mechanical forces on the bones stimulate bone formation and help build up a greater peak bone mass. In older people exercise can help reduce the rate of bone loss, although the level of activity should be realistically tailored to capacity with increasing age.

A number of nutraceuticals have been used to improve bone health, including melatonin, carnitine, polyunsaturated fattys acids (PUFAs), conjugated linoleic acid (CLA) and phytoestrogens from soy and flax.

Melatonin

Melatonin is synthesised by the pineal gland in a cyclical fashion over 24 hours, with most released during the hours of darkness (5–25 µg secreted daily[7]). One of the main roles of this hormone is to regulate the sleep–wake cycle (see Chapter 10) in response to changes in daylight detected by the retina.

There is also variation in the total amount of melatonin found in the body over the lifespan, the greatest quantities being found around ages 1–3 years followed by a rapid decline by old age.[7] It is for this reason that melatonin has been implicated as a protective nutraceutical against degenerative conditions associated with old age, including osteoporosis. Bone formation/resorption cycles are also thought to follow a circadian pattern which might in part be modulated by the cyclical secretion of melatonin.

Melatonin occurs naturally in various fruits and vegetables, although only in very small quantities compared with those in the human body As a consequence, impractically large quantities of melatonin-containing foods would have to be eaten in order to obtain significant physiological concentrations.

In vitro research has suggested that the primary modes of action of melatonin is as an antioxidant that neutralises the action of toxic free radicals which cause cellular damage.[8] As it is a highly lipophilic molecule it is able to readily penetrate lipid membranes of cells and exert its effects on intracellular enzymes, such as through inhibition of oxidases. The relevance of this to bone health is that osteoclasts utilise oxygen radicals including superoxide, hydroxyl and peroxyl to initiate the resorption of bone matrix, and so melatonin may halt this activity.[1]

Another mechanism of melatonin may be its binding to various intracellular receptors relevant to bone cell regulation and physiology. A number of *in vitro* and animal studies have been carried out that support this function. Melatonin may itself have a local hormone action on bone, as there is evidence for its synthesis by both rat and human bone marrow cells.[9,10] High concentrations of both melatonin and enzymes involved in its synthesis have been found in cultures of rat osteoblast precursors.[11]

Application of exogenous melatonin to these types of cell lines led to their differentiation into fully mature osteoblasts which secreted measurable amounts of bone formation markers such as osteocalcin. A similar action was observed *in vitro* in human osteoblast cultures in a dose-related manner, together with increased secretion of bone collagen precursors. Melatonin may therefore act in a paracrine manner through modulation of the RANK ligand/OPG receptor–ligand signalling pathways that link osteoblast and osteoclast activities described above.

There have also been studies investigating the effects of melatonin in whole animals. Providing four-week-old mice with exogenous melatonin led to significant increases in bone mineral density (36%) and thickness of trabeculae (19%), together with reduction in serum markers of bone resorption compared with a control group.[13] Therefore melatonin may act by inhibiting resorption rather than promoting formation.

The effects of melatonin on bone may also be mediated through the presence or absence of oestrogens, particularly as there is a decline in melatonin levels following the menopause. A number of studies have investigated this effect further by measuring melatonin effects in ovariectomised (OVX) rodents, which serve as a model of the human postmenopausal state.

A detailed study then examined how melatonin influenced bone metabolism markers and bone mineral density in OVX mice in the presence or absence of oestrogen supplementation.[15] In some cases melatonin augmented the effects of oestrogen in OVX mice with regard to lowering of urine deoxypyrolidine, serum phosphate and serum alkaline phosphatase. Oestradiol and melatonin together also reduced the loss of bone mineral density seen after OVX to a greater extent than either given alone. It therefore appears from this study that melatonin may require a certain quantity of oestrogens in order to maximise its bone-protecting action.[15]

GH is implicated in bone formation, particularly in longitudinal growth during childhood and adolescence through promotion of cartilage synthesis and bone cell precursor differentiation. In one study eight young male volunteers were administered doses of 0.05, 0.5 and 5 mg of melatonin, and serum GH levels were measured at regular intervals for up to 150 minutes afterwards. Compared with a group receiving placebo, GH levels were found to increase for doses of 0.5 mg melatonin and greater.[16]

As yet, the mode of action of melatonin is unclear. It may be through a direct paracrine effect on bone cells as a free radical scavenger or via receptors. Alternatively it may be via indirect effects through modulating the action of systemic hormones with known roles in bone metabolism, including oestrogens and GH.

Melatonin appears to have minimal toxicity at standard doses of 0.3–15 mg daily.[7] Its potential as a nutraceutical for bone health warrants further study, particularly in clinical trials.

L-Carnitine

L-Carnitine acts as a cofactor in the oxidative metabolism of fatty acids. It is synthesised in the kidney and liver, and is found in the greatest quantities in skeletal and cardiac muscle. It can also be obtained from the diet from meat and dairy produce, with typical intakes being 100–200 μmol daily.[7]

With ageing there is gradual decline in the ability to efficiently generate energy necessary for anabolic processes, including the protein-synthesising activity of osteoblasts. L-Carnitine is necessary as a carrier molecule for the transport of acyl and acetyl groups from fatty acids across the mitochondrial membrane. There is evidence of a decline in both the total levels of this molecule in muscle tissue and also its carrier activity with advancing age, which suggests its link with senile reduction in bone synthesis.[17]

Endogenous dehydroepiandrosterone (DHEA) is thought to affect levels of L-carnitine through promoting the expression of carnitine-synthesising enzymes.[18]

An *in vitro* study on cultured pig osteoblast-like cells examined the action of L-carnitine and DHEA on fatty acid oxidation and osteoblast activation.[18] Cells treated with high concentrations of L-carnitine (with or without DHEA) were found to have evidence of increased oxidative respiration and markers of bone formation, namely collagen and alkaline phosphatase. However, the concentrations of L-carnitine necessary to induce these changes were considerably greater than those known to occur naturally in tissues, which suggest that there may be additional factors *in vivo* that are needed for its efficient use.

In vitro studies of human osteoblast cell cultures have investigated a second mechanism for L-carnitine involvement in bone metabolism, based on the expression of insulin-like growth factor-I (IGF-I).[17] IGF is one of the paracrine factors which mediates osteoblast differentiation and proliferation. Its effects are further fine-tuned via its binding to IGF-binding proteins (IGFBPs). So far, up to six of these proteins have been identified as being expressed in bone tissue, each having different effects on IGF and suggesting a highly sophisticated mechanism of regulation. For example binding to IGFBP-2 inactivates IGFs and leads to decreased osteoblast function, whereas IGFBP-3 binding enhances IGF actions.

Administration of L-carnitine or an isovalyl fumarate derivative to the osteoblasts may have influenced function through altering IGFBP expression, measured as an increase in mRNA levels. The main changes were found to be an increase in IGFBP-3 mRNA (an activator of IGF action) and decrease in IGFBP-5 expression (an inhibitor of IGF action). L-Carnitine and its derivative were therefore both able to stimulate osteoblast proliferation (measured as an increase in markers of bone formation, including collagen), although the isovalyl form was found to be more efficient, showing a maximal effect at concentrations ten-fold less than those of carnitine.

The studies described have only investigated *in vitro* models and so their findings are of limited value in terms of the use of L-carnitine and DHEA as supplements for bone health. L-Carnitine is used medically, however, at doses of up to 400 mg/kg daily in cases of carnitine deficiency with few serious side-effects.[7]

Polyunsaturated fatty acids

Dietary fat intake, predominantly from saturated fatty acid sources commonly found in animal fats, is thought to be detrimental to bone mineral density, leading to a greater risk of fracture. A recent epidemiological study of almost 15 000 people (the NHANES III trial[19]) found an inverse relationship between bone mineral density and fat intake in postmenopausal women, and a further study found a similar relationship with fracture risk.[20]

There is evidence from intervention studies that providing supplements of unsaturated fatty acids can prevent loss in bone mineral density. Elderly women with established osteoporosis were provided with a γ-linolenic acid (GLA), eicosapentaenoic acid (EPA) and docosahexaenoic acid (DHA) supplement. When compared with a control group receiving coconut oil (containing saturated fatty acids) there was reduced bone loss at the spine and hip.

Animal models have also suggested that n-3 and n-6 PUFAs may have a beneficial effect on bone strength, although if given in excess were found to lead to bone marrow damage through oxidation (DHA supplements)[21] and loss of bone strength in ageing rats (GLA supplements).[19] This suggests that optimal concentrations of PUFAs may differ with stages of the life cycle.

There are a number of postulated mechanisms as to how PUFA supplements may promote bone health. PUFAs constitute part of the structures of lipid bilayers of cell membranes and can be enzymatically converted into important mediators of inflammation and bone metabolism, notably the prostanoids.

As components of lipid bilayers, certain PUFAs may influence the structure and function of intestinal brush borders and membranes of kidney tubules. As a consequence this may have an impact on calcium absorption from the gut and renal reabsorption from the urine. One study found that providing fish oil supplements altered intestinal membrane structure such that calcium absorption was enhanced.[22] An increase in n-6:n-3 PUFA intake ratio may have a negative effect on bone formation due to an increase in PGE_2 over PGE_1 formation, resulting in increased bone resorption through the mechanisms described above. In recent times there has been a gradual substitution of saturated animal fats for polyunsaturated plant oils in foods, although many of these substitutes are of the n-6 rather than n-3 type. This means that many diets at present have an n-6:n-3 imbalance by up to 30 times in favour of n-6, which may also be detrimental to health. As a result there is a suggestion that eating PUFA-rich oils (found in large quantities in fish oils and flaxseed) may help to re-address this imbalance and promote bone formation.

PUFAs, in particular DHA and EPA, can block the formation of PGE_2 through competition with arachidonic acid for their synthetic enzyme COX-2. Studies of their direct effects on *in vitro* cultures of bone cells showed evidence of reduced osteoclast differentiation and bone resorption. In addition, EPA-treated osteoblasts were found to promote alkaline phosphatase enzyme expression.[5] Studies in intact animal models have further supported this role, with evidence of increased bone formation markers seen in rats[26] and piglets[25] fed *n*-3 PUFAs.

Studies have been carried out *in vitro* to examine the effects of PUFAs and their derivatives on Cbfa-1 expression, which is involved in fetal bone development.[23] Cultured osteoblast-like cells from rat fetuses when treated with arachidonic acid and EPA demonstrated an increase in expression probably mediated through prostaglandins.

As in the case of melatonin there have also been studies on OVX-treated rats, where it was found that an EPA supplement administered for 35 days arrested the decline in bone strength due to lack of oestrogens, even at minimal calcium levels.[27] These results also suggest there may be a synergistic interaction of *n*-3 PUFAs with oestrogen in preventing bone loss, possibly via the transcription factor mechanism described above. This suggests that *n*-3 PUFAs may be of value as post-menopausal supplements.

It is also thought that *n*-6 GLA supplementation may be of benefit for elderly people by favouring formation of PGE_1 in favour of PGE_2. The reason for this is that the higher levels of GLA shift fatty acid metabolism toward PGE_1 formation in favour of arachidonic acid and PGE_2, since the synthetic desaturase enzyme of the latter step has a low activity. There is also evidence from rat studies that a second enzyme involved in conversion of linoleic acid to GLA shows reduced activity with age and therefore can lead to less PGE_1 formation.[28]

Certain fatty acids may also exert their effects via GH. In addition to acting as a promoter of bone formation, GH can also stimulate the breakdown of body fat stores, leading to a raised serum free fatty acid concentration. A diet rich in fats may have a negative feedback effect on GH secretion, which was found experimentally in humans given high fat meals over 28 weeks,[29] and so may in turn lead to reduction in bone formation, especially as its levels are already low in the elderly.

PUFAs may promote bone health, either directly through influencing the metabolism of prostanoid precursors involved in bone homeostasis, or indirectly via GH action.

However the situation is further complicated by the fact that different types of PUFA have differential effects, and that their effects may relate to age and development of the subject. Therefore more research is necessary to determine which fatty acids and what n-3 to n-6 ratio would provide maximal benefit as a nutraceutical supplement.

Conjugated linoleic acid

In vivo rat studies have investigated dietary supplements of CLA on bone mineralisation and markers of bone turnover. Overall, results showed an increase in overall bone mineral content measured as body ash content.[30]

It has been proposed that as with the case of n-3 PUFAs, CLA may affect the synthesis of prostaglandins through competition with n-6 PUFA substrates for COX-2, with reduction in formation of detrimental PGE_2. A study on human *in vitro* osteoblast-like cell lines confirmed significantly reduced PGE_2 and raised osteocalcin secretion,[31] although this effect depended on which specific isomeric form of CLA was administered. Reasons for differences in response to different isomers may relate to how they are metabolised and transported in the blood, therefore influencing how readily they can be taken up by bone tissue.

In a study in which rats were fed with CLA, it was shown to enhance calcium absorption by bone and this effect was enhanced if it was co-administered with n-3 PUFAs.[32] It therefore appears that age, dietary PUFA ratios and isomeric forms of CLA may be important factors in its effectiveness and therefore in its use as a nutraceutical.

In a randomised double-blind intervention trial of CLA versus a placebo in 60 healthy adult males (aged between 39 and 64 years), results showed no significant effect on a wide range of serum and urinary markers of bone metabolism. The lack of any meaningful findings was suggested as being due to use of a less active isomeric form of CLA, or that the doses used were much lower than those used in the above animal studies.

A double-blind study of adult type 2 diabetics using either CLA or n-6 PUFAs (derived from safflower) after eight weeks found a decrease in serum concentrations of the hormone leptin.[33] This is a CNS-secreted neuroendocrine factor with a central role in appetite and lipid metabolism, and is proposed as a local regulatory factor in bone-promoting osteoblast activity.

More studies are necessary to determine whether CLA has any potential effect on osteoblast or osteoclast functioning and whether it is of any value in bone health.

Soy isoflavones

The use of soy phytoestrogens to treat menopausal symptoms, including osteoporosis, has been recently reviewed,[34] and several large-scale epidemiological studies and clinical trials have been carried out in the area of bone health. The major dietary sources are soybean, which contains isoflavones, and flaxseed, which contains lignans.[35]

Soy isoflavones are thought to be most promising in their role as supplements in preventing and treating postmenopausal osteoporosis, because of their similarity in structure to oestradiol and therefore as potential replacements for oestrogen deficiency. As a result, most studies with phytoestrogens have restricted themselves to female subjects during or after the menopause.

These compounds are able to act as weak agonists at oestrogen receptors, specifically the beta type located on osteoblast membranes. As they are lipophilic molecules they can readily traverse cell membranes and bind to cytoplasmic ERs which go on to act as transcription factors. This leads to increased gene expression of alkaline phosphatases and osteocalcin (bone formation factors), OPG (an inhibitor of osteoclast activity) and IGF (a promoter of osteoblast activity), resulting in reduced bone resorption and increased bone formation. Their particular attractiveness over other forms of oestrogen replacement is that they have no activity at the alpha form of oestrogen receptors located in the breast and uterus, so have none of the adverse effects on these tissues associated with standard hormone replacement therapy (HRT).[36]

Experiments with cultures of osteoblast-like cells have found evidence of direct responses to administered isoflavones, although at levels much greater than would be obtained in a normal diet. Examples of the effects noted include increased alkaline phosphatase and collagen synthesis activity in mouse osteoblasts administered genestein or daidzein.[37] The positive effects of soy isoflavones in reducing the loss of bone mineral density (BMD) as well as in promoting bone formation over resorption have been reviewed.[38] Similar studies with female rats have shown that providing flax lignans in the diet was able to promote bone strength early in development.[39]

Epidemiological studies have shown strong evidence that soy isoflavones have a positive effect on BMD. These were borne out by the fact that far lower rates of osteoporosis and fractures have been observed in East Asian women compared with their Western counterparts even when corrected for height and weight. Soy has been part of the East Asian diet far longer than in the West, with daily soy protein consumption being significantly greater (55 g daily noted in Japanese women).[35]

A prospective cohort study of over 24 000 postmenopausal Chinese women aged 40–70 years used evidence of clinical fracture as the main measure of comparison with soy consumption, because it is considered more appropriate than markers of bone formation.[40] The main findings after a 4-year follow-up were that high soy intakes correlated with a significantly reduced risk of postmenopausal fractures, particularly in the first few postmenopausal years. This is of interest as this is where bone loss rates are thought to be greatest and suggests this to be the optimal time to use soy supplements.

Clinical intervention trials have also been carried out using isoflavone extracts and have demonstrated varying levels of significance. Reduction in loss of bone marrow density and changes in biochemical markers were variably reported.[34]

Most intervention studies focused on soy isoflavones, but one study attempted to compare soy isoflavones with flaxseed lignan supplementation in a group of 46 postmenopausal women over 16 weeks. They were randomly assigned a soy, flax or wheat placebo muffin daily.[41] Results found that only flax appeared to have significant effects on serum alkaline phosphatase concentrations. This may be explained by the fact that flaxseed oil is also a rich source of α-linolenic acid (ALA), one of the beneficial n-3 PUFAs associated with bone health described above.

Studies have attempted to determine which isoflavones in particular are likely to have the greatest effect in preventing bone loss, with many proposing genistein. However, an in vivo rat study has shown evidence that daidzein may be the most active.[42] This may, however, be mediated through its metabolism by the body. Following ingestion there is initial hydrolysis of their sugar moiety by enzymes of the intestinal brush border, enabling their ready absorption in to the bloodstream. Within peripheral tissues daidzein is enzymatically converted to equol, which has been demonstrated in rats to have twice the oestrogenic actions of its parent molecule.[43]

In addition to isoflavone content there may also be additional beneficial actions of soy protein in that it can replace animal sources in the diet. As described above, animal proteins interfere with the process of calcium reabsorption by the kidneys, and thus indirectly lead to reduced bone formation.

Further studies are therefore needed to determine beneficial doses of phytoestrogens, with current recommendations being 40–100 mg of isoflavones daily,[35] based on a standard East Asian dietary intake. It has been suggested that phytoestrogens may have adverse effects on the uterus and fertility in animals due to their oestrogen-like actions, although at the doses suggested they are thought to be safe.[44] Overall, phytoestrogens appear to show the most promise of all the nutraceuticals so far described, although they have only been investigated in pre- and postmenopausal osteoporosis.

Conclusions

Due to the shortcomings of current treatments for osteoporosis, there is a strong argument for patients taking a more active role either in preventing the onset of osteoporosis through healthy diet and exercise from a young age, or use of individualised nutraceutical therapies for prevention and treatment.

Although there is some promise being generated about the compounds considered in this chapter, prevention of osteoporosis still appears likely to be a better option than cure.[45]

References

1. Ferguson N. *Osteoporosis in Focus*, 1st edn. London: Pharmaceutical Press, 2004.
2. Tanna N. Osteoporosis and its treatment. *Pharm J* 2005; 275: 521–522.
3. World Health Organization Scientific Group on the Prevention and Management of Osteoporosis. *Prevention and Management of Osteoporosis: Report of a World Health Organization Scientific Group*. Geneva: WHO, 2003.
4. Goldring S R. Inflammatory mediators as essential elements in bone remodeling. *Calc Tissue Int* 2003; 73: 97–100.
5. Watkins B A, Li Y, Lippman H E, Feng S. Modulatory effect of omega-3 polyunsaturated fatty acids on osteoblast function and bone metabolism. *Prostaglandins Leukot Essent Fatty Acids* 2003; 68: 387–398.
6. National Osteoporosis Society. *What is Osteoporosis?* December 2005. http://www.nos.org.uk/osteo.asp (accessed 09 June 2006).
7. Rapport L, Lockwood B. *Nutraceuticals*, 1st edn. London: Pharmaceutical Press, 2002.
8. Cardinali D P, Ladizesky M G, Boggio V *et al*. Melatonin effects on bone: experimental facts and clinical perspectives. *J Pineal Res* 2003; 34: 81–87.
9. Conti A, Conconi S, Hertens E *et al*. Evidence for melatonin synthesis in mouse and human bone marrow cells. *J Pineal Res* 2000; 28: 193–202.
10. Tan D X, Manchester L C, Reiter R J *et al*. Identification of highly elevated levels of melatonin in bone marrow: its origin and significance. *Biochim Biophys Acta* 1999; 1472: 206–214.

11. Roth J A, Kim B G, Lin W L, Cho M I. Melatonin promotes osteoblast differentiation and bone formation. *J Biol Chem* 1999; 274: 22041–22047.
12. Fernandes G, Lawrence R, Sun D. Protective role of *n*-3 lipids and soy protein in osteoporosis. *Prostaglandins Leukot Essent Fatty Acids* 2003; 68: 361–372.
13. Koyama H, Nakade O, Takada Y *et al.* Melatonin at pharmacologic doses increases bone mass by suppressing resorption through down-regulation of the RANKL-mediated osteoclast formation and activation. *J Bone Mineral Res* 2002; 17: 1219–1229.
14. Suzuki N. Hattori A. Melatonin suppresses osteoclastic and osteoblastic activities in the scales of goldfish. *J Pineal Res* 2002; 33: 253–258.
15. Ladizesky M G, Boggio V, Albornoz L E *et al.* Melatonin increases estradiol-induced bone formation in ovariectomized rats. *J Pineal Res* 2003; 34: 143–151.
16. Forsling M L, Wheeler M J, Williams A J. The effect of melatonin administration on pituitary hormone secretion in man. *Clin Endocrinol* 1999; 51: 637–642.
17. Colucci S, Mori G, Vaira S *et al.* L-Carnitine and isovaleryl L-carnitine fumarate positively affect human osteoblast proliferation and differentiation in vitro. *Calcif Tissue Int* 2005; 76: 458–465.
18. Chiu K M, Keller E T, Crenshaw T D, Gravenstein S. Carnitine and dehydroepiandrosterone sulfate induce protein synthesis in porcine primary osteoblast-like cells. *Calcif Tissue Int* 1999; 64: 527–533.
19. Corwin R L. Effects of dietary fats on bone health in advanced age. *Prostaglandins Leukot Essent Fatty Acids* 2003; 68: 379–386.
20. Kato I, Toniolo P, Zeleniuch-Jacquotte A *et al.* Diet, smoking and anthropometric indices and postmenopausal bone fractures: a prospective study. *Int J Epidemiol* 2000; 29: 85–92.
21. Umegaki K, Hashimoto M, Yamasaki H *et al.* Docosahexaenoic acid supplementation-increased oxidative damage in bone marrow DNA in aged rats and its relation to antioxidant vitamins. *Free Radic Res* 2001; 34: 427–435.
22. Coetzer H, Claasen N, van-Papendorp D H, Kruger M C. Calcium transport by isolated brush border and basolateral membrane vesicles: role of essential fatty acid supplementation. *Prostaglandins Leukot Essent Fatty Acids* 1994; 50: 257–266.
23. Marie P J. Cellular and molecular alterations of osteoblasts in human disorders of bone formation. *Histol Histopathol* 1999; 14: 525–538.
24. Weiler H A, Fitzpatrick-Wong S C. Modulation of essential (*n*-6):(*n*-3) fatty acid ratios alters fatty acid status but not bone mass in piglets. *J Nutr* 2002; 132: 2667–2672.
25. Watkins B A, Li Y, Allen K G *et al.* Dietary ratio of (*n*-6)/(*n*-3) polyunsaturated fatty acids alters the fatty acid composition of bone compartments and biomarkers of bone formation in rats. *J Nutr* 2000; 130: 2274–2284.
26. Sakaguchi K, Morita I, Murota S. Eicosapentaenoic acid inhibits bone loss due to ovariectomy in rats. *Prostaglandins Leukot Essent Fatty Acids* 1994; 50: 81–84.
27. Lorenzini A, Bordoni A, Spano C *et al.* Age-related changes in essential fatty

acid metabolism in cultured rat heart myocytes. *Prostaglandins Leukot Essent Fatty Acids* 1997; 57: 143–147.

28. Bhathena S J, Berlin E, Judd J T *et al*. Effects of n3 fatty acids and vitamin E on hormones involved in carbohydrate and lipid metabolism in men. *Am J Clin Nutr* 1991; 54: 684–688.

29. Park Y, Albright K J, Liu W *et al*. Effect of conjugated linoleic acid on body composition in mice. *Lipids* 1997; 32: 853–858.

30. Cusack S, Jewell C, Cashman K D. The effect of conjugated linoleic acid on the viability and metabolism of human osteoblast-like cells. *Prostaglandins Leukot Essent Fatty Acids* 2005; 72: 29–39.

31. Kelly O, Cusack S, Jewell C, Cashman K D. The effect of polyunsaturated fatty acids, including conjugated linoleic acid, on calcium absorption and bone metabolism and composition in young growing rats. *Br J Nutr* 2003; 90: 743–750.

32. Doyle L, Jewell C, Mullen A *et al*. Effect of dietary supplementation with conjugated linoleic acid on markers of calcium and bone metabolism in healthy adult men. *Eur J Clin Nutr* 2005; 59: 432–440.

33. Belury M A, Mahon A, Banni S. The conjugated linoleic acid (CLA) isomer, t10c12-CLA, is inversely associated with changes in body weight and serum leptin in subjects with type 2 diabetes mellitus. *J Nutr* 2003; 133: 257S–260S.

34. Kotecha N, Lockwood B. Soy-relieving the symptoms of menopause and fighting osteoporosis. *Pharm J* 2005; 275: 483–487.

35. Jones M. Soya and osteoporosis. *NutraCos* 2003; 26–28.

36. Chen Y M, Ho S C, Lam S S, Ho S S *et al*. Soy isoflavones have a favorable effect on bone loss in Chinese postmenopausal women with lower bone mass: a double-blind, randomized, controlled trial. *J Clin Endocrinol Metab* 2003; 88: 4740–4747.

37. Dang Z C, Papapoulos S, Lowik C. Phytoestrogens enhance osteogenesis and concurrently inhibit adipogenesis. *J Nutr* 2002; 132: 617S.

38. Setchell K D, Lydeking-Olsen E. Dietary phytoestrogens and their effect on bone: evidence from in vitro and in vivo, human observational, and dietary intervention studies. *Am J Clin Nutr* 2003; 78: 593S–609S.

39. Ward W E, Yuan Y V, Cheung A M, Thompson L U. Exposure to purified lignan from flaxseed (*Linum usitatissimum*) alters bone development in female rats. *Br J Nutr* 2001; 86: 499–505.

40. Zhang X, Shu X O, Li H *et al*. Prospective cohort study of soy food consumption and risk of bone fracture among postmenopausal women. *Arch Intern Med* 2005; 165: 1890–1895.

41. Brooks J D, Ward W E, Lewis J E *et al*. Supplementation with flaxseed alters estrogen metabolism in postmenopausal women to a greater extent than does supplementation with an equal amount of soy. *Am J Clin Nutr* 2004; 79: 318–325.

42. Picherit C, Coxam V, Bennetau-Pelissero C *et al*. Daidzein is more efficient than genistein in preventing ovariectomy-induced bone loss in rats. *J Nutr* 2000; 130: 1675–1681.

43. Setchell K D. Absorption and metabolism of soy isoflavones-from food to dietary supplements and adults to infants. *J Nutr* 2000; 130: 654S–655S.

44.   Barnes S. Phyto-oestrogens and osteoporosis: what is a safe dose? *Br J Nutr* 2003; 89: S101–S108.
45.   Appleton D, Lockwood B. Building bones with nutraceuticals. *Pharm J* 2006; 277: 78–83.

12

Respiratory health

There are many diseases that affect the pulmonary system. The main disorders of respiratory function are asthma, chronic obstructive pulmonary disease (COPD), allergic rhinitis and cough. These disorders can result from a number of different factors, including changes to the airway smooth muscle tone, vascular congestion of the upper respiratory tract and/or mucus plugging. Airway smooth muscle tone affects the airway resistance and depends on the balance of various neuro-humoral efferent pathways.[1] In respiratory disorders the condition of the mucosa and the activity of the glands contribute towards increased airway resistance, with other mediators playing crucial roles.[2]

Complementary and alternative medicine (CAM) can be used alone or in conjunction with conventional treatment to treat a whole range of symptoms. A survey of practitioners in the USA that specifically addressed CAM and its use in asthma showed diet and nutritional approaches to be the most prevalent CAM therapies prescribed by both conventional physicians and CAM practitioners to asthmatic patients.[3] In recent years, many medical professionals have been approached by their patients, especially asthmatics, with claims of improvement in health due to these unorthodox practices. In a UK survey of CAM use by patients with asthma the majority of patients (59%) had tried at least one type of CAM treatment. Most patients, in particular those with severe asthma, perceived CAM treatments to be helpful and thought they could form an integral part of their therapy.[4] CAM is also used by 33% of children with asthma in the UK.[5] The major applications for nutraceuticals in this area are in asthma and COPD.

Asthma

A recent health review based on reports from the European Community Respiratory Health Survey of Asthma Prevalence in Adults and the International Study of Asthma and Allergies in Childhood[6] shows that the prevalence of asthma and other allergic disorders is increasing worldwide. Since 1980, asthma prevalence has increased dramatically, especially in children. Overall, asthma prevalence among people aged 0–17 years increased by approximately 5% each year from 1980 to 1995. Asthma affects ~4–5% of the population of developed countries. Among children, asthma is the most common chronic disease and leading cause of disability in the developed world, rseulting in frequent need for medical intervention.[7] There are many reasons underlying this current trend, including increased exposure to allergens and pollution, a predisposition to respiratory viral infections and a lack of exposure to microbial antigens during childhood.[8]

Polyunsaturated fatty acids

Polyunsaturated fatty acids (PUFAs) have a potential role in asthma because they are substrates for inflammatory mediators. *n*-3 and *n*-6 Fatty acids are metabolised through a common pathway and compete for acylation sites in cellular phospholipids. *n*-6 Fatty acids are converted to linoleic acid, which undergoes desaturation to become γ-linolenic acid (GLA). GLA is elongated to dihomo γ-linolenic acid (DGLA), which is desaturated to arachidonic acid. *n*-3 Fatty acids, on the other hand, are converted to α-linolenic acid (ALA), which then becomes stearidonic acid. This is converted into *n*-3 arachidonic acid and finally eicosapentaenoic acid (EPA), which is the precursor of docosahexaenoic acid (DHA).[9] Fatty acids need to be obtained from the diet because humans do not generally have the enzymatic capability to synthesise these essential nutrients directly.

There is growing evidence that an increase in *n*-6 and a decrease in *n*-3 fatty acids in the diet may have led to an increase in allergic sensitisation, which may in turn account for changes in the prevalence of asthma. The anti-inflammatory properties of *n*-3 and the proinflammatory properties of *n*-6 fatty acids suggest that dietary trends have predisposed some individuals to inflammatory disorders.[10] It may be that the ratio of *n*-6:*n*-3, rather than the absolute amount, is the most important factor.

Epidemiological studies of various populations have shown that a high dietary intake of marine fatty acids or fish is associated with lower incidence of inflammatory diseases such as rheumatoid arthritis and asthma.[11,12] Inuit populations have a very high dietary intake of fish and a low incidence of inflammatory conditions. In the modern Western world diets are deficient in fish, which may have contributed to the increased prevalence of asthma. The active PUFA components of fish are thought to be *n*-3 fatty acids, EPA and DHA. An association between diet (consumption of fish more than once a week) and airway disease in children (reduced risk of developing airway hyperresponsiveness (AHR)) was explored in the light of these epidemiological studies. Diet was assessed using a food frequency questionnaire, which asked about the child's eating habits over that past year and if the child took any supplements. The extent of airway disease was assessed by respiratory symptoms and response to exercise. After adjusting for confounders such as sex, atopy and smoking in the household it was concluded that children who ate fresh, oily fish were at a significantly reduced risk of current asthma. Fish consumption may also prevent against developing asthma.[13]

A study of 1601 young adults was performed to find out whether people with and without asthma consumed different quantities of PUFAs. A number of methods, including respiratory and food frequency questionnaires (indirect markers of fat intake), skin prick testing, lung function tests and plasma fatty acid levels (direct markers) were used in this study. DGLA, an immediate precursor to arachidonic acid, was positively associated with current asthma. It is biologically plausible that the increased precursor pool is a risk factor for the promotion of asthmatic airway inflammation through the generation of proinflammatory mediators. It warrants further research, including intervention studies to determine a cause–effect relationship and to verify the role of fatty acids in asthma. This study found no association between *n*-3 intake and asthma, which has been suggested in other studies.[14]

In several countries there are regional differences in the prevalence of allergic disease. This can be associated with varied consumption of fatty acids. In Germany following reunification there was a lower incidence of atopic disease in the east and a higher lifetime prevalence of asthma in the west.[15] These findings suggest differences may be due to disparity in allergic sensitisation. In one study, the prevalence of the specific immunoglobulin E (IgE) to house dust mite was fivefold higher in Leuna in the west compared with Duisburg in the east.[16] These asthma prevalence studies need to be compared with those concerning food intake to determine if differences are due to diet. There are few studies of food intake in Germany prior to unification, but one project in relation to cardiovascular disease involved middle-aged men keeping a 3-day record of their food intake. It found that there was a much lower intake (35% compared with 67%) of PUFAs in the east because margarine was not readily available. The higher intake of linoleic acid in margarine may possibly be linked to a higher incidence of asthma in the west at the time of reunification.[17]

A study carried out in children that combined dietary manipulation and n-3 supplementation demonstrated a significant improvement in peak expiratory flow rate (PEFR) and asthma medication use.[18] It remains to be seen if these results can be replicated using different populations. The nutrients in our food interact with each other and thus provide better benefits when consumed in food rather than as isolated ingredients in supplements. Intervention studies have been carried out to determine the role of supplementation but the results are conflicting: some demonstrate the beneficial effects these supplements can have on the disease but others show no clinical improvement, despite known changes in inflammatory cell functions.[18] There are also difficulties in selecting the nature and duration of the intervention. Much of the interest surrounding n-3 supplements and their use in asthma began when the neutrophil was considered to have an important role in the pathogenesis of asthma. The most profound anti-inflammatory effects of these fatty acids are on neutrophil function and mediator generation. Currently, eosinophilis and mast cells are thought to be more important and n-3 PUFAs do not show evidence of having a significant effect on these.[19]

A Cochrane Review was carried out on several randomised controlled trials that used an n-3 PUFA supplement.[19] The beneficial effects of supplementation are controversial because data from these studies are conflicting. No overall consistent effect was found on any of the analysable outcomes: forced expiration volume per second (FEV_1), peak expiratory flow (PEF), asthma symptoms, medication use or bronchial hyperactivity. Nine different studies were analysed in this review: seven parallel design and two crossover studies. Four of the parallel studies and both crossover studies used PEF as a marker. When the parallel studies were combined, significant improvement in PEF was suggested, but it may have been the significant heterogeneity between the studies that caused this change. The two crossover studies also used asthma symptoms to monitor change in the condition. Both used an n-3 supplement and an olive oil placebo but only one study reported an improvement in symptoms, the other reported no change. Four of the parallel studies considered asthma medication use. When data from all the studies were pooled, no overall change occurred but one of these studies did demonstrate a significant decline in medication use.[18]

Another study used a supplement containing both EPA and GLA. This was a double-blind, randomised, controlled trial of 29 children with bronchial asthma in a long-term treatment hospital. This strictly controlled environment minimised the effects of environmental allergens and diet. This study also ran for a longer period than most trials, covering a 10-month period. Many beneficial effects were seen during this time, demonstrating that supplementation can be beneficial. Patients used less medication, their asthma scores were lower, they had a greater acetylcholine threshold and they had significantly higher EPA plasma levels.[20]

The role of oxidants and antioxidants in asthma

Oxidant generation is part of the normal metabolism of many types of cells and is critical for cell homeostasis. To protect itself against exposure to these noxious oxidants, the lung has a well-developed antioxidant system.[21] There is a significant amount of evidence for the presence of increased oxidative stress in asthma, indicating the potential role of oxidants in the pathogenesis of asthma, particularly during exacerbations. Asthmatic patients represent a classical case study where the cellular level of free radicals is basically high and increased further during an exacerbation.

Antioxidant nutraceuticals

If reactive oxygen species (ROS) participate in airway disease, then modulation of antioxidant defence by supplementation could protect against oxidant damage and be a useful adjuvant in the complex management of the disease. The use of antioxidant supplements has led to inconsistent results but has been shown to be beneficial in combating oxidative stress.[22] Some recent studies found that supplementation reduces oxidant-related decrement in lung function in asthmatic subjects, especially in those with a genetically determined increased susceptibility to oxidant stress.[23]

Coenzyme Q10

Coenzyme Q10 (Co Q10) scavenges free radicals and is an important marker of antioxidant potential. A recent study investigated levels of Co Q10, α-tocopherol and β-carotene in plasma and whole blood, as well as the levels of malandialdehyde, a marker of end-stage lipid peroxidation, and eosinophil cationic protein (ECP), a marker of inflammation, in people with asthma. The study found no correlation between concentrations of ECP, levels of the compounds and pulmonary function tests, but the concentration of Co Q10 was considerably reduced in subjects with asthma compared with the healthy population, whereas the level of ECP was significantly increased. This suboptimal concentration of Co Q10 in people with asthma may highlight the need for supplementation.[24] Protective effects on pulmonary function have been demonstrated in animal experiments but there is limited information regarding humans.[25] Controlled studies are required to determine whether this supplement is clinically relevant.

Lycopene

Lycopene also has the ability to destroy free radicals that form when the body metabolises oxygen. It appears to suppress the attack of cellular oxygen and ROS, slow down the formation of more radicals and therefore prevent destruction of the lipophilic parts of the cell.[26] A study assessing the acute effects of lycopene on AHR was carried out in patients with exercise-induced asthma (EIA). Patients taking the lycopene supplement (30 mg/day) showed an elevated serum lycopene level. Pulmonary function was measured at rest and following physical exercise. Those on the placebo experienced a significant reduction in their post-exercise FEV_1 of more than 15%. Fifty-five per cent of those taking lycopene were significantly protected against EIA and did not experience this FEV_1 reduction.[27]

α-Lipoic acid

α-Lipoic acid is a naturally occurring antioxidant has been used clinically for the treatment of oxidant-induced diseases because it has many beneficial characteristics. It directly scavenges free radicals, has metal chelating activity, recycles antioxidants, accelerates glutathione synthesis and modulates the activity of transportation factors such as nuclear factor kappa B (NFκB).[28] The mechanism of action may be related to anti-oxidant suppressed activity of NFκB in lung tissues but the amount of ROS in alveolar macrophages was not significantly different in treated and untreated patients. Another possible mechanism is direct intervention with intracellular inflammatory signalling pathways. The therapeutic activity of this supplement has not been determined in humans but it has been tested in a mouse model of asthma. It was found that asthmatic mice receiving this supplement had a significantly reduced AHR, a lower proportion of the inflammatory eosinophilis in bronchoalveolar lavage, appreciably improved pathologic lesion scores, significantly reduced ovalbumin-specific immunoglobulin E, interleukin 4 (IL-4) and IL-5 and intracellular ROS concentration and reduced NFκB DNA-binding activity. This supplement effectively suppressed allergic inflammation in the mouse model, which supports the hypothesis that oxidative stress plays an important role in asthmatic airway inflammation.[28]

Pycnogenol

Pycnogenol, a bioflavonoid mixture extracted from pine bark, is anti-allergic, antiviral and anti-inflammatory. It also has a potent antioxidant effect, scavenging free radicals as well as enhancing endogenous anti-oxidant systems.[29] Clinical trials have been carried out using this supplement with positive results. A randomised, double-blind, placebo-controlled, crossover study involving 26 patients with varying asthma severity was conducted. Adults taking this supplement responded favourably, in contrast to those using the placebo, and had significantly reduced serum leukotrienes.[30] Another study was conducted in children. This randomised, placebo-controlled, double-blind study involved 60 subjects (6–18 years) with mild to moderate asthma using the supplement for three months. Those who took Pycnogenol had significantly more improvement in pulmonary functions and asthma symptoms and found that they could reduce their use of inhaler medication. These beneficial changes may be due to the significant reduction in leukotrienes, analysed in urine.[31]

Other respiratory conditions

COPD is another pathological state that increases airway resistance, but unlike asthma, COPD is chronic and progressive, usually being caused by cigarette smoking. COPD consists of two conditions: chronic bronchitis and emphysema. Chronic bronchitis is characterised by inflammation and thickening of the airway lining which reduces airway diameter and can lead to destruction of the normal tissue. Along with inflammation there is a high rate of mucus secretion, which exacerbates airway obstruction and often promotes secondary infection. Symptoms include coughing, wheezing and breathlessness. Emphysema is distension and damage of lung tissue beyond the respiratory bronchioles. There are no definitive conventional therapies for COPD, which leads many patients to explore adjunctive complementary approaches.[32] As in asthma, a diet rich in fruit and vegetables may be beneficial because higher levels of antioxidants, measured by dietary assessment and serum biomarkers, are associated with improved lung function.[33] A study of

2349 smokers and ex-smokers concluded that the level of DHA in plasma is inversely related to the odds of having COPD.[34]

Another respiratory condition, allergic rhinitis, is also on the rise in the Western world. In the USA it affects 40% of children under 6 years and 20% of the adult population and is another trigger of asthma.[35] Allergic rhinitis is characterised by continuous or periodic nasal congestion, sneezing, pruitis of the conjunctiva, nasal mucosa and oropharynx, dark circles under the eyes and fatigue. Epidemiological data, which are so abundant for asthma, are lacking for this condition but theoretically they will benefit from the same nutritional considerations.

Two unexpected applications for nutraceuticals in respiratory disorders have been reported. The efficacy of methylsulfonylmethane (MSM) in the treatment of seasonal allergic rhinitis (SAR) has been assessed in one open-label trial involving 50 subjects with either medically diagnosed SAR or minimum 2 years history of suffering from SAR. MSM 2600 mg was taken orally for 30 days, and responses to treatment were measured by a seasonal allergy symptom questionnaire. By day 7, upper and total respiratory symptoms were significantly reduced, and by day 14 energy levels of subjects were increased, and all improvements were maintained until the day 30 completion.[36]

Other effects of nutraceuticals on respiratory conditions

A pilot study on the effects of chondroitin sulfate on snoring have also been published. Seven subjects were given 8 mg (from a 3% solution) via nasal instillation, resulting in a decrease in snoring compared with placebo.[37]

Soy sauce (*shoyu*) is a fermented soy product, containing both isoflavones and polysaccharides. The polysaccharide fraction has been shown to exert antiallergenic activity both *in vivo* and *in vitro* and has been evaluated as a treatment for seasonal allergic rhinitis. In a randomised double-blind trial patients were treated with 600 mg of polysaccharides daily, over four weeks, and symptom scores for sneezing, nasal stuffiness and impact on everyday life was found to be significantly improved compared with the placebo group.[38]

Conclusion

Despite the theoretical basis for the use of these supplements in respiratory conditions, the complex and sometimes contradictory nature of evidence from both epidemiological and intervention studies prevents any clear conclusions being drawn at this stage. To date, there are no reliable, prospective, multifaceted, dietary intervention clinical trials that test data derived from epidemiologic, cross-sectional and case–control studies. There is a need for further studies to be carried out before we can reach a definite outcome. These studies need to be longer, use larger and more diverse subject populations and measure more outcomes such as exacerbation frequency, hospital admissions and quality of life.

It has been suggested that susceptible populations should increase their fruit, vegetable and *n*-3 fatty acid intake, and limit their *n*-6 intake as well as their exposure to allergens and tobacco smoke. This primary prevention strategy may achieve a 50% reduction in the prevalence of asthma.[39] Patients who already have asthma and other respiratory conditions may also benefit from these changes. Diet modification may become one of the initial steps in the management of asthma. If people with respiratory disorders want to incorporate nutraceuticals such as lycopene and *n*-3 into their diet they do have a very safe profile. The main importance in the treatment of respiratory conditions is that patients are well educated about the proper management of their condition. Improved dietary education has been shown to reduce asthma morbidity and mortality. The use of certain nutraceuticals such as those discussed may be beneficial in supplementing nutritionally poor diets, or in patients excessively challenged with allergens.

References

1. Page C, Curtis M J, Sutter M C *et al. Integrated Pharmacology*, 2nd edn. Edinburgh: Mosby, 1997.
2. Rang H P, Dale M M, Ritter J M, Moore P K. *Pharmacology*, 5th edn. London: Churchill Livingstone, 2003.
3. Davis P A, Gold E B, Hackman R M. The use of CAM for the treatment of asthma in the US. *J Invest Allergol Clin Immunol* 1998; 8: 73–77.
4. Ernst E. Complementary therapies for asthma: what patients use. *J Asthma* 1998; 35: 667–671.
5. Ernst E. Use of complementary therapies in childhood asthma. *Pediatr Asthma Allergy Immunol* 1998; 12: 29–32.
6. Anderson H R, Butland B K. Trends in prevalence and severity of childhood asthma. *BMJ* 1994; 308: 1600–1604.
7. Centers for Disease Control. Disabilities among children aged 17 years: VS, 1991–2. *MMWR Morb Mortal Wkly Rep* 1995; 44: 609–613.
8. Kay A B. Allergy and allergic disease. *N Engl J Med* 2001; 344: 30–36.
9. Smit H A, Grievink L, Tabak C. Dietary influences on chronic obstructive lung disease and asthma: a review of the epidemiological evidence. *Proc Nutr Soc* 1999; 58: 309–319.

10. Kelley D S. Modulation of human immune and inflammatory response by dietary fatty acids. *Nutrition* 2001; 17: 669–673.

11. Schwartz J. The relationship of dietary fish oil intake to level of pulmonary function in the first National Health and Nutrition Survey. *Eur Respir J* 1994; 7: 1821–1824.

12. Peat J K. Factors associated with bronchial hyperresponsiveness in Australian adults and children. *Eur Respir J* 1992; 5: 921–929.

13. Hodge L, Salome C M, Peat J K *et al.* Consumption of oily fish and childhood asthma risk. *Med J Austr* 1996; 164: 137–140.

14. Woods R K, Raven J M, Walters E H *et al.* Fatty acid levels and risk of asthma in young adults *Thorax* 2004; 59: 105–110.

15. von Mutius E, Martinez F D, Fritzsh C *et al.* Prevalence of asthma and atopy in two areas of East and West Germany. *Am J Respir Crit Care Med* 1994; 149: 358–364.

16. Klein K, Dathe R. Allergies: a comparison between two schools in East and West Germany. *Allergy* 1992; 47: 259.

17. Winkler G, Holtz H, Doring A. Comparison of food intakes of selected populations in former East and West Germany: results from the MONICA Projects Erfurt and Augsburg. *Ann Nutr Metab* 1992; 36: 219–234.

18. Hodge L, Salome C M, Hughes J M *et al.* Effect of dietary intake of omega 3 and omega 6 on severity of asthma in children. *Eur Respir J* 1998; 11: 361–365.

19. Thein F C K, Woods R, Abramson M J. Dietary marine fatty acids for asthma in adults and children. *The Cochrane Library* 2004; 3.

20. Surette M E, Koumenis I L, Edens M B *et al.* Inhibition of leukotriene biosynthesis by a novel dietary fatty acid formulation in patients with atopic asthma: a randomized, placebo-controlled, parallel-group, prospective trial. *Clin Ther* 2003; 25: 972–979.

21. Comhair S A, Erzurum S C. Antioxidant responses to oxidant-mediated lung diseases. *Am J Physiol Lung Cell Mol Physiol* 2002; 283: L246–L255.

22. Romieu I, Sienra-Monge J J, Ramirez-Aguilar M *et al.* Antioxidant supplementation and lung functions among children with asthma exposed to high levels of air pollutants. *Am J Respir Crit Care Med* 2002; 166: 703–709.

23. Remieu I, Sienra-Monge J J, Ramirez-Aguilar M *et al.* Genetic polymorphism of GSTMI and antioxidant supplementation influence lung function in relation to ozone exposure in asthmatic children in Mexico City. *Thorax* 2004; 59: 8–10.

24. Gazdik F, Gvozdjakova A, Nadvornikova R *et al.* Decreased levels of coenzyme Q(10) in patients with bronchial asthma. *Allergy* 2002; 57: 811–814.

25. Fujimoto S, Kurihara N, Hirata K, Takeda T. Effects of coenzyme Q10 administration on pulmonary function and exercise performance in patients with chronic lung diseases. *Clin Invest* 1993; 71: S162–S166.

26. Klebanov G I, Kapitanov A B, Teselkin Yu O *et al.* The antioxidant properties of lycopene. *Membr Cell Biol* 1998; 12: 287–300.

27. Neuman I, Nahum H, Ben-Amotz A. Reduction of exercise-induced asthma oxidative stress by lycopene, a natural antioxidant. *Allergy* 2000; 55: 1184–1189.

28. Packer L. alpha-Lipoic acid: a metabolic antioxidant which regulates NF-kappa B signal transduction and protects against oxidative injury. *Drug Metab Rev* 1998; 30: 245–275.
29. Bayeta E, Lau B H S. Pycnogenol inhibits generation of inflammatory mediators in macrophages. *Nutr Res* 2000; 20: 249–259.
30. Hosseini S, Pishnamazi S, Sadrzadeh S M *et al*. Pycnogenol((R)) in the management of asthma. *J Med Food* 2001; 4: 201–209.
31. Lau B H S, Riesen S. Pycogenol as an adjunct in the management of childhood asthma *J Asthma* 2004; 41: 825–832.
32. Jones K L, Robbins R A. Alternative therapies for chronic bronchitis. *Am J Med Sci* 1999; 318: 96–98.
33. Hu G, Cassano P A. Antioxidant nutrients and pulmonary function: the Third National Health and Nutrition Examination Survey (NHANES III). *Am J Epidemiol* 2000; 151: 975–981.
34. Shahar E, Boland L, Folson A *et al*. Docosahexenoic acid and smoking-related COPD. *Am J Respir Crit Care Med* 1999; 159: 1780–1785.
35. Naclerio R, Solomon W. Rhinitis and inhalant allergens. *JAMA* 1997; 278: 1842–1848.
36. Barrager E, Veltmann J R Jr, Schauss A G, Schiller R N. A multicentered, open label trial on the safety and efficacy of methylsulfonylmethane in the treatment of seasonal allergic rhinitis. *J Altern Comp Med* 2002; 8: 167–173.
37. Lenclud C, Chapelle P, Van Muylem A *et al*. Effects of chondroitin sulfate on snoring characteristics: a pilot study. *Curr Ther Res* 1998; 59: 234–243.
38. Kobayashi M, Matsushita H, Tsukiyama R *et al*. Shoyu polysaccharides from soy sauce improve quality of life for patients with seasonal allergic rhinitis: a double-blind placebo-controlled clinical study. *Int J Mol Med* 2005; 15: 463–467.
39. Peat J K. Prevention of asthma. *Eur Respir J* 1996; 9: 1545–1555.

13

Women's health

In addition to a number of specific menstrual problems that affect women, there are various other health-related problems. The menopause is signalled by a woman's last menstrual period and is defined as the permanent cessation of menstruation resulting from loss of ovarian follicular activity.[1]

Menopausal symptoms

Following the menopause many women experience a decrease in the quality of life. The major symptoms associated with the postmenopausal period are:

- Vasomotor symptoms
- Vaginal symptoms
- Cognitive problems
- Breast cancer
- Cardiovascular disease
- Osteoporosis.

The most common vasomotor symptoms displayed by women during the menopause are hot flushes, night sweats and palpitations. Psychological problems experienced include sleep deprivation, forgetfulness, difficulty concentrating and depression. Many women also suffer from vaginal dryness, leading to loss of libido. These symptoms are all linked to the declining and erratic production of oestrogen by the ovaries.[2]

Menopausal symptoms, especially hot flushes, have been reported to vary in incidence levels between women in different countries. In East Asia (e.g. Japan and China), only 10–20% of women experience hot flushes in the perimenopausal period, compared with 70–80% of women in Western countries such as the UK and Denmark.[3] This may possibly be a result of the high proportion of soy isoflavones consumed in the traditional East Asian diet, which may have an influence on the body's response to the changing hormone levels at menopause. It has been estimated that Japanese women consume 50–200 mg of isoflavones daily, whereas the typical Western diet contains <1 mg/daily. These findings have encouraged research on the potential benefits of soy isoflavones on menopausal symptoms. A survey carried out in the USA into the use of nutraceuticals found that 7.4% of women questioned used soy products for perimenopausal symptoms.[4]

Conventional treatment

Hormone replacement therapy (HRT) is commonly prescribed for the relief of menopausal symptoms and for protection against bone loss and ischaemic heart disease. However, reports in the media on the long-term effects of HRT have deterred women from using it due to the associated risks with breast cancer, myocardial infarctions and strokes. Studies have suggested that the risk of breast cancer in patients using HRT increases over time, and the relative risk has been stated as 1.3–2.4 times after 5 years of therapy.[5] As a result, increasing numbers of women have turned to complementary and alternative medicines for relief from their menopausal symptoms.

The major goup of nutraceuticals used for women's problems include phytoestrogens such as soy isoflavones and flax lignans. In addition, there is limited evidence for the use of resveratrol and other nutraceuticals.

Soy isoflavones

The main isoflavones in soybeans are genistein and daidzein and their respective β-glycosides, genistin and daidzin. Genistein occurs at higher levels than daidzein in soybeans and soy products. There are also small amounts of glycitein and its glycoside glycitin.[6]

The isoflavones are present in the bound form as glycosides in plants, but when the sugar residue is removed, for example during metabolism, these compounds become activated.[7] Both the metabolite and parent compound are liable to absorption.

Ingestion of the isoflavonoid glycoside results in rapid hydrolysis in the oral cavity to yield the aglycone, but it has been reported that there is a greater than 20-fold interindividual variation in this hydrolysis.[8] Ingestion of 50 mg of isoflavone leads to levels of 50–800 ng/mL in the plasma, and peak concentration has been found to occur 6–8 hours after a dose of 100 mg.[9] The effect of the food matrix consumed alongside the isoflavonoid is likely to be important in determining the distribution.

Since the chemical structure of isoflavones is similar to that of oestrogen it is not surprising that they bind and interact with the oestrogen receptor (ER), predominantly the ERβ form of the receptor, and thereby exert a weak oestrogenic effect. However, the isoflavones generally have much lower binding affinities to oestrogen receptors than oestradiol. The ER-binding abilities of a number of phytoestrogens have been evaluated.[11] The comparable levels are shown in Table 10.1.

The soy metabolite equol has been found to have the same order of affinities for ERα and ERβ as genistein, as opposed to daidzein from which it is derived.[12] The flax lignan metabolites enterolactone and enterodiol and resveratrol have been reported to possess the same affinities for ER as the red clover isoflavones, <0.01% that of oestradiol.[12,13]

In addition, phytoestrogens have been shown to have lower potential to stimulate alkaline phosphatase production in bone cells than oestradiol.[14]

The structural differences between oestrogens and isoflavones may explain why isoflavones have more selective effects in different oestrogen-responsive tissues. Bone contains only ERβ, but ERα and ERβ are both located in the vascular system, the placenta, the uterus and in breast tissue.[15] Isoflavones (particularly genistein) have greater affinity for ERβ as opposed to ERα and this may explain why they have positive effects on the central nervous system, blood vessels and bone, whilst having little or no effect on breast and endometrial tissue. The different affinities of isoflavones to ERα and ERβ, and the different tissue distribution of these two oestrogen receptors, could possibly offer an explanation as to the inconsistent effects of isoflavones that have been reported on menopausal symptoms and osteoporosis.

Mechanisms of action

Soy isoflavones have been shown to reduce menopausal symptoms, but the exact mechanism of action is yet to be determined. Several studies have hypothesised possible mechanisms.

Oestrogen receptors bind to endogenous oestrogens and isoflavones, as well as to other environmental oestrogen-like molecules. When isoflavones reach the target tissue, they cross the cell membrane by passive diffusion, bind to ERs in the cytosol and form an isoflavone–ER complex. This complex then translocates into the nucleus for activation of the oestrogen response element (ERE), which is involved in the regulation of DNA-directed mRNA synthesis and the production of new proteins.[16] Therefore, by this mechanism isoflavones may bind to ERs and so directly affect transcription of oestrogen-regulated gene products. In order to act as phytoestrogens isoflavones require 2–4 hydroxyl groups in fixed positions, and methylation of these reduces oestrogenic activity. The 2-position of the benzyl ring in the isoflavonoids gives them greater activity than other flavonoids.[17]

Another explanation is that isoflavones act through their antioxidant effects. The antioxidant properties of isoflavones are associated with the presence of hydroxyl groups at positions 4' and 5' on the aromatic ring.[18] Furthermore, there appears to be a positive synergy between phytoestrogens and other antioxidants.[19] This may be important in disease processes that involve oxidative stress, for example, in reducing low-density lipoprotein (LDL) oxidation in atherosclerosis. Apart from protecting lipid-carrying proteins, phytoestrogens may also prevent the oxidation of critical enzymes in the signal transduction pathways through protection of cysteine groups. This property is not, however, governed by their oestrogen-like structures, but rather their antioxidant properties, suggesting that the overall effect of isoflavones may appear to be like that of an oestrogen or an anti-oestrogen.[16]

Some isoflavones, such as genistein, can also bind with membrane receptors and function as tyrosine kinase inhibitors,[16] which are involved in protein phosphorylation during cell proliferation. In this way, isoflavones can influence the cell cycle and metabolism through second messengers in the cytoplasm.[16] In addition, genistein inhibits DNA topoisomerase II and ribosomal S6 kinase, both of which may lead to protein-linked DNA strand breaks in cancerous cells.[7]

Studies have shown an increase in the amount 17β-oestradiol in the presence of isoflavones, which suggests that isoflavone supplementation increases oestrogen levels. They may have an indirect effect due to isoflavones acting on sex hormone-binding globulin.[20] Isoflavones might compete with oestrogens for this protein.

Importance of the metabolite equol

Equol (see Figure 2.25) is not found in soy but is a product of intestinal bacterial metabolism of diadzein,[21] one of the main isoflavones in soyfoods. It is not, however, a metabolite of either genistein or glycitein. Equol possesses oestrogenic activity, having affinity for both oestrogen receptors.

Equol is not produced in adults who lack the intestinal bacteria required to metabolise diadzein in soy products, and it has been estimated that only 30–50% of the population are able to produce equol. Infants and germ-free animals are unable to produce equol, and antibiotic therapy inhibits its production. It has been proposed that the ability to make equol may be important to the effectiveness of soy protein diets when employed in the treatment or prevention of hormone-dependent conditions. The failure to distinguish those subjects who are 'equol-producers' from 'non-equol producers' in previous clinical studies could possibly explain the variance in reported data on the health benefits associated with soy.[21]

A recent investigation into the stereochemistry of equol has shown that the S-enantiomer is the exclusive product of human intestinal bacterial synthesis from soy isoflavones. The S-form has high affinity for ERβ, whereas R-equol is relatively inactive.[22]

Evidence for activity

One double-blind, placebo-controlled trial of four months' duration suggested that soy isoflavone (100 mg per day) treatment may be a safe and effective alternative therapy for many menopausal symptoms.[23] In that particular study it was noted that genistein and daidzein plasma concentrations peak 6–8 hours after ingestion, so it was suggested that 33.3 mg should be administered every 8 hours.

Four large-scale critical analyses of many of the published clinical trials on the use of soy products for treatment of menopausal symptoms have been published. Clearly, a number of studies have failed to demonstrate a reduction of menopausal symptoms.[24-27] The data are summarised in Table 13.1.

It has been reported that the placebo effect has appeared at levels of 50–60% in these trials.[26] The variability seen in the table is caused by a number of factors: different products and foods contain varying levels of isoflavones, the optimum dose of isoflavones is not known,

Table 13.1 Summary of clinical trials using soy products for treatment of menopausal symptoms

Trials included	Number showing positive effects	Number showing negative effects
10[24]	4	6
8 on soy foods[25]	1	7
5 on soy extract[25]	2	2
8[26]	3	5
13[27]	Overall benefit	

formulated products may not contain stated levels, and variability and deficiencies in reporting of outcomes exist in the original data.[25] To put some of the claimed benefits into context, a 15% reduction in hot flushes may only represent one less flush per day in patients experiencing 10–12 incidents daily.[5]

No beneficial effects on genital atrophy can be expected, and have not been reported, but vaginal dryness variably improved.[25]

Even though many clinical trials have been conducted, the understanding of the potential health benefits of soy isoflavones is far from complete. The lack of clarity in determining any potential benefit of soy is most significantly due to methodological variation in trials. The most important factors include the menopausal status of the participating women, dosage of soy (i.e. isoflavone content) and the outcome measures that have been used to test the efficacy.

Trials carried out have ranged from 6 to 24 weeks' duration,[24] making it difficult to compare the findings directly. The vast majority of the trials do not state specific compositions of their soy treatment, and therefore it is not possible to make conclusions on specific isoflavone quantities. Equally, the quality of the soy product used or the bioavailability of the isoflavone content may not have been assessed. Furthermore, as mentioned earlier, there is great variability in the ability to metabolise daidzein to its metabolite equol[21] between individuals. The isoflavone content of trials materials needs to be used at standardised levels to determine the most effective dose.

Plant sources that are rich in isoflavones, such as soy, flax and grape products, also contain other compounds that may have the potential to interact with phytoestrogens, interfering with their activity and bioavailability. Consideration must therefore be given to these compounds as well. In addition, some phytoestrogens may act as oestrogen agonists or oestrogen antagonists depending on their structure and concentration. Isoflavones have been shown to have oestrogen agonist effects in low endogenous oestrogen concentrations and oestrogen antagonist effects in a more oestrogenic environment.[28] Thus you would expect isoflavones to have oestrogenic effects after the onset of menopause due to the low endogenous oestrogen concentration, and oestrogen antagonist effects before the onset of menopause when the endogenous oestrogen concentration is high. The oestrogen antagonist activity of phytoestrogens may be partially explained by their competition with endogenous 17β-oestradiol for the oestrogen receptors.[7]

Overall, there appears to be some evidence to substantiate the use of soy to alleviate menopausal symptoms. In addition there appear to be no safety concerns with soy products in short-term use.[29,30] The main adverse effects of soy products reported are gastrointestinal disturbances such as nausea. However, allergy to soy has been noted[29] and several randomised controlled trials suffered from unpalatability of the treatment, especially in studies that involved soy drinks. In one study 10 out of 263 woman volunteers dropped out for this reason.[31] This is important because if patients are not able to tolerate soy they are less likely to be compliant.

Use of soy foods

There is now a wide range of soy foods readily available for those who wish to increase the phytoestrogens in their diet, specifically to alleviate menopausal symptoms. In addition to this, isoflavones are now directly extracted from soya and red clover for use as an additive to non-soya foods.

It is yet to be determined whether split doses of isoflavones over 24 hours would be more effective than a single daily dose of isoflavones.

The published studies on menopausal symptoms and osteoporosis have examined different quantities of soy or isoflavones, making it difficult to make direct comparisons and hence dose recommendations. Reports on the efficacy of soy isoflavones in reduction of menopausal symptoms suggest that an average dose is approximately 50 mg of isoflavones per day. There are few data on suitable dose levels for other known phytoestrogens. Much of the justification regarding the selection of a dose of 50 mg isoflavones/day (0.5–1.0 mg/kg body weight per day) is based on the presumed average intake of isoflavones in adults in China, Japan and Taiwan. Toxicity studies of human subjects suggest that purified isoflavones are safe at doses at least twice as high as used in reported studies.[16]

Traditional soyfoods have an isoflavone-to-protein ratio of approximately 1:300; therefore, consuming 15 g soy protein will result in consuming approximately 50 mg isoflavones. These amounts of soy protein and isoflavones are provided by approximately two servings of traditional soyfoods and are likely to be efficacious for those diseases for which soy is proven to be beneficial.[6]

Cardiovascular disease

Epidemiological evidence suggests that women with high consumption of phytoestrogens, particularly soy isoflavones, have less cardiovascular disease. Although there is much published research on the cardiac benefits of soy isoflavones, little of it relates specifically to menopausal women. Soy protein is the subject of the US Food and Drug Administration (FDA) approved model health claim that '25 grams of soy protein a day, as part of a diet low in saturated fat and cholesterol, may reduce the risk of heart disease', but it is not clear what role the constituent isoflavones play. A large meta-analysis on the effects of soy protein is understood to be the stimulus for the FDA claim. In this work, the significant mean decreases in total cholesterol (9%), LDL–cholesterol (13%) and triglycerides (11%) and a small non-significant reduction in high-density lipoprotein–cholesterol (HDL-C) were reported.[32] Studies involving isoflavone supplements containing little or no soy protein for menopausal women have tended to yield only negative findings.[33] Studies involving combinations of isoflavones and soy protein in pre- and postmenopausal women showed modest but consistent effects on lipoprotein profiles.[34,35] The situation regarding direct cardiovascular effects is confused due to a number of trials showing no effect.[33]

A recent longitudinal study investigated the effects of soy consumption in nearly 46 000 middle-aged and elderly women in Shanghai, over a period of 2–3 years. Researchers found that there was an inverse association between consumption of soy foods and both systolic and diastolic blood pressure.[36]

Cognitive function

Evidence that postmenopausal women suffer cognitive decline is thought to be associated with decreased oestrogen levels, and soy has been suggested as an alternative to HRT after controversial evidence that HRT leads to increased risk of breast cancer, and that the cognitive benefits of HRT may actually be reversed over long-term usage.[37] There is limited evidence, however, to substantiate the benefits of soy isoflavones. One trial involving 53 postmenopausal women over six months showed a significant improvement in one of five cognitive tests, insignificant improvement in two tests and no improvement in the rest.[38] Other work using low levels of isoflavone (60 mg) over short time periods (12 weeks) has been reported to increase memory, pattern recognition and mental flexibility.[37] Another trial carried out with young subjects over a ten-week period found that a dose of 100 mg per day of total isoflavones caused significant cognitive improvements in both young men and women, in both short- and long-term memory, but also in mental flexibility.[39]

Osteoporosis

The continual loss of bone in the elderly is a natural process associated with ageing. Women have a higher incidence of osteoporotic fractures than men due to their lower peak bone mass, but in addition, the abrupt decrease in oestrogen secretion in postmenopausal women accelerates bone loss.[7] Soyfoods and isoflavones have received considerable attention for their potential in preventing and treating osteoporosis.

Conventional pharmaceutical treatment of osteoporosis involves medicines that either inhibit bone resorption, such as oestrogens, calcitonin or bisphosphonates, or stimulate bone formation, such as fluorides, parathyroid fragments and anabolic steroids.[40]

The role of soy-containing phytoestrogens in bone health is an area of growing interest and is based on observational studies among Asian women showing that a higher consumption of phytoestrogens is associated with higher values of bone mineral density and consequently a lower incidence of osteoporotic fractures.

Human investigations

Large-scale epidemiological evidence has recently been published. A large prospective cohort study of soy food consumption and risk of bone fracture in postmenopausal women has been carried out involving 24 403 women in Shanghai. Over 4.5 years the level of consumption of soy protein and isoflavones was found to be possibly associated with a reduction in bone fracture, particularly in the early years following menopause.[41] Data from human studies are limited, and have shown contradicting results. Clinical trials in postmenopausal and peri-menopausal women that have analysed bone mass change and bone mineral density have demonstrated that isoflavones can significantly increase bone mineral density at the lumbar spine.[42,43] The studies of up to 24 weeks' duration are of only limited relevance, because bone remodelling cycle can take as long as 80 weeks.[44] It would therefore be premature to assume that soy with isoflavones has a significant long-term bone-sparing effect or that soy reduces bone fractures of the spine. Longer studies of 2–3 years' duration are required for realistic evidence.

Some studies have suggested that isolated soy protein may have a protective role in bone maintenance[45] and that daily supplementation of soybean isoflavones (61.8 mg) for four weeks is associated with a significant reduction in the excretion of bone resorption markers (pyridinoline and deoxypyridinoline).[46] In postmenopausal women diets rich in soyfoods have resulted in significant increases in serum osteocalcin concentrations.[43]

However, other researchers have reported that soy supplementation over a three-month period did not produce any significant changes in two markers of bone resorption and that soy protein isolate containing high concentrations of isoflavones was not protective against bone loss in early menopausal women.[47]

Trials have shown a greater response to oestrogen treatments in the spine than in the hip due to the higher content of trabecular bone in the spine.[48] Trabecular bone is known to have a higher turnover rate than cortical bone that is found in the hip. Thus the lumbar spine, which is relatively high in trabecular bone, should be more sensitive to compounds that are thought to affect remodelling, such as oestrogens and phytoestrogens.[48]

In a recent study, daily administration of 54 mg genistein reduced postmenopausal bone mineral loss at the femoral neck and lumbar spine as effectively as HRT with 1 mg per day of oestrogen.[49] These findings add to the existing evidence that soy intake may be beneficial for bone conservation in postmenopausal women. However, further longer term randomised control trials are needed to find the optimal dosages most effective in maintaining bone mass.

Mechanism of action on bone cells

Researchers have reviewed several studies on isoflavones that include possible mechanisms of action to explain the beneficial effect of phytoestrogens on bone loss.[20] These mechanisms include prevention of calcium loss, beneficial effects on osteoblasts, and influences on the secretion of calcitonin that suppress bone resorption. Both genistein and daidzein suppress osteoclast activity by a number of possible mechanisms, including induction of apoptosis, activation of protein tyrosine phosphatase, inhibition of cytokines, changes in intracellular calcium and membrane depolarisation, all of which are involved in bone turnover.[50]

Oestrogen receptors (only ERβ) have been found in osteoblasts. The phytoestrogen–ER complex may bind to EREs and may thus cause alteration in the production of certain proteins.

Bone remodelling is the function of the activity of both osteoblasts and osteoclasts. Osteoblasts respond to changes in the activity of osteoclasts, the bone-resorbing cells.[50] Osteoblasts are responsible for secreting bone formation-related proteins, such as alkaline phosphatase and osteocalcin. Besides this osteoblasts are also capable of synthesising many other cytokines such as IL-6 and osteoprotegerin. These cytokines have been demonstrated to have critical roles in the regulation of osteoclast differentiation and activities.[51] Isoflavones may, therefore, have indirect effects on osteoclasts by mediating cytokine production in osteoblasts.

Additional components in soy

There are additional components in soy products that may also be responsible for the prevention of bone loss or stimulating bone formation. The main ones are calcium and vitamin K_2 (menatetrenone). Vitamin K_2 is present in fermented soybeans (also known as tofu) and is known to both stimulate bone formation and prevent bone loss.[52] A significant correlation has been found between bone mineral density, the number of years since the onset of menopause and consumption of fermented soybeans. This suggests that the effects of calcium, vitamin K_2 and isoflavones might be synergistic.[53] Fermented soybeans are consumed in higher quantities in eastern than in western Japan, correlating with epidemiologic data that show a lower incidence of osteoporotic bone fractures in eastern rather than in western Japan.[53] This might indicate that consumption of fermented soybeans is required to achieve the synergistic effects of calcium, vitamin K_2 and isoflavone, rather than consuming isolated isoflavone extracts from soy.

Ipriflavone

Ipriflavone is a synthetic isoflavonoid that has been studied in numerous clinical trials. It is non-oestrogenic and is mainly used in treating osteoporosis. Approximately 10% of ipriflavone is metabolised first to daidzein, consequently acting as a prodrug, and then to five other products (Figure 13.1).[5]

Ipriflavone, 200 mg three times daily, has been shown to produce statistically significant increases in bone mineral density and markers of bone metabolism.[54] It also causes increased calcium uptake in the duodenum, which may explain its activity, but some trials have shown no benefits from therapy. In one trial 13% of subjects developed subclinical

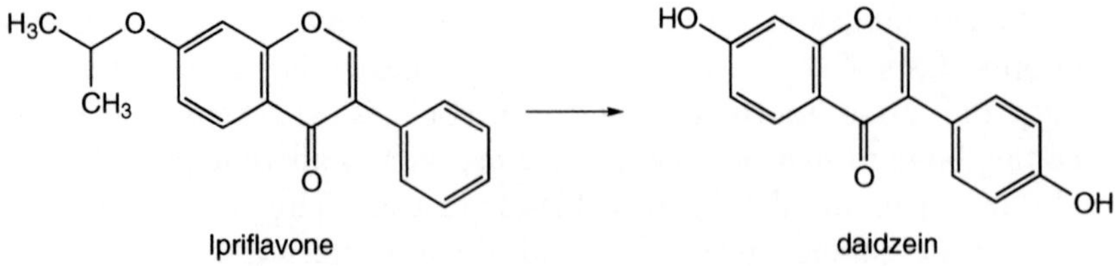

Figure 13.1 Structures of ipriflavone and its metabolite daidzein.

lymphocytopenia.[55] Although its mechanism of action is still not fully understood, both *in vivo* and *in vitro* studies indicate that the drug inhibits osteoclast-mediated bone resorption, and stimulates bone formation in some systems.[56]

Red clover and other isoflavones

Red clover has lower isoflavone levels than soy but is widely available, with more than eight preparations are available in Austria. It has been claimed to have similar benefits to soy in osteoporosis[17] and 80 mg isoflavone/day has been reported to produce a 44% reduction in hot flushes.[17,57] However, one study investigating 82 and 57 mg of isoflavones per day, found no significant difference between red clover and placebo on both hot flushes and other menopausal symptoms.[58] It has been claimed that obese women benefit more with this therapy, as they tend to have higher levels of endogenous oestrogens.[58] Reduced breast cancer, prostate cancer and ovarian cancer risks have been reported,[17] but insignificant effects have been shown on lipoprotein levels.[59]

Formononetin and biochanin A are efficiently demethylated to daidzein and genistein respectively (Figure 13.2).[60] This may explain their similarity in action to the soy isoflavones.

Safety issues concerning isoflavones

The long-term safety of isoflavones, either mixed with soy protein or as purified supplements, remains to be examined in human subjects. Risks of long-term effects of therapeutic soy use are largely unknown although epidemiological data do not seem to indicate that serious problems exist.[3]

Human studies with isoflavones suggest that doses ranging from 1 to 16 mg/kg body weight are reasonably safe.[16] At the higher doses being

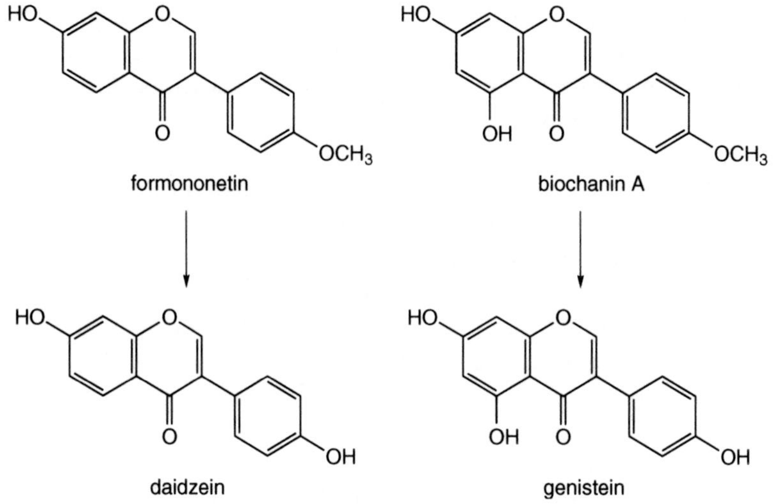

Figure 13.2 Formononetin, biochanin and their metabolites.

recommended for prevention of bone loss in postmenopausal women, little concern has been raised about adverse effects. Genistein at high doses such as 600 mg per day has been shown *in vitro* to inhibit cell growth and induce apoptosis.[61] In addition, some reproductive disturbances, such as uterotropic effects, have been reported in animals fed a diet rich in isoflavones or other phytoestrogens.[62]

The amounts of isoflavones consumed in standard food products such as tofu is generally regarded as safe but the higher quantities in supplements used over long periods is a concern to many researchers. There has been one report that high level male tofu users have actually suffered cognitive impairment and brain atrophy in late life.[63]

Flax lignans

Flaxseed contains a number of lignans that are phytoestrogenic. The major one is seicoislariciresinol, which occurs as the diglucoside. Both seicoislariciresinol and matairesinol may be converted to enterodiol and enterolactone by intestinal microflora. The importance of the metabolites enterolactone and enterodiol has yet to be elucidated.

In one study into menopausal symptoms, supplementation of women's diets with 40 g/day of flaxseed was shown to produce a decrease in the number of hot flushes, and attenuated menopausal symptoms.[64] The effect of flaxseed on bone metabolism has been studied, and a number of biochemical markers of osteoclastic activity measured, such as bone mass change,[64] but no effects have been observed.[65] A number of researchers have investigated the effects of flax on menopausal symptoms. One randomised controlled trial reported that eating flaxseed for two months had the same effect as using HRT on mild menopausal symptoms, but was unable to improve the cholesterol profile in hypercholesterolaemic women.[66] A number of trials not comparing effects to HRT have produced variable results, sometimes confounded by the concomitant presence of soy isoflavones in the diet. Some have confirmed the positive benefits of flax on hot flushes and vaginal dryness, and it is likely that consumption of 40 g/day or more of flaxseed is required to elicit beneficial effects, whereas 25 g is insufficient.[65]

The relationships between bone mineral density and urinary excretion of lignan metabolites, particularly enterolactone, have been studied, but conflicting results have been obtained, showing both beneficial effects and negative effects on bone mineral density.[65] Flaxseed supplementation (25 g) has been shown to modify oestrogen metabolite excretion in urine by more than 25 g of soy, and this outcome appears with a concomitant increase in urinary lignan excretion, but no negative effect on bone cell metabolism was detected.[67]

In a study of postmenopausal women in the Netherlands, a high intake of flax phytoestrogens, of the order of 0.5 mg/day, was associated with a higher probability of intact cognitive function, particularly in women with longer postmenopausal timespans, from 20 to 30 years. It was thought that these may act via a number of routes, by increasing vascular compliance, interference with tyrosine kinase-dependent mechanisms and induction of synaptogenesis in the hippocampus.[68]

Flax has been shown to cause a reduction in LDL/HDL-C levels, but n-3 PUFAs, particularly α-linolenic acid, in flax may be responsible for this activity.

Resveratrol

Physiological levels of resveratrol are obtained from wine, up to 15 mg/L, and have been shown to have antioxidant, anticancer activity and to be cardioprotective.[13] Dosage forms of 10–200 mg are available, but no specified dosage has been established.

Resveratrol is oestrogenic, and binds to ERα and ERβ with 1:7000 the activity of oestradiol.[13] Increases in bone density in ovariectomised rats[69] and postmenopausal women have been reported.[70] The effects of a resveratrol-containing grape extract have been shown to reduce LDL-C in pre- and postmenopausal women.[71]

Other nutraceuticals

There is limited evidence that evening primrose oil, tea and the pine bark extract Pycnogenol may also exert beneficial effects on menopausal symptoms. One randomised, double-blind, placebo-controlled study investigated the effects of a 4 g daily dose of evening primrose oil (360 mg GLA) on menopausal hot flushing, and concluded that there was no benefit over placebo.[72] The effect of tea drinking on bone mineral density was surveyed in 1256 women in the UK, and it was found that drinkers of English tea had higher bone mineral density levels than those who did not. It was concluded that tea drinking may protect against osteoporosis in older women.[73] The use of Pycnogenol, 30–60 mg daily, has been claimed to help patients with endometriosis, premenstrual cramps and abdominal pain after supplementation for 2–4 weeks.[74]

Although black cohosh has been investigated for its effects on menopausal symptoms and statistically significant improvement of symptoms has been reported compared with placebo, it does not act as a phytoestrogen.[75]

Conclusions

There is a growing body of literature on the subject of phytoestrogens that suggests that they may provide substantial health benefits for treating menopausal symptoms. Phytoestrogens of dietary origin can be a significant contributor of oestrogens that may have health effects that are especially relevant to women's health due to hormone-associated diseases. The plant isoflavones share structural similarities with endogenous oestrogens and *in vitro* studies have shown that the iso-flavones can bind to oestrogen receptors. Functionally, it appears that the phytoestrogens may exert both oestrogenic and anti-oestrogenic effects, depending on circulating levels of endogenous sex hormones.

Although the purity, potency and effectiveness of the soy extracts are not well established, they are popularly believed to be safe and effective for the treatment of menopausal symptoms. It is clear, however, that much research is required to clearly define the pharmacological effect of dietary isoflavones and that future studies need to be of longer duration and carried out using standardised quantities and structurally characterised mixtures of compounds, or with isolated phytoestrogens.

References

1. Walker R, Edwards C. *Clinical Pharmacy and Therapeutics*, 3rd edn. London: Churchill Livingstone, 2003.
2. Cornwell T, Cohick W, Raskin I. Dietary phytoestrogens and health. *Phytochemistry* 2004; 65: 995–1016.
3. Scambia G, Mango D, Signorile P G. Clinical effects of a standardized soy extract in postmenopausal women: a pilot study. *Menopause* 2000; 7: 105–111.
4. Newton K M, Buist D S M, Keenan N L *et al*. Use of alternative therapies for menopause symptoms: results of a population-based survey. *Obstet Gynecol* 2002; 100: 18–25.
5. Glazier M G, Bowman M A. A review of the evidence for the use of phytoestrogens as a replacement for traditional estrogen replacement therapy. *Arch Intern Med* 2001; 161: 1161–1172.
6. Messina M J. Soy foods and soybean isoflavones and menopausal health. *Nutr Clin Care* 2002; 5: 272–282.
7. Tham D M, Gardner C D, Haskell W L. Potential health benefits of dietary phytoestrogens: a review of the clinical, epidemiological, and mechanistic evidence. *J Clin Endocrinol Metab* 1998; 83: 2223–2235.
8. Walle T, Browning A M, Steed L L *et al*. Flavonoid glucosides are hydrolyzed and thus activated in the oral cavity in humans. *J Nutr* 2005; 135: 48–52.
9. Rowland I, Faughnan M, Hoey L *et al*. Bioavailability of phyto-oestrogens. *Br J Nutr* 2003; 89: S45–S58.
10. Setchell K D, Cassidy A. Dietary isoflavones: biological effects and relevance to human health. *J Nutr* 1999; 129: 758S–767S.
11. Kuiper G G J M, Lemmen J G, Carlsson B *et al*. Interaction of estrogenic chemicals and phytoestrogens with estrogen receptor β. *Endocrinology* 1998; 139: 4252–4263.
12. Safford B, Dickens A, Halleron N *et al*. A model to estimate the oestrogen receptor mediated effects from exposure to soy isoflavones in food. *Regulat Toxicol Pharmacol* 2003; 38: 196–209.
13. Wolter F, Stein J. Biological activities of resveratrol and its analogs. *Drugs of the Future* 2002; 27: 949–959.
14. Routledge E J, White R, Parker M G, Sumpter J P. Differential effects of xenoestrogens on coactivator recruitment by estrogen receptor (ER) alpha and ERbeta. *J Biol Chem* 2000; 275: 35986–35993.
15. Zittermann A, Geppert J, Baier S *et al*. Short-term effects of high soy supplementation on sex hormones, bone markers, and lipid parameters in young female adults. *Eur J Nutr* 2004; 43: 100–108.
16. Chen X, Anderson J J B. Isoflavones and bone: Animal and human evidence of efficacy. *J Musculoskel Neuron Interaction* 2002; 2: 352–359.
17. Beck V, Rohr U, Jungbauer A. Phytoestrogens derived from red clover: an alternative to estrogen replacement therapy? *J Steroid Biochem Mol Biol* 2005; 94: 499–518.
18. Barnes S. Phyto-oestrogens and osteoporosis: what is a safe dose? *Br J Nutr* 2003; 89: S101–S108.

19. Hwang J, Sevanian A, Hodis H N. Synergistic inhibition of LDL oxidation by phyto-oestrogens and ascorbic acid. *Free Radic Biol Med* 2000; 29: 79–89.
20. Kurzer M S, Xu X. Dietary phytoestrogens. *Annu Rev Nutr* 1997; 17: 353–381.
21. Setchell K D, Brown N M, Lydeking-Olsen E. The clinical importance of the metabolite equol – a clue to the effectiveness of soy and its isoflavones. *J Nutr* 2002; 132: 3577–3584.
22. Setchell K D R, Clerici C, Lephart E D et al. S-Equol, a potent ligand for estrogen receptor β, is the exclusive enantiomeric form of the soy isoflavone metabolite produced by human intestinal bacterial flora. *Am J Clin Nutr* 2005; 81: 1072–1079.
23. Han K K, Soares J M, Haidar M A. Benefits of soy isoflavone therapeutic regimen on menopausal symptoms. *Obstet Gynecol* 2002; 99: 384–394.
24. Huntley A L, Ernst E. Soy for the treatment of perimenopausal symptoms – a systematic review. *Maturitas* 2004; 47: 1–9.
25. Krebs E E, Ensrud K E, MacDonald R, Wilt T J. Phytoestrogens for treatment of menopausal symptoms: a systematic review. *Obstet Gynecol* 2004; 104: 824–836.
26. Kronenberg F, Fugh-Berman A. Complementary and alternative medicine for menopausal symptoms: a review of randomized, controlled trials. *Ann Intern Med* 2002; 137: 805–813.
27. Messina M, Hughes C. Efficacy of soyfoods and soybean isoflavone supplements for alleviating menopausal symptoms is positively related to initial hot flush frequency. *J Med Food* 2003; 6: 1–11.
28. Cooper C W, Aihie A. Osteoporosis: recent advances in pathogenesis and treatment. *Q J Med* 1994; 87: 203–209.
29. St. Germain A, Peterson C T, Robinson J G. Isoflavone-rich or isoflavone-poor soy protein does not reduce menopausal symptoms during 24 weeks of treatment. *Menopause* 2001; 8: 17–26.
30. This P, De La Rochefordiere A, Clough K. Phytoestrogens after breast cancer. *Endocrin Rel Cancer* 2001; 8: 129–134.
31. Alekel D L, Germain A S, Peterson C T. Isoflavone-rich soy protein isolate attenuates bone loss in the lumbar spine of perimenopausal women. *Am J Clin Nutr* 2000; 72: 844–852.
32. Anderson J W, Johnstone B M, Cook-Newell M. Meta-analysis of the effects of soy protein intake on serum lipids. *N Engl J Med* 1995; 333: 276–282.
33. Phipps W R, Duncan A M, Kurzer M S. Isoflavones and postmenopausal women: a critical review. *Treatment Endocrinol* 2002; 1: 293–311.
34. Merz-Demlow B E, Duncan A M, Wangen K E et al. Soy isoflavones improve plasma lipids in normocholesterolemic, premenopausal women. *Am J Clin Nutr* 2000; 71: 1462–1469.
35. Wangen K E, Duncan A M, Xu X, Kurzer M S. Soy isoflavones improve plasma lipids in normocholesterolemic and mildly hypercholesterolemic post-menopausal women. *Am J Clin Nutr* 2001; 73: 225–231.
36. Yang G, Shu X-O, Jin F et al. Longitudinal study of soy food intake and blood pressure among middle-aged and elderly Chinese women. *Am J Clin Nutr* 2005; 81: 1012–1017.

37. Hill C E, Dye L. Phytoestrogens and cognitive performance: a review of the evidence. *Curr Top Nutraceut Res* 2003; 1: 203–212.

38. Kritz-Silverstein D, Von Muhlen D, Barrett-Connor E, Bressel M A B. Isoflavones and cognitive function in older women: the SOy and Postmenopausal Health In Aging (SOPHIA) Study. *Menopause* 2003; 10: 196–202.

39. File S E, Jarrett N, Fluck E *et al.* Eating soya improves human memory. *Psychopharmacology* 2001; 157: 430–436.

40. Kotecha N, Lockwood B. Soy-relieving the symptoms of menopause and fighting osteoporosis. *Pharm J* 2005; 275: 483–487.

41. Zhang X, Shu X-O, Li H *et al.* Prospective cohort study of soy food consumption and risk of bone fracture among postmenopausal women. *Arch Intern Med* 2005; 165: 1890–1895.

42. Atkinson C, Compston J E, Day N E. The effects of phytoestrogen isoflavones on bone density in women: a double-blind, randomized, placebo-controlled trial. *Am J Clin Nutr* 2004; 79: 326–333.

43. Heaney R P. The bone-remodeling transient: implications for the interpretation of clinical studies of bone mass change. *J Bone Miner Res* 1994; 9: 1515–1523.

44. Potter S M, Baum J A, Teng H. Soy protein and isoflavones: their effects on blood lipids and bone density in postmenopausal women. *Am J Clin Nutr* 1998; 68: 1375S–1379S.

45. Uesugi T, Fukai Y, Yamori Y. Beneficial effects of soybean isoflavone supplementation on bone metabolism and serum lipids in postmenopausal Japanese women: a four-week study. *J Am Coll Nutr* 2002; 21: 97–102.

46. Dalais F S, Ebeling P R, Kotsopoulos D. The effects of soy protein containing isoflavones on lipids and indices of bone resorption in postmenopausal women. *Clin Endocrinol* 2003; 58: 704–709.

47. Erdman J W, Stillman R J, Boileau R A. Provocative relation between soy and bone maintenance. *Am J Clin Nutr* 2000; 72: 679–680.

48. Recker R, Lappe J, Davies K. Characterization of perimenopausal bone loss: a prospective study. *J Bone Miner Res* 2000; 15: 1965–1973.

49. Ho S C, Woo J, Lam S. Soy protein consumption and bone mass in early postmenopausal Chinese women. *Osteoporosis Int* 2003; 14: 835–842.

50. Setchell K, Lydeking-Olsen E. Dietary phytoestrogens and their effect on bone: evidence from in vitro and in vivo, human observational, and dietary intervention studies. *Am J Clin Nutr* 2003; 78: 593S–609S.

51. Simonet W S, Lacey D L, Dunstan C R. Osteoprotegerin: a novel secreted protein involved in the regulation of bone density. *Cell* 1997; 89: 309–319.

52. Somekawa Y, Chiguchi M, Ishibashi T. Use of vitamin K_2 (menatetrenone) and 1,25-dihydroxyvitamin D_3 in the prevention of bone loss induced by leuprolide. *J Clin Endocrinol Metab* 1999; 84: 2700–2704.

53. Orimo H, Hashimoto T, Yoshimora N. Nationwide incidence survey of femoral neck fracture in Japan. *J Bone Miner Metab* 1997; 15: 100–106.

54. Agnusdei D, Bufalino L. Efficacy of ipriflavone in established osteoporosis and long-term safety. *Calc Tissue Int* 1997; 61: S23–S27.

55. Alexandersen P, Toussaint A, Christiansen C *et al.* Ipriflavone in the treatment of postmenopausal osteoporosis: a randomized controlled trial. *JAMA* 2001; 285: 1482–1488.

56. Anderson J J, Garner S C. Phytoestrogens and bone. *Baillière's Clin Endocrinol Metab* 1998; 12: 543–557.

57. van de Weijer P H M, Barentsen R. Isoflavones from red clover (Promensil) significantly reduce menopausal hot flush symptoms compared with placebo. *Maturitas* 2002; 42: 187–193.

58. Tice J A, Ettinger B, Ensrud K *et al*. Phytoestrogen supplements for the treatment of hot flashes: the isoflavone clover extract (ICE) study. A randomized controlled trial. *JAMA* 2003; 290: 207–214.

59. Howes J B, Sullivan D, Lai N *et al*. The effects of dietary supplementation with isoflavones from red clover on the lipoprotein profiles of post menopausal women with mild to moderate hypercholesterolaemia. *Atherosclerosis* 2000; 152: 143–147.

60. Tolleson W H, Doerge D R, Churchwell M I *et al*. Metabolism of biochanin A and formononetin by human liver microsomes in vitro. *J Agric Food Chem* 2002; 50: 4783–4790.

61. Sandy J, Davies M, Prime S. Signal pathways that transduce growth factor-stimulated mitogenesis in bone cells. *Bone* 1998; 23: 17–26.

62. Messina M J, Persky V, Setchell K D. Soy intake and cancer risk: a review of the in vitro and in vivo data. *Nutr Cancer* 1994; 21: 113–131.

63. White L R, Petrovitch H, Ross G W *et al*. Brain aging and midlife tofu consumption. *J Am Coll Nutr* 2000; 19: 242–255.

64. Westcott N D, Muir A D. Flax seed lignan in disease prevention and health promotion. *Phytochem Rev* 2003; 2: 401–417.

65. Ward W E. Effect of flaxseed on bone metabolism and menopause. In: Thomson L U, Cunnane S C, ed. *Flaxseed in Human Nutrition*, 2nd edn. Champaign, IL: AOCS Press, 2003: 319–332.

66. Lemay A, Dodin S, Kadri N *et al*. Flaxseed dietary supplement versus hormone replacement therapy in hypercholesterolemic menopausal women. *Obstet Gynecol* 2002; 100: 495–504.

67. Brooks J D, Ward W E, Lewis J E *et al*. Supplementation with flaxseed alters estrogen metabolism in postmenopausal women to a greater extent than does supplementation with an equal amount of soy. *Am J Clin Nutr* 2004; 79: 318–325.

68. Franco O H, Burger H, Lebrun, *et al*. Higher dietary intake of lignans is associated with better cognitive performance in postmenopausal women. *J Nutr* 2005; 135: 1190–1195.

69. Liu Z P, Li W X, Yu B *et al*. Effects of trans-resveratrol from *Polygonum cuspidatum* on bone loss using the ovariectomized rat model. *J Med Food* 2005; 8: 14–19.

70. Bagchi D, Preuss H G, Bagchi M, Stohs S J. Phytoestrogen, resveratrol and women's health. *Res Commun Pharmacol Toxicol* 2000; 5: 107–121.

71. Zern T L, Wood R J, Greene C *et al*. Grape polyphenols exert a cardioprotective effect in pre- and postmenopausal women by lowering plasma lipids and reducing oxidative stress. *J Nutr* 2005; 135: 1911–1917.

72. Chenoy R, Hussain S, Tayob Y *et al*. Effect of oral gamolenic acid from evening primrose oil on menopausal flushing. *BMJ* 1994; 308: 501–503.

73. Hegarty V M, May H M, Khaw K-T. Tea drinking and bone mineral density in older women. *Am J Clin Nutr* 2000; 71: 1003–1007.

74. Rohdewald P. A review of the French maritime pine bark extract (Pycnogenol), a herbal medication with a diverse clinical pharmacology. *Int J Clin Pharmacol Ther* 2002; 40: 158–168.

75. Viereck V, Emons G, Wuttke W. Black cohosh: just another phytoestrogen? *Trends Endocrinol Metab* 2005; 16: 214–221.

14

Weight management

Obesity

In the UK, as in many other developed countries, there is an increasing obesity epidemic. Between 1993 and 2003 the number of clinically obese individuals almost doubled. Numbers of clinically obese men rose from 13% to 23%, and women from 16% to 23%.[1] A further 44% of men and 33% of women in the UK are classed as clinically overweight.[1] Childhood obesity has also become a major issue, prompting the UK government to aim new policies at curbing the increase of unhealthy children[2] following a recent TV series highlighting the role of convenience food in the growing childhood obesity epidemic.[3]

Obesity is not only a major health problem, it also causes concern for individuals for cosmetic reasons, and the enormous variety of dieting supplements and popularity of weight loss clubs show how weight loss has become a multimillion pound industry. In the USA, the number one health issue (as reported by 40% of the population) is the need to lose weight for reasons of appearance.[4] Two-thirds of Americans (representing 138 million adults) also report that they have used some method to maintain or manage their weight during 2004.[4]

Strategies for weight loss

Low carbohydrate diets are just one example from the long list of diets on offer for those wanting to lose weight. The popularity of the Atkins diet, the Glycaemic Index (GI) diet and meal replacement diets such as Slimfast, are examples of the many routes people are willing to try in order to achieve weight loss.

Clubs and organisations where group support and encouragement are available alongside a diet regime are also popular. Weight Watchers, an international slimming organisation that has 6000 classes weekly in the UK and claims to have helped around 30 million dieters to lose weight,[5] and Slimming World, which has recently joined forces with

NHS Primary Care Trusts to aid dieters,[6] are examples of such organisations.

Supplements for weight loss are numerous. People generally prefer to seek a shortcut to weight loss, so the demand for such supplements, which often claim to give fast results, is huge. Coupled with the fact that many of these products can be marketed as food supplements with relatively little regulatory controls, the market is rapidly expanding.[7]

The universally acknowledged way to lose weight is a calorie controlled diet with increased physical activity, as most healthcare professionals advise.[8] Diet alone is useful, but for long-term maintenance of body weight, exercise is critical, helping prevent the cyclical effect of rapid weight gain after a period of dieting.[9] Self-monitoring and other behavioural interventions can also enhance weight loss.[8]

Conventional pharmaceutical treatments such as the lipase inhibitor orlistat are also available for weight loss, but only on prescription. Orlistat works by blocking fat absorption but has unpleasant and common side-effects of faecal incontinence and flatulence.[10]

Nutraceuticals

Nutraceuticals are a growing sector of the supplements market for weight loss, and there are a wide variety of products, formulated into capsules or tablets, or even incorporated into foods or convenience style foods such as snack bars. Several nutraceuticals currently being marketed as aids to weight loss have been the subject of scientific and medical research. The major examples include L-carnitine and acetyl-L-carnitine, dehydroepiandrosterone (DHEA), green tea and conjugated linoleic acid (CLA).

L-Carnitine and acetyl-L-carnitine

L-Carnitine is an endogenous product found in the kidneys and liver that can also be obtained by intake of dairy products and red meat in the diet. It is a co-factor in the process of fat oxidation for cellular energy production.[11] Fat oxidation in muscle tissue is reduced in obesity due to a reduction of L-carnitine-mediated enzyme activity.[12] It is for this reason that carnitine is purported to be of benefit in obese people by increasing fat oxidation,[13] and explains why it is often promoted as a 'fat burner'. However, it has not been tested for its effectiveness or safety over prolonged periods of time.

One study found that rats fed L-carnitine supplementation in combination with an energy-restricted diet had the same weight loss and body composition as rats fed an energy-restricted diet alone.[14] Results showed both groups lost considerable amounts of weight and had a marked reduction in body fat, but there were no significant differences between the control group and the treated group.

L-Carnitine was shown to drastically reduce body fat in a study of basketball players, although it did not cause a significant fall in overall body mass.[15] The study was investigating L-carnitine as an ergogenic aid for reducing body fat in already lean athletes. A cohort of 12 basketball players were supplemented with L-carnitine for eight weeks and compared with a control group. In the supplemented group there were significant improvements in speed, jumping ability and Vo_2 max (maximal oxygen uptake), and an average 21% fall in body fat. However, there was no significant difference in overall reduction of body mass between the two groups.

A review of common dietary supplements for weight loss concluded that there was insufficient or conflicting evidence for L-carnitine, and that despite no evidence of adverse effects, no trials demonstrated L-carnitine's effectiveness as a supplement for weight loss. The review suggested that doctors should caution patients that L-carnitine has so far not been proven useful for weight loss, but if a patient wanted to use the supplement, then doctors should monitor them for any positive or negative effects.[16]

Acetyl-L-carnitine has similar roles to L-carnitine, and is used by athletes as a metabolic source of L-carnitine. It is synthesised by mitochondria and found in the brain, kidney and liver. Claims have been made that supplementation with acetyl-L-cartinine can increase energy and help weight loss.[17] Acetyl-L-carnitine is capable of restoring mitochondrial energy production, so it is believed to increase general metabolic activity as well. It is for these reasons that acetyl-L-carnitine is purported to increase ambulatory activity and increase metabolism, although animal studies show mixed results, with one study showing an improvement in metabolic function of rats supplemented with acetyl-L-carnitine,[17] and another study showing that acetyl-L-carnitine prevented weight loss in rats.[18] There is no scientific evidence for weight loss in humans with acetyl-L-carnitine.

Dehydroepiandrosterone

DHEA is an adrenal hormone found naturally in the body. Blood levels of DHEA in humans peak at around the age of 20, and decrease rapidly after 25 years of age. DHEA plays a role in receptor and enzyme adaptations that are thought to favour increased fat oxidation and decreased fat deposition.[19] Administration of DHEA to rats has led to a decrease in their visceral fat accumulation, and also resulted in a lower increase of body fat with advancing age.[19] For human consumption DHEA is only available on prescription in the UK, but is widely available for sale on the Internet. It is marketed as a 'thermogenic' compound with the ability to burn fat and also to help maintain fat loss.[18]

One study concluded that inefficient energy utilisation and obesity in rats was corrected with DHEA treatment.[20] DHEA was administered to obese prediabetic OLETF rats for a 17-day period, during which the rats sustained significant weight loss. This loss was partly attributed to enhanced utilisation of energy ingested. It was suggested that DHEA corrected deficient expression levels of uncoupling protein 1 (UCP-1) in brown adipose tissue in these rats, which contributed to more efficient energy utilisation and hence weight loss.

A study of the effects of DHEA in humans concluded that compared with a placebo, DHEA induced significant decreases in abdominal fat in elderly men and women.[19] In a randomised, double-blind, placebo-controlled six-month trial of men and women over 65 years, a daily dose of 50 mg DHEA reduced visceral and subcutaneous fat significantly. The volunteers in this study were included if their weight had been stable for the previous year. During the study volunteers were asked not to alter their usual diet or activity levels. No significant adverse effects were reported with the DHEA supplements. It was suggested that DHEA acts as a peroxisome proliferator-activated receptor α (PPARα) agonist, which have been shown to reduce fat stores in muscle and reduce obesity. DHEA also increased the concentration of circulating insulin-like growth factor I (IGF-I) within the body, which has been shown in previous studies to reduce abdominal fat.

More research is needed to assess the side-effect profile of DHEA, and there are inherent dangers involved in unsupervised use of these steroids. Long-term studies are also needed with DHEA to assess the effects of increased IGF-I levels, and the effect of changes in oestradiol and testosterone levels on the body, as this supplement could be taken for long periods of time if found to be effective.

Green tea

The claimed benefits of drinking green tea and taking green tea supplements are becoming more widely discussed, with the lay media and articles on the Internet extolling their claimed health benefits. Green tea contains catechin polyphenols, which have been shown to inhibit catechol-O-methyltransferase (COMT), an enzyme responsible for the degradation of noradrenaline, which itself has an important role in the control of thermogenesis and fat metabolism.[21]

Tea catechins have been shown to cause loss of appetite, which might involve neuropeptides other than leptins, since (—)-epigallocatechin gallate (EGCG) is effective in reducing the body weight of both lean and obese (leptin receptor-negative) rats. However, the body weight loss has been found to be reversible, and the animals regain body weight when EGCG administration is stopped. The *in vitro* thermogenic effect of green tea extract on adipose tissue can be mimicked by EGCG, giving credence to the belief that EGCG is the important component of green tea.[22]

It has been recommended that the use of green tea for weight loss should be cautioned and closely monitored in patients that choose to take it, as product quality and efficacy is uncertain, although adverse effects are not likely if the equivalent of five cups daily is not exceeded.[16]

A small study of ten male adults indicated that green tea extract significantly increased 24-hour energy expenditure, measured by indirect calorimetry while in a respiratory chamber.[21] This was a crossover study in which the ten volunteers were assigned one of three treatments (a placebo, green tea extract or the equivalent amount of caffeine to that in the green tea extract) on three occasions. Treatment with the placebo or the caffeine did not have any significant effects on energy expenditure. These results rule out the hypothesis that caffeine alone is responsible for the increased energy expenditure. The major limitation of this study, aside from its small sample size, is that it did not actually measure body weight as a parameter, as it was only carried out for a period of 24 hours at any one time. However, the authors do suggest that green tea extract has good potential to influence body weight and body composition due to its promotion of fat oxidation and thermogenic properties. An important observation of the study was that there was no increase in heart rate, as is seen with other substances that increase energy expenditure such as ephedrine and other sympathomimetic drugs. This means that the risk of adverse cardiovascular effects is greatly reduced.

Another study on the effects of green tea for weight maintenance after weight loss showed that weight maintenance over a 13-week period, after a 7.5% body weight loss, was not affected by green tea consumption.[23] This randomised, parallel and placebo-controlled trial included 104 participants and was undertaken over a four-week weight loss period, followed by a 13-week weight maintenance period. Overweight and moderately obese men and women volunteers were recruited. The study attempted to try to find a solution to the common problem of cyclical weight loss and regain, and the issue of long-term weight maintenance that is obviously required if patients are to maintain the benefits of their initial weight loss. Overall results showed that the body weight regained (as a percentage of body weight lost) by the green tea and placebo groups was not significantly different. Hunger and satiety were also the same in the two groups, and there were no metabolic differences. The same study[23] showed that the high habitual caffeine consumers had higher weight gain in the 13 weeks than low habitual caffeine consumers. Habitual caffeine consumption did not differ between the green tea and the placebo group. This result could indicate that the green tea supplement was only effective when habitual caffeine intake was low (or that a much increased dose was needed if caffeine intake was high). The authors suggested that saturation of the ability of green tea to further stimulate noradrenaline-related mechanisms of weight loss may be important, as caffeine and green tea both produce some of their effects through this mechanism. This seems to contradict the previous study[21] that claimed it was the catechins exerting the effect on fat metabolism and thermogenesis, not the caffeine. However, caffeine may be exerting its effect via a different mechanism.

No side-effects were reported in any of the studies. As green tea is consumed by a large number of people worldwide with few reported adverse effects, it would appear to be relatively safe. Green tea could be incorporated into an everyday Western lifestyle without necessitating the trouble of buying and taking tablets and capsules. However, some people may be unable to palate the astringent taste of green tea, in which case supplements may be preferred.

Conjugated linoleic acid

CLA is a collective term used to describe a mixture of positional and geometric dienoic linoleic acid isomers with conjugated double bonds. In dietary supplements, various combinations of the different isomers are found. CLA isomers can be obtained from normal dietary components such as dairy and meat products.

A review of 13 randomised, placebo-controlled trials in humans concluded that there was little evidence to support the proposition that CLA reduced body weight or promoted repartitioning of body fat in humans.[24] It only reviewed trials that had lasted for longer than four weeks, and concluded that the CLA isomer *trans*-10, *cis*-12 may produce liver hypertrophy and insulin resistance. The authors recommended that

CLA supplementation should be cautioned before studies with further data to clarify this situation were published.

Studies in rodents have shown that adminstration of CLA can significantly reduce body fat and lower body weight.[24-27] However, in human studies, results have been mixed. One review article found that of all the 13 studies reviewed, none showed any evidence for significant reduction in body weight and only two showed significant fat-lowering effects.[25] It has been noted that the body fat-lowering effect of CLA is due to the *trans*-10, *cis*-12 isomer[25,26] (but that over 90% of human CLA intake from food is from the *cis*-9, *trans*-11 isomer[25]).

A further review concluded that although CLA reduced weight gain and fat deposition in rodents, the effects in humans are less significant and often inconsistent.[26] The different mechanisms thought to be responsible for the activity of CLA are increasing energy expenditure, reduced fat cell size, increasing apoptosis of fat cells, and the inhibition of lipogenesis in the liver or increasing fat oxidation. Side-effects of CLA that have been found are the negative effect on insulin sensitivity and glycaemic control, and the development of fatty liver and spleen. However, these side-effects have so far only been shown in rodents.[27] This indicates that further reliable data are required before a clear judgement can be made on the use of CLA for weight management in humans. The safety of CLA was investigated in a trial on rats in which the equivalent of 30 times the human dose was used, and no adverse effects were observed.[27] Several human trials have been reported in which no adverse effects occurred when high-quality CLA was taken at doses of 3–6 g per day.

One year-long study into the effects of CLA on body fat mass concluded that long-term supplementation of CLA in healthy over-weight adults significantly reduced body fat mass.[28] This randomised, double-blind, placebo-controlled study, with no diet or lifestyle restrictions placed on the volunteers, showed a slight reduction in body mass index and body weight in the CLA group, whereas there was no change in the placebo group. Adverse effects were mainly mild or moderate gastrointestinal symptoms. A high compliance and low dropout rate of volunteers also showed CLA was well tolerated. A later trial by the same team assessed the effect of CLA supplementation at 3.4 g/day over 12 months, and found a 6–8% reduction in body fat mass.[29]

A further review found that there were insufficient data to support the use of CLA for weight loss in humans, and that overall quality, safety and efficacy of CLA is uncertain.[16] It recommended that doctors should caution patients about the use of CLA, and closely monitor those who took the supplement, as efficacy and safety have not been proven.

A further recent study concluded that the metabolic effects of CLA are complex and still not well understood.[30] This is partly due to the lack of knowledge regarding the mechanisms of CLA at a molecular level, and the lack of controlled studies on the different isomers of CLA. Another study found that there was no effect on body weight and body mass index in volunteers taking CLA for a 12-week period, but that CLA in a dose of 3.4 g per day was safe.[31] The most recent trial involving 122 obese subjects and the same daily dose over a period of one year concluded that CLA did not prevent weight or fat mass regain.[32] Further studies are required in order to make a clear judgement on the efficacy of CLA as a weight loss aid.

Conclusions

Of all the nutraceuticals reviewed, DHEA seems the most likely candidate for producing actual weight loss, as opposed to alteration of body composition. It has shown weight loss effects in both animal and human studies. In some countries, however, supply is restricted as is the case in the UK, and consequently it is not legally available for self-medication. L-Carnitine has demonstrated potential as an ergogenic aid, but there is little firm evidence to support its use for weight loss. Green tea has also shown little evidence for ability to cause weight loss, although studies have shown it can increase energy expenditure, so further long-term trials are needed to assess whether it can have effects on body weight over an extended period of time. Green tea also seems to have a better safety profile than the other nutraceuticals reviewed. CLA has been shown to have variable ability to reduce body fat in humans. Although it has shown weight loss effects in rodents, it has not yet been demonstrated to cause weight loss in humans.

So far, the studies that have been published do not go far enough in establishing the long-term safety and efficacy of these nutraceuticals. It is critically important in supplements that are likely to be taken long term that safety is established. It is also important that the efficacy of these nutraceuticals is established in large human studies with actual body weight loss as a parameter, as opposed to energy expenditure or body fat loss with no overall weight loss.

Despite the promise and lure of nutraceutical supplements and crash diets, consumers can never expect dramatic weight loss and long-term maintenance of a lower body weight unless they reduce their calorie intake and take some form of exercise. For those individuals with a body mass index indicative of clinical obesity (30 kg/m^2 and above), medical intervention for weight loss must be considered to reduce the risk of weight-related health problems such as type 2 diabetes and cardio-vascular disease.

Even if nutraceutical supplementation is only a psychological prop or placebo to aid weight loss, alongside diet or lifestyle changes, it may be helpful because if there is an overall weight loss then that will be beneficial to the patient's health. One argument frequently claimed for the use of supplements is that when patients have tried and failed on other weight-loss programmes and various diets, their weight may have become a serious health threat, so that any possible aid to weight loss becomes worth trying. The risks of any dieting aids must obviously be balanced against the benefits of weight loss and the reduction of the health risks of remaining overweight.

With the huge range of products available, pharmacists and nutri-tionists are at the forefront when it comes to explaining and justifying the relative merits of the various weight loss supplements available, alongside offering basic diet and lifestyle advice to customers, and knowing when to direct them to their GP if medical intervention is required. Such professional advice is necessary to weigh up and evaluate the clinical evidence of different products, as opposed to the possibility of inaccurate and often unreliable information supplied by the media and on the Internet. However, a lack of quality data obviously impacts on the ability of the pharmacist to offer good quality advice. Further trials are needed for these nutraceuticals to establish a greater degree of knowledge on their potential contribution to weight loss.

References

1. National Statistics. Health Highlights. www.statistics.gov.uk/cci/nugget.asp?id=1049 (accessed 27 March 2005).
2. Fister K. UK government puts children at centre of plan to improve the country's health. *BMJ* 2005; 330: 618.
3. Spence D. Jamie's school dinners. *BMJ* 2005; 330: 678.
4. Marra J. The state of dietary supplements. *Nutraceuticals World* September 2004; 50–57.
5. Weight Watchers. About us; history and philosophy. http://www.weightwatchers.co.uk/about/his/history.aspx (accessed 6 June 2006).
6. Slimming on Referral. Tackling obesity in primary care. http://www.slimming-on-referral.com/public_home.asp (accessed 6 June 2006).
7. Mason P. OTC Weight control products. *Pharm J* 2002; 269: 103–105.

8. Noel P H, Pugh J A. Management of overweight and obese adults. *BMJ* 2002; 325: 757–761.

9. Grubbs L. The critical role of exercise in weight control. *Nurse Pract* 1993; 18: 20–22.

10. *British National Formulary Number 52*. London: BMJ Publishing and RPS Publishing, 2006.

11. Kelly G S. L-Carnitine: therapeutic applications of a conditionally-essential amino acid. *Altern Med Rev* 1998; 3: 345–360.

12. Kim J Y, Hickner R C, Cortright R L *et al.* Lipid oxidation is reduced in obese human skeletal muscle. *Am J Physiol Endocrinol Metab* 2000; 279: 1039–1044.

13. Dyck D J. Dietary fat intake, supplements and weight loss. *Can J Appl Physiol* 2000; 25: 495–523.

14. Brandsch C, Eder K. Effect of L-carnitine on weight loss and body composition of rats fed a hypocaloric diet. *Ann Nutr Metab* 2002; 46: 205–210.

15. Zajac A, Waskiewicz K, Nowak K. The influence of L-carnitine supplementation on body fat content, speed, explosive strength and VO_2 max in elite athletes. *Biol Sport* 2001; 18: 127–135.

16. Saper R, Eisenberg D, Phillips R. Common dietary supplements for weight loss. *Am Fam Physician* 2004; 70: 1734–1738.

17. Wadsworth F, Lockwood B. Combined alpha-lipoic acid and acetyl-L-carnitine supplementation. *Pharm J* 2003. 270; 587–589.

18. Lolic M, Fiskum G, Rosenthal R. Neuroprotective effects of acetyl-L-carnitine after stroke in rats. *Ann Emerg Med* 1997; 29: 758–765.

19. Villareal D, Holloszy J. Effect of DHEA on abdominal fat and insulin action in elderly women and men. *JAMA* 2004; 292: 2243–2248.

20. Ryu J, Kim S, Kim C *et al.* DHEA administration increases brown fat uncoupling protein 1 levels in obese OLETF rats. *Biochem Biophys Res Commun* 2003. 303; 726–731.

21. Dulloo A, Duret C, Rohrer D *et al.* Efficacy of a green tea extract rich in catechin polyphenols and caffeine in increasing 24-h energy expenditure and fat oxidation in humans. *Am J Clin Nutr* 1999; 70: 1040–1045.

22. Kao Y-H, Hiipakka R A, Liao S. Modulation of obesity by a green tea catechin. *Am J Clin Nutr* 2000; 72: 1232–1233.

23. Kovacs E, Lejeune M, Nijs I, Westerterp-Plantenga M. Effects of green tea on weight maintenance after body-weight loss. *Br J Nutr* 2004; 91; 431–437.

24. Larsen T, Toubro S, Astrup A. Efficacy and safety of dietary supplements containing CLA for the treatment of obesity: evidence from animal and human studies. *J Lipid Res* 2003; 44: 2234–2241.

25. Terpstra A. Effect of conjugated linoleic acid on body composition and plasma lipids in humans: an overview of the literature. *Am J Clin Nutr* 2004; 79: 352–361.

26. Wang Y, Jones P. Conjugated linoleic acid and obesity control: efficacy and mechanisms. *Int J Obesity* 2004; 28: 941–955.

27. Pariza M. Perspective on the safety and effectiveness of conjugated linoleic acid. *Am J Clin Nutr* 2004; 79: 1132S–1136S.

28. Gaullier J-M, Halse J, Hoye K *et al.* Conjugated linoleic supplementation for

1 y reduces body fat mass in healthy overweight humans. *Am J Clin Nutr* 2004; 79: 1118–1125.

29. Gaullier, J-M, Halse J, Hoye K *et al*. Supplementation with conjugated linoleic acid for 24 months is well tolerated by and reduces body fat mass in healthy, overweight humans. *J Nutr* 2005; 135: 778–784.

30. Riserus U, Smedman A, Basu S, Vessby B. Metabolic effects of conjugated linoleic acid in humans: the Swedish experience. *Am J Clin Nutr* 2004; 79: 1146–1148.

31. Berven G, Bye A, Hals O *et al*. Safety of conjugated linoleic acid (CLA) in overweight or obese human volunteers. *Eur J Lipid Sci Technol* 2000; 102: 455–462.

32. Larsen T M, Toubro S, Gudmundsen O, Astrup A. Conjugated linoleic acid supplementation for 1 y does not prevent weight or body fat regain. *Am J Clin Nutr* 2006; 83: 606–612.

15

Skin health

The skin is the largest organ in the human body, and its primary function is to act as a barrier to protect the body from damage caused by outside forces, contaminants, microorganisms and radiation exposure. Exposure of the skin to UV light has the potential to induce the formation of reactive oxygen species (ROS) and free radicals which can damage organelles and modify the structures of important molecules such as proteins, lipids and genetic material. Sunlight, particularly UVB (wavelength 290–320 nm), is responsible for sunburn, but also causes cellular damage. UVA light (wavelength 320–400 nm) burns less than UVB, but is able to penetrate deep into the dermis unlike UVB, which is capable of penetrating only as far as the boundary between the epidermis and the dermis. UVA light makes up the majority of sunlight, and is absorbed by a wide range of molecules, which can become photosensitisers, and can do more damage to the skin due to its greater ability to penetrate. Environmental pollutants such as ozone and oxides of nitrogen and sulfur are also able to produce free radicals in the skin, thereby also risking skin damage.[1] Although formed in the outer layers of the epidermis, these radicals induce damage in deeper layers in a manner similar to UV light.

A number of nutraceuticals have been claimed to exhibit useful activities in the area of skin health, including proanthocyanidins and the pine bark extract Pycnogenol, carotenoids, polyunsaturated fatty acids (PUFAs), tea, soy, glucosamine and melatonin.

Grape seed proanthocyanidin extract

The protective effect of grape seed proanthocyanidin extract (GSPE) against UVB-promoted photo-oxidation of PUFAs has been studied in micelles. As a result it was suggested that GSPE could be used as an adjuvant in skin protection from sunlight damage.[2] One per cent GSPE formulated into a skin cream and applied 30 minutes prior to UVA/UVB radiation, has been reported to produce a 9% increase in sun protection factor, which was suggested to result from the scavenging of oxygen free radicals.[3] GSPE was found to be effective in reducing the hyperpigmentation of women with chloasma, and was maximally effective after six months, but no further improvements were reported after this period.[4] The proprietary product Pycnogenol has also been researched in this role: UV radiation-induced erythema in human volunteers was reduced after oral supplementation with 1.10 mg/kg body weight.[5] Further research on the effects of UV radiation from sunlight exposure in women found that supplementation with 25 mg Pycnogenol three times daily for 30 days resulted in approximately 38% decrease in skin area affected by melasma (cutaneous hyperpigmentation).[6]

Carotenoids

Lutein has been widely marketed as a filter for high-energy blue light with particular benefits for human eyes (see Chapter 7), but this perceived property may also benefit skin, and it is available in a range of topical and oral formulations. Epidemiological evidence has found a link between diets rich in lutein and other carotenoids, and reduction of incidence of melanoma in humans, and animal work has been used to investigate a number of UV-induced effects.[1] It has been claimed that it can also reduce UVA- and UVB-induced erythema caused by reactive oxygen species. Supplementation with lutein has been shown to result in its deposition in the skin, and carotenoid supplementation (containing mainly carotene plus 0.12 mg lutein) has been shown to result in less erythema in human subjects in response to UV irradiation. Work with mice showed that those supplemented with lutein had significantly fewer tumours of smaller size after irradiation with UVB light.[7] Long-term supplementation with a carotenoid mixture (β-carotene, lutein, lycopene, 8 mg each) over 12 weeks was reported to ameliorate UV-induced erythema in humans.[8]

Polyunsaturated fatty acids

The topical use of PUFAs in cosmetics and topical skin formulations is restricted due to the formation of malodorous secondary oxidation products. Research into the topical application of fish oil has shown a statistically significant improvement in erythema and scaling, and marked improvement in plaque thickness. A fish oil concentrate has been shown to benefit patients suffering from atopic dermatitis.[9] Atopic eczma has been treated with evening primrose oil, due to the 9% content of γ-linolenic acid (GLA). Although this had a product licence as a medicine until November 2002, this has now been withdrawn. Early meta-analysis of placebo-controlled studies found insignificant effects compared with controls,[10] but a later analysis revealed an improvement in atopic eczema.[11] One further trial evaluated skin parameters in healthy elderly people after supplementation with 360–720 mg GLA (from borage oil) daily, over two months. Cutaneous layer function was improved by 11%, and dry skin reduced by 14–42%.[12]

Tea

Since tea catechins inhibit UV-induced skin cancers in experimental animal models, it is thought that they may have application as treatments for skin ailments.[13] A number of formulated skin preparations, including sunscreens, contain tea extracts as they are believed to have a soothing effect on the skin as well as acting as antioxidants.[14] Black tea polyphenols have been shown to protect against UVB-induced erythema, an inflammation response in mouse and human skin, and (—)-epigallocatechin gallate (EGCG) and (—)-epicatechin gallate (ECG) inhibit 5α-reductase present in skin, which is associated with androgen-dependent dermatological disorders such as acne.[15] Sebum production from the male human forehead is also inhibited by topical application of EGCG, suggesting its possible use for acne treatment.[13]

Reports concerning protection from UV radiation may allow for improved formulations of sunscreens. Photocarcinogenesis treatment with EGCG has been investigated in mice. Significant reduction in tumours has been reported after topical, but not oral application. EGCG is believed to act through a mechanism other than inhibition of photo-immunosuppression.[16]

Soy isoflavones

Many cosmetic products contain hyaluronic acid, a natural glycoamino-glycan normally present in skin, which is known to hydrate the skin, allowing it to appear smoother. A number of *in vitro* studies have shown that genistein and daidzein can stimulate hyaluronic acid production in the skin.[17] Genistein has been reported to inhibit skin cancer and cutaneous ageing induced by UV light in mice, and also photodamage and associated discomfort in humans. It is thought that the mechanism of action involves protection of oxidative and photodynamically damaged DNA, downregulation of UVB-activated signal transduction cascades, and antioxidant activity.[18]

Coenzyme Q10

Ageing and photoageing are associated with an increase in cellular oxidation, possibly caused by declining levels of coenzyme Q10 (Co Q10). Topical application of Co Q10 has been shown to penetrate into viable layers of the epidermis and to reduce the level of oxidation, resulting in a reduction in wrinkle depth. It has also been found to be effective against UVA-mediated oxidative stress in human keratinocytes, and to prevent oxidative DNA damage.[19]

Glucosamine

Although the major use of glucosamine in the Western world is in the area of joint health, numerous patents and publications have appeared in Japan and Korea on its application for skin problems. Oral glucosamine has been shown to improve skin dryness and smoothness,[20] and a significant reduction in wrinkles and fine lines was reported in one group of women.[21]

Another nutraceutical used to treat osteoarthritis, methylsulfonyl-methane (MSM), is also widely used for improvement of skin, nails and hair, but there is only anecdotal and no published evidence to substantiate these uses.

Melatonin

Topical application of melatonin either alone or in combination with vitamins C and E has been shown to reduce UV-induced skin erythema after topical application 30 minutes before exposure.[22]

Activity of nutraceuticals on hair growth

Stimulation of hair growth is the 'holy grail' for cosmetic scientists, but as yet there is little clear evidence for the use of nutraceuticals in this area. Many plant extracts have been investigated for possible use. One report surveyed 1000 plant extracts in an *in vitro* test system. GSPE was the most successful product, causing growth of hair follicle cells in mice at a level of 230% compared with controls. The most active fraction of

GSPE was the catechin and epicatechin polymers of 3.5 average polymerisation.[23]

The possibility of soy has been considered, based on the premise that its antiandrogenic effects may reverse androgen-mediated disorders such as hair loss. Men with male pattern baldness have been shown to have higher levels of circulating 5α-dihydrotestosterone (DHT), which binds to androgen receptors in hair follicles. Hair loss treatments have been produced to block DHT, but no evidence has yet been published for the effects of soy on this.[24] The possibility of soy having an effect are based upon its effect in prostate cancer, which is controlled by androgens, thus fuelling speculation that flax lignans may also have an effect.

Spermidine has recently been investigated, particularly for telogen effluvium, a common form of alopecia, which is often caused by prescription medicines and stress. A clinical trial using 0.5 mg oral supplementation for two months was shown to reduce the symptoms compared with controls.[25]

References

1. Roberts R L, Barnes H T. Lutein. Part 1 – Natural support for healthy skin *Agrofood* 2004; 15: 49–52.
2. Carini M, Facino R, Maffei A G *et al*. The protection of polyunsaturated fatty acids in micellar systems against UVB-induced photo-oxidation by procyanidins from *Vitis vinifera* L., and the protective synergy with vitamin E. *Int J Cosmet Sci* 1998; 20: 203–215.
3. Bagchi D, Bagchi M, Stohs S J *et al*. Free radicals and grape seed proanthocyanidin extract: importance in human health and disease prevention. *Toxicol* 2000; 148: 187–197.
4. Yamakoshi J, Sano A, Tokutake S *et al*. Oral intake of proanthocyanidin-rich extract from grape seeds improves chloasma. *Phytother Res* 2004; 18: 895–899.
5. Saliou C, Rimbach G, Moini H *et al*. Solar ultraviolet-induced erythema in human skin and nuclear factor-kappa-B-dependent gene expression in keratinocytes are modulated by a French maritime pine bark extract. *Free Radic Biol Med* 2001; 30: 154–160.
6. Ni Z, Mu Y, Gulati O. Treatment of melasma with Pycnogenol. *Phytother Res* 2002 16: 567–571.
7. Alves-Rodrigues A, Shao A. The science behind lutein. *Toxicol Lett* 2004; 150: 57–83.
8. Heinrich U, Gartner C, Wiebusch M *et al*. Supplementation with β-carotene or a similar amount of mixed carotenoids protects humans from UV-induced erythema. *J Nutr* 2003; 133: 98–101.
9. Shukla V K S, Bhattacharya K. Novel introduction of omega 3 oils for enhancing the value of cosmeceuticals. *NutraCos* 2004; 3: 20–22.

10. Morse P F, Horrobin D F, Manku M S *et al.* Meta-analysis of placebo-controlled studies of the efficacy of Epogam in the treatment of atopic eczema. Relationship between plasma essential fatty acid changes and clinical response. *Br J Dermatol* 1989; 121: 75–90.

11. Kerscher M J, Korting H C. Treatment of atopic eczema with evening primrose oil: rationale and clinical results. *Clin Invest* 1992; 70: 167–171.

12. Brosche T, Platt D. Effect of borage oil consumption on fatty acid metabolism, transepidermal water loss and skin parameters in elderly people. *Arch Gerontol Geriatr* 2000; 30: 139–150.

13. Liao S, Kao Y H, Hiipakka R A. Green tea: biochemical and biological basis for health benefits. *Vitamin Hormone* 2001; 62: 1–94.

14. Wang H, Provan G, Helliwell K. The functional benefits of flavonoids: the case of tea. *Phytochem Funct Foods* 2003: 128–159.

15. Dufresne C J, Farnworth E R. A review of latest research findings on the health promotion properties of tea. *J Nutr Biochem* 2001; 12: 404–421.

16. Gensler H L, Timmermann B N, Valcic S *et al.* Prevention of photocarcino-genesis by topical administration of pure epigallocatechin gallate isolated from green tea. *Nutr Cancer* 1996; 26: 325–335.

17. Miyazaki K, Hanamizu T, Iizuka R, Chiba K. Genistein and daidzein stimulate hyaluronic acid production in transformed human keratinocyte culture and hairless mouse skin. *Skin Pharmacol Appl Skin Physiol* 2002; 15: 175–183.

18. Wei H, Saladi R, Lu Y *et al.* Isoflavone genistein: photoprotection and clinical implications in dermatology. *J Nutr* 2003; 133: 3811S–3819S.

19. Hoppe U, Bergemann J, Diembeck W *et al.* Coenzyme Q10, a cutaneous antioxidant and energizer. *BioFactors* 1999; 9: 371–378.

20. Kajimoto O, Suguro S, Takahashi T. Clinical effects of glucosamine hydrochloride diet for dry skin. *Nippon Shokuhin Kagaku Kogaku Kaishi* 2001; 48: 335–343.

21. Murad H Tabibian M P. The effect of an oral supplement containing glucosamine, amino acids, minerals, and antioxidants on cutaneous aging: a preliminary study. *J Dermatol Treat* 2001; 12: 47–51.

22. Dreher F, Gabard B, Schwindt D A, Maibach H I. Topical melatonin in combination with vitamins E and C protects skin from ultraviolet-induced erythema : a human study *in vivo. Br J Dermatol* 1998; 139: 332–339.

23. Takahashi T, Kamiya T, Yokoo Y. Proanthocyanidins from grape seeds promote proliferation of mouse hair follicle cells in vitro and convert hair cycle in vivo. *Acta dermato-vener* 1998; 78: 428–432.

24. Theobald H E. Soya helps prevent hair loss-or does it? *Nutr Bull* 2004; 29: 177–179.

25. Rinaldi F, Sorbellini E, Bezzola P, Marchioretto D I. Biogena based food supplement: hair growth enhancer. *Nutrafoods* 2003; 2: 1–7.

16

Oral health

Dental caries is a common chronic disease involving the interation between teeth, food and bacteria. The major bacteria are believed to be *Streptococcus mutans* and *S. sobrinus*, although several other types are also involved. Three stages have been outlined in caries: adherence of bacteria to the teeth, formation of glycocalyx due to synthesis of a sticky branched glucan by the action of the bacterial enzyme glucosyl transferase (GTase) on sucrose, and accumulation of plaque, which is a biofilm. In the dental plaque there is continuing acid production by the bacteria, which are able to metabolise carbohydrates in acid medium, and the acid demineralises the enamel of the teeth.[1]

In a number of countries fluoride is added to drinking water to reduce the incidence of caries, and to add confusion to the arguments relating to the dental benefits of tea drinking, tea leaves are rich in fluoride.

Tea

Epidemiological evidence from tea plantation areas in Japan shows that schoolchildren from these areas have a lower incidence of caries than those from other areas.[2] The relevance of this finding is debatable.

The major constituents of teas are polyphenolic catechins and theaflavins, which exist as either monomers or polymers in green and black teas respectively, and are both well known to be inhibitory and bactericidal against *Streptococcus* spp. The minimum inhibitory concentration of tea polyphenols against cariogenic bacteria was reported to be 0.25–1.0 mg/mL and a green tea extract (20 mg/mL) has been shown to reduce the number of *S. mutans* from 10^7 to 10^2 after 3 minutes. (—)-Epigallocatechin gallate (EGCG) and (—)-epicatechin gallate (ECG) (monomeric catechins present in both green and black tea) were found to inhibit adherence of streptococci to teeth at 50 µg/mL or less.[2] They bind to bacterial surface proteins of the bacteria, induce aggregation, and inhibit the enzymic activity of glucosyl transferase. Both teas inhibit salivary and streptococcal amylase, overall producing reduction in plaque.[1] Green tea, EGCG and ECG were shown to inhibit the growth of cariogenic bacteria by inhibiting the adherence and growth of bacteria on the tooth surface, as well as glucan synthesis by streptococci. In addition, tea flavour components, indole and delta-cadinene, have been reported to have a synergistic effect on the inhibition of *S. mutans*, and EGCG also inhibits the growth and adherence of *Porphyromonas gingivalis*, which is responsible for periodontal disease.[3]

Extract of oolong tea has been shown to retard growth and reduce the rate of acid production by *S. mutans*. Extracts were also found to decrease cell surface hydophobicity and adherence of *S. mutans* to saliva-coated hydroxyapatite.[4] Recently, a specific polyphenol from oolong tea was shown to demonstrate strong anti-GTase activity and to inhibit experimental caries.[4] Results showed that this polyphenol may inhibit bacterial adherence to dental surfaces by reducing the hydrophobicity of *S. mutans*. The total tea extract itself may inhibit the caries-inducing activity of *S. mutans* by reducing the rate of acid production.[5]

Studies in animals have shown that tea consumption reduces caries, and it has been associated with lower caries levels in humans. Adults rinsing their mouth with black tea ten times daily for 7 days were reported to have a significantly less pronounced pH reduction, lower plaque index and fewer colonies of *S. mutans* and total oral streptococci in plaque, but not saliva.[6] Further trials have been carried out in children and volunteers, using a variety of teas and control treatments. Comparisons between the trials are difficult, but generally there appears to be an increase in caries inhibition.[6]

Tea extracts have been added to chewing gum and sweets in order to reduce caries, as well as deodorise the breath,[7] and it has been suggested that both black and green tea leaves can be used as a slow release source of polyphenols in the mouth for reducing caries.[8] Halitosis is mainly caused by food and bacterial proteins in the mouth, which are degraded by enzymes to produce volatile odorous sulfides, particularly methylmercaptan. The deodorising effect of tea catechins, particularly EGCG, is brought about by a chemical reaction, effectively neutralising the methylthio group of the methylmercapten.[9]

Proanthocyanidins such as the tea catechins are present in a number of other plant sources and have been tested for anti-GTase activity, but catechin and epicatechin were found to have the highest activity. Importantly, enzymic metabolites of these two, with lower molecular weights, showed high GTase inhibitory activity, suggesting that the activity of tea may be due to human metabolites, as opposed to the endogenous plant constituents.[10]

Pycnogenol

Chewing gum containing 5 mg Pycnogenol produced a 50% reduction in bleeding in patients with gingival inflammation after use of six chewing gums/day for 14 days. The trial showed that Pycnogenol was capable of reducing gingival bleeding and no increase in plaque formation was evident compared with control patients who did not brush their teeth.[11]

Coenzyme Q10

A deficiency in coenzyme Q10 (Co Q10) in gingival biopsy tissue from patients with advanced periodontal disease suggested possible benefits from Co Q10 supplementation. A double-blind trial involving 18 patients, eight of whom took 25 mg Co Q10 twice daily, showed improvement in a number of parameters associated with periodontal disease, such as calculus and plaque levels.[12]

References

1. Hamilton-Miller J M T. Anti-cariogenic properties of tea (*Camellia sinensis*). *J Med Microbiol* 2001; 50: 299–302.
2. Wang H, Provan G, Helliwell K. The functional benefits of flavonoids: the case of tea. *Phytochem Funct Foods* 2003; 128–159.
3. Muroi H, Kubo I. Combination effects of antibacterial compounds in green tea flavor against *Streptococcus mutans*. *J Agric Food Chem* 1993; 41: 1102–1105.
4. Matsumoto M, Minami T, Sasaki H et al. Inhibitory effects of oolong tea extract on caries-inducing properties of mutans streptococci. *Caries Res* 1999; 33: 441–445.
5. Matsumoto M, Hamada S, Ooshima T. Molecular analysis of the inhibitory effects of oolong tea polyphenols on glucan-binding domain of recombinant glucosyltransferases from *Streptococcus mutans* MT8148. *FEMS Microbiol Lett* 2003; 228: 73–80.
6. Wu C D, Wei G-X. Tea as a functional food for oral health. *Nutrition* 2002; 18: 443–444.
7. Liao S, Kao Y H, Hiipakka R A. Green tea: biochemical and biological basis for health benefits. *Vitamins Hormones* 2001; 62: 1–94.
8. Lee M-J, Lambert JD, Prabhu S et al. Delivery of tea polyphenols to the oral cavity by green tea leaves and black tea extract. *Cancer Epidemiol Biomarkers Prev* 2004; 13: 132–137.

9. Rao T P, Okubo T, Chu D-C, Juneja L R. Pharmacological functions of green tea polyphenols. *Performance Funct Foods* 2003; 140–167.

10. Mitsunaga T. Anti-caries activity of bark proanthocyanidins. *Basic Life Sci* 1999; 66: 555–573.

11. Kimbrough C, Chun M, dela Roca G, Lau B H S. Pycnogenol chewing gum minimizes gingival bleeding and plaque formation. *Phytomedicine* 2002; 9: 410–413.

12. Wilkinson E G, Arnold R M, Folkers K. Bioenergetics in clinical medicine. VI. adjunctive treatment of periodontal disease with coenzyme Q10. *Res Commun Chem Path Pharmacol* 1976; 14: 715–719.

17

Enhancement of sporting performance

Nutraceutical supplementation is thought to enhance athletic performance, and this is widely perceived to give athletes a competitive edge
without compromising their health. Although scientific evidence of their
effectiveness is variable, the popularity of ergogenic nutraceuticals is
rising. By 1999, expenditure on sports nutritional products was
estimated to be US$927 million per annum in the USA, and 9% of this
figure was accounted for by dietary supplements. The largest companies
involved in this market are now subsidiaries of pharmaceutical
companies.[1]

Nutraceuticals are believed to increase performance either by
renewing or increasing energy stores in the body or by modifying the
biochemical changes contributing to fatigue. One of the major reasons
for use of nutraceuticals by athletes is to avoid the disadvantages of using
drugs, particularly the anabolic steroids, namely the risk of detection
and suspension and the often serious side-effects associated with their
use. Four of the most popular supplements currently used by athletes to
directly enhance their performance are creatine, carnitine, acetyl-L-
carnitine and octacosanol, and there are many others for which less
positive evidence is available, for example conjugated linoleic acid
(CLA), dehydroepiandrosterone (DHEA), ornithine α-ketoglutarate,
melatonin and antioxidants such as coenzyme Q10 (Co Q10).

Creatine

The use of creatine is widespread among athletes and body builders. It
is currently legal to market it, it does not contravene current doping
regulations and it is readily available over the counter in healthfood
shops.[2] The popularity of creatine is such that 86% of high school
athletes in the USA have been reported to purchase supplies.[3]

Creatine is synthesised endogenously in the kidneys and to a small
extent in the pancreas and liver, and it is distributed throughout the body
via the bloodstream. Exogenous creatine is most probably actively

absorbed from the gastrointestinal tract. The mechanisms of action of creatine in human energy production, via phosphocreatine and ATP regeneration, have been reviewed.[4] Creatine facilitates an increase in anaerobic work capacity and muscle mass when taken in conjunction with resistance training and improvements in the rate of phospho-creatine resynthesis are mainly responsible for improvements in acute work capacity, although the effects on muscle protein synthesis are less clear.[5] The effects of creatine supplementation on performance and training adaptations have been extensively reviewed.[6]

Reviewing a trial on sprinting performance after supplementation with 5 g/day for 5 days, it was concluded that despite elevated free creatine, total creatine and phosphocreatine levels in the muscle for up to four weeks after supplementation, this had no effect on intermittent sprinting performance. Creatine was shown to produce variable results in repeated 6- to 30-second bouts of maximal stationary cycling sprints, but data regarding its ergogenic effect on mass-dependent activities such as running and swimming were unreliable. It was shown that ingestion of 20 g of creatine over 5 days led to an increase in both total muscle creatine and phosphocreatine regeneration in five of the eight subjects during the 2nd minute of recovery from intense muscle contraction. Short-duration, high-intensity exercise activities showed improvements with both 21-day low-dose supplementation (7.7 g/day) and high loading dose (25 g/7 days) followed by 5 g/day.[6]

In a study on the effect of creatine supplementation (6 g/day) in endurance sports, it was concluded that creatine improves performance in endurance athletes but only if they are required to sprint during an aerobic bout. Studies involving high-intensity exercise are more promising. In a study of nine subjects carrying out two bouts of 30-second maximal isokinetic cycling before and after ingestion of 20 g of creatine monohydrate per day for 5 days, a total increase in work production (by approximately 4%) and a reduction in ATP loss after supplementation was recorded.[7]

Three meta-analyses on the use of creatine in sporting activity have been carried out. In one investigation in which 16 studies were included it was concluded that oral creatine supplementation combined with resistance training increased the maximal weight that young men could lift. There was insufficient evidence to substantiate claims for other measures of strength, such as cycle ergometry, sprint peak power, or isokinetic dynamometer peak torque, or that creatine improved strength in women or older individuals.[8] In the other investigation of 18 studies, it was concluded that creatine augmented lean body mass (0.36% per week), and produced strength gains with resistance training (1.09% per week). [9] In the last investigation, 100 studies were included, and the major conclusions reported were: body composition changes were greater with loading-only regimens as opposed to maintenance regimens, effect sizes were greater for laboratory-based tasks than for field-based tasks, and there were no differences in effect sizes between males and females, or trained and untrained subjects. The overall conclusion was that effect sizes were greater for lean body mass following short-term creatine supplementation, repetitive laboratory-based exercises and upper body exercise, and creatine does not appear to be effective in improving running and swimming performances. Another important conclusion was that the efficacy of creatine was not consistent for all variables and populations studied.[10]

Over 300 research studies have evaluated the effects of creatine supplementation on exercise capacity and muscle indicators. Approximately 70% of the studies report significant results: compared with placebo results show up to 5–15% improvement in maximal power and strength, work performed during sets of maximal effort muscle contractions and during repetitive sprinting, and 1–5% improvement during single-effort sprinting.[6] Results regarding effectiveness also vary according to athletic ability (amateur or professional), creatine dosage regimen (loading or non-loading) and type of exercise (high intensity or endurance). Lastly, one report of the effectiveness of creatine supplementation at 8 g/day for 5 days in reducing mental fatigue caused by mathematical calculations has appeared.[4]

Relatively minor side-effects have been reported following creatine supplementation, such as diarrhoea, cramps and loss of appetite,[3] weight gain, headaches, tendon injury and occasional gastrointestinal disturbances,[11] but it may also cause electrolyte imbalance, which can lead to dehydration. A far more serious problem has recently been reported concerning unregulated creatine supplements which were found to contain substances banned by the International Olympic Committee, effectively negating any claim to legality normally associated with nutraceuticals.[12]

One of a number of studies to report increased intramuscular phosphocreatine levels after supplementation showed that concomitant intake of caffeine at a level of 0.5 mg/kg completely inhibited the beneficial effect.[13]

Carnitine

Carnitine is used as an ergogenic aid predominantly by body builders due to the perception that it boosts their stamina and energy, and helps them to lose weight, as a result of increased fat oxidation.[14]

Carnitine is synthesised in the kidneys, liver and brain. It can also be obtained from exogenous sources such as meats and other foods from animal sources. It is an essential component of cells and carnitine deficiency, although rare, can require supplementation. L-Carnitine is the naturally occurring isomer and 98% of the body's supply is found in skeletal muscle.[14]

L-Carnitine has an essential role in the metabolism of fatty acids to produce energy.[4] A deficiency could impair the oxidation of fatty acids and lead to muscle fatigue, and it is possible that L-carnitine supplementation could improve the oxidation of fatty acids and increase energy levels. One report concerning 110 top athletes showed that L-carnitine increased endurance and enhanced performance in strength sports (rowing, kayaking, weightlifting, etc.). The subjects carried out six trials using either single-dose supplementation or supplementation over three weeks. The authors claimed that increased free L-carnitine permitted a larger quantity of free fatty acids to enter mitochondria and hence be more extensively used as an energy source.[15] Another study looked at the effects of oral L-carnitine supplementation on physical performance and metabolism of endurance-trained athletes. Although levels of all L-carnitine fractions increased, there was no change in plasma concentrations of carbohydrate or fat metabolites. Also, there was no change in marathon running time. Acute L-carnitine supplementation does not improve the performance of endurance-trained athletes, nor their recovery.[16] Similarly, a study on L-carnitine supplementation of 2 g/day for two and four weeks showed negligible enhancement of performance in untrained men and women when cycling to exhaustion.[17]

These studies would suggest that neither acute nor chronic supplementation over a period of weeks leads to enhanced performance. However, in another study of ten moderately trained males cycling to exhaustion after acute administration of 2 g of L-carnitine 1 hour before exercise, it was reported that L-carnitine supplementation increased time to exhaustion, resulting in improved endurance.[18] One investigation on the effects of 200 mg carnitine daily for eight weeks on the performance of male basketball players reported significant reduction in body fat, allowing for improvement in maximal oxygen uptake, speed and power.[19]

Studies with positive results are few. One report showed an increase in maximal oxygen uptake in national class walkers following L-carnitine supplementation of 4 g/day for two weeks, but only six subjects were used in the study.[20] Improved performance in other sports, such as football and ice-hockey, have been reported. A review of the literature available on L-carnitine as an ergogenic aid concluded that available data did not support the use of L-carnitine administration to improve exercise performance in healthy persons.[21] An increase in plasma carnitine levels has been recorded after supplementation, but increases in skeletal muscle carnitine have not been shown to increase. Seven further published papers on the effects of carnitine on athletic performance have revealed no positive outcomes.[22]

Other applications for carnitine supplementation in aerobic sport include prevention of muscle damage during strenuous exercise, particularly in untrained athletes, and also in enhancement of performance in athletes suffering from chronic renal failure and peripheral vascular disease.[1,14]

Few side-effects have been reported with normal dosing with carnitine. Those that have been mentioned are mainly gastrointestinal disturbances.

Acetyl-L-carnitine

Acetyl-L-carnitine is currently marketed as an ergogenic aid in the UK and the USA. Its ergogenic properties are claimed to include increasing energy, aiding weight loss, boosting immune function and lowering cholesterol. Acetyl-L-carnitine is available from dietary sources such as meat and dairy products but is also found throughout the central nervous system, where it is involved in synthesis of the neurotransmitter acetylcholine and in the liver and kidneys.[23]

As is the case with L-carnitine, acetyl-L-carnitine is involved in energy production via fatty acid metabolism. Although there is less evidence that acetyl-L-carnitine is an effective ergogenic aid,[23] some manufacturers of acetyl-L-carnitine claim that it is more effective than L-carnitine due to its increased bioavailability. This has not yet been confirmed. Although there is little biochemical evidence to support the manufacturers' claims that acetyl-L-carnitine is an ergogenic aid, it is still widely used by athletes to supplement their diet.

Octacosanol

Octacosanol is not a major endogenous body component and is rarely found in dietary materials, but it is thought to improve cardiac function, stamina, strength and reaction time and is thus used by athletes as an ergogenic aid. It has also been reported to have cholesterol-lowering properties when in combination with other fatty alcohols in policosanol.[14]

It has been suggested that an action on nerve tissue could be responsible for the role of octacosanol in the development of muscle and strength, as an increase in the efficiency of the nervous system would facilitate speed and strength production as well as activation of more muscle fibres during contraction.[4]

One study on the effect of octacosanol (1 mg daily for eight weeks) on reaction time, chest strength and grip strength, showed an increased reaction time to visual stimuli and increased grip strength. Chest strength, endurance, and reaction time to auditory stimulus were unaffected.[24] More investigation into the effects of octacosanol needs to be carried out before claims of its ergogenicity can be confirmed. Octacosanol appears to be safe, as no side-effects were reported even after long-term supplementation at levels of 20 mg/day.[4]

Conjugated linoleic acid

CLA is often used to aid in weight loss, and therefore it is of no surprise that some athletes have shown interest in using it as an adjunct to their normal physical and dietary programmes. Studies involving athletes have been carried out on resistance-trained males and novice body builders. Supplementation with 3.6 g/day CLA produced no benefits for the resistance-trained males in body mass, percentage fat or lean mass, but there was a small improvement in strength performance in exercise tests. However, in the body builders supplemented with 7.2 g/day CLA there was enhanced strength and body mass without increase in body fat.[25] A more recent trial carried out with both male and female resistance-trained athletes failed to show any benefit with supplementation (54% CLA, 7 g/day).[26]

Other nutraceuticals

Acute administration of 50 mg DHEA and chronic administration of 150 mg/day did not increase serum testosterone levels in young men, but strength and lean body mass were found to improve significantly with resistance training, as reported in one study.[27]

Although ornithine α-ketoglutarate (OKG) is widely promoted as a supplement for athletes and bodybuilders, there is little scientific and medical literature available on its benefits. OKG is a salt formed from one molecule of α-ketoglutarate and two molecules of ornithine, and is a precursor of many metabolites involved in cell propagation and tissue repair.[14] It is involved in a number of metabolic pathways, and synthesis of amino acids in muscle, liver and lung tissue, and is used for treatment of burns and post-surgery trauma.[14] The literature concerning the effects of ornithine on athletes has been reviewed.[28] It appears to have variable effects on serum growth hormone levels, beneficial effects being observed at dosage levels of 170 mg/kg, but unacceptable levels of diarrhoea and stomach cramps, and no effect seen at lower doses. OKG supplementation did not increase training volume or intensity, or muscle mass, or levels of growth hormone.

Melatonin has been suggested to be beneficial to athletic performance. The claimed hypothermic effects in hot environments and athletic performance variables had not until recently been substantiated by research data.[29] A significant reduction in rectal temperature of 0.25°C has been reported after supplementing athletes with 2.5 mg melatonin prior to 66 minutes of exercise under moderate heat stress.[30] The demonstrable beneficial effects in sleep adjustment may indirectly help affected athletes, for example overcoming the effects of jet lag and other sleeping disorders, but there are no data on the role melatonin plays in exercise training problems such as amenorrhoea and over-training syndrome.

Co Q10 is an example of a nutraceutical for which there is little direct evidence in the area of improvement of sporting performance. It is known to be antioxidant due to its free radical scavenging activity, and it stimulates oxygen uptake and exercise performance in cardiac patients. One report on the effects of supplementation with 60 mg twice daily during intense exercise revealed increased cell damage due to increased plasma creatine kinase.[30]

There is no doubt that nutraceutical ergogenic aids are safer than the more traditional drugs abused in sports, but they may not be as effective. Of the four major compounds described, creatine appears to have the most potential in terms of performance enhancement. It is also freely available for legitimate use by athletes, and this is reflected by its popularity. Claims of the potential ergogenicity of carnitine and its acetyl ester, however, seem to be based on their known biochemical mechanisms and not on clinical research. In contrast, claims about the ergogenicity of octacosanol are based on relatively few clinical studies and its mechanism of action has not been identified. Limited evidence exists for the direct effects of CLA, DHEA, OKG, melatonin and Co Q10.

Although most nutraceticals supplemented in sport are used specifically to improve strength, energy levels and lean body mass, others are used for protection of the immune system during the trauma of exercising. For example, coenzyme Q10 and Pycnogenol and the major joint health products, glucosamine, chondroitin, methylsulfonylmethane (MSM) and S-adenosyl methionine (SAMe), are widely used either for recovery from injury or as a preventive measure.

Conclusion

Undoubtedly, properly manufactured nutraceuticals will be safer than poorly manufactured illegal drugs, but there is as yet no large body of evidence substantiating their unequivocal benefits. A recent systematic and critical evaluation of their benefits concluded that the majority of studies supported the use of carnitine for 'maintenance of or improvements in physical performance', creatine for 'maintenance of or improvements in muscle mass, strength, protein synthesis or anaerobic exercise performance' and CLA for 'improvements in body fat loss or leanness'.[32]

References

1. Turpin A A, Feliciano J, Bucci L R. Nutritional ergogenic aids: introduction, definitions and regulatory issues. *Nutr Ergogenic Aids* 2004; 3–17.
2. Mason P. *Dietary Supplements*, 2nd edn. London: Pharmaceutical Press, 2001.
3. Smith J, Dahm D L. Creatine use among a select population of high school athletes. *Mayo Clin Proc* 2000; 75: 1257–1263.
4. Marsland L, Lockwood B. Ergogenic nutraceuticals in sport – mechanisms, effectiveness and safety. *Nutrafoods* 2004; 1: 23–34.
5. Paddon-Jones D, Borsheim E, Wolfe R R. Potential ergogenic effects of arginine and creatine supplementation. *J Nutr* 2004, 134: 2888S–2894S.
6. Kreider R B. Effects of creatine supplementation on performance and training adaptations. *Mol Cell Biochem* 2003; 244: 89–94.
7. Casey A, Constantin-Teodosiu D, Howell S *et al.* Creatine ingestion favourably affects performance and muscle metabolism during maximal exercise in humans. *Am J Physiol* 1996; 271: E31–E37.
8. Dempsey R L, Mazzone M F, Meurer L N. Does oral creatine supplementation improve strength? A meta-analysis. *J Fam Pract* 2002; 51: 945–951.
9. Nissen S L, Sharp R L. Effect of dietary supplements on lean mass and strength gains with resistance exercise: a meta-analysis. *J Appl Physiol* 2003; 94: 651–659.
10. Branch J D. Effect of creatine supplementation on body composition and performance: a meta-analysis. *Int J Sport Nutr Exerc Metab* 2003; 13: 198–226.

11. Juhn M S, Tarnopolsky M. Oral creatine supplementation and athletic performance: a critical review. *Clin J Sport Med* 1998; 8: 286–297.
12. Maughan R J, King D S, Lea T. Dietary supplements. *J Sport Sci* 2004; 22: 95–113.
13. Vandenberghe K, Gillis N, Van Leemputte M *et al*. Caffeine counteracts the ergogenic action of muscle creatine loading. *J Appl Physiol* 1996; 80: 432–437.
14. Rapport L, Lockwood B. *Nutraceuticals*. London: Pharmaceutical Press, 2002.
15. Dragan G I, Vasiliu A, Georgescu E, Eremia N. Studies concerning chronic and acute effects of L-carnitine in elite athletes *Physiologie* 1989; 26: 111–129.
16. Colombani P, Wenk C, Kunz I *et al*. Effects of L-carnitine supplementation on physical performance and energy metabolism of endurance-trained athletes: a double-blind crossover field study. *Eur J Appl Physiol Occup Physiol* 1996; 73: 434–439.
17. Greig C, Finch K M, Jones D A, Cooper M. The effect of oral supplementation with L-carnitine on maximum and submaximum exercise capacity. *Eur J App Physiol* 1987; 56: 457–460.
18. Siliprandi N, DiLisi F, Pieralisi G *et al*. Metabolic changes induced by maximal exercise in human subjects following L-carnitine administration. *Biochim Biophys Acta* 1990; 1034: 17–21.
19. Zajac A, Waskiewicz Z, Nowak K. The influence of L-carnitine supplementation on body fat content, speed, explosive strength and VO$_2$ max in elite athletes. *Biol Sport* 2001; 18: 127–135.
20. Marconi C, Sassi G, Carpinelli A, Cerretelli P. Effects of L-carnitine loading on the aerobic and anaerobic performance of endurance athletes. *Eur J Appl Physiol Occup Physiol* 1985; 54: 131–135.
21. Brass E P, Hiatt W R. The role of carnitine and carnitine supplementation during exercise in man and in individuals with special needs. *J Am Coll Nutr* 1998; 17: 207–215.
22. Moffat R J, Chelland, S A. Carnitine. *Nutr Ergogenic Aids* 2004; 61–79.
23. Wadsworth F, Lockwood B. Combined alpha-lipoic acid and acetyl-l-carnitine supplementation. *Pharm J* 2003; 270: 587–589.
24. Saint John M, McNaughton L. Octacosanol ingestion and its effects on metabolic responses to sub-maximal cycle ergometry, reaction time and chest and grip strength. *Int Clin Nutr Rev* 1986; 6: 81–87.
25. Whigham, L D, Cook M E, Atkinson R L. Conjugated linoleic acid: implications for human health. *Pharmacol Res* 2000; 42: 503–510.
26. von Loeffelholz C, Kratzsch J, Jahreis G. Influence of conjugated linoleic acids on body composition and selected serum and endocrine parameters in resistance-trained athletes. *Eur J Lipid Sci Technol* 2003; 105: 251–259.
27. Brown G A, Vukovich M D, Sharp R L *et al*. Effect of oral DHEA on serum testosterone and adaptations to resistance training in young men. *J Appl Physiol* 1999; 87: 2274–2283.
28. Robertson T D. Ornithine, ornithine alpha-ketoglutarate and taurine. *Nutr Ergogenic Aids* 2004; 197–206.
29. Atkinson G, Drust B, Reilly T, Waterhouse J. The relevance of melatonin to sports medicine and science. *Sports Med* 2003; 33: 809–31.

30. Atkinson G, Holder A, Robertson C *et al.* Effects of melatonin on the thermo-regulatory responses to intermittent exercise. *J Pineal Res* 2005; 39: 353–359.
31. Malm C, Svensson M, Joeberg B *et al.* Supplementation with ubiquinone-10 causes cellular damage during intense exercise. *Acta Physiol Scand* 1996; 157: 511–512.
32. Turpin A A, Talbott Sh M, Feliciano J, Bucci L R.. Systematic and critical evaluation of benefits and possible risks of nutritional ergogenic aids. *Nutr Ergogenic Aids* 2004; 469–504.

18

Animal health

Nutraceuticals are a section of the supplements market that is becoming increasingly popular within the veterinary profession. They have been described by the North American Veterinary Nutraceutical Council as a 'non-drug substance that is produced in a purified or extracted form and administered orally to provide agents required for normal body structure and function with the intent of improving the health and well-being of animals'.[1] These products are widely available and can be purchased in many forms, including capsules, tablets, powders and are often included in animal feeds. A number of nutraceuticals are currently being used in the prevention and treatment of common diseases in animals, including cardiovascular disease, osteoarthritis, periodontal disease, cognitive dysfunction and cancer, with clinical trials providing evidence of their efficacy in a variety of animal species.

Cardiovascular disease

Polyunsaturated fatty acids

Although mammals are able to synthesise saturated fatty acids themselves, they are unable to produce n-6 and n-3 polyunsaturated fatty acids (PUFAs)[2] so need to obtain them from their diet. Both n-6 and n-3 fatty acids are required for cell membrane phospholipids and to act as substrates for various enzymes, which make them important for skin and hair texture, joint, cardiovascular, eye and mental health. The most commonly ingested n-6 PUFA is linoleic acid, which is found in seeds, nuts and vegetable oils. The n-3 PUFA α-linolenic acid (ALA) is also readily available in animal meat and vegetable oils. These essential fatty acids are also precursors for longer chain polyunsaturated fatty acids: linoleic acid is converted to arachidonic acid by the action of a desaturase enzyme,[2] and ALA is converted to eicosapentaenoic acid (EPA) and docosahexaenoic acid (DHA) by the same enzyme.[3] As a result, any cardioprotective benefit seen from the supplementation of ALA is believed to be due to the formation of EPA within the body .

Fish oils are known to be rich in both DHA and EPA, with both DHA and arichidonic acid also found in high concentrations in the many mammalian organs, including the brain, where it is vital for normal functioning.[4]

Arachidonic acid and DHA are synthesised in the liver, where desaturation of the dietary components takes place. In most mammals arachidonic acid is produced in sufficient quantities to support normal functioning of tissues and reproduction. However, in some animals, such as cats, the production of both arachidonic acid and ALA is insufficient and they may require supplementation.[5] Studies have shown that some animals are in a state of DHA deficiency, with low levels seen in early life. Rats show decreased memory skills and learning ability when deficient in DHA, which can be reversed if the diet is supplemented. This phenomenon is also apparent in puppies.[3] The effects of supplementing the feline diet with 0.12 g/day of EPA and 0.19 g/day DHA have been investigated. A shift in the n-6:n-3 ratio of long-chain PUFAs was observed, which was reflected in total fatty acids and phospholipids.[3] This is especially useful for animals such as the cat, where deficiencies are regularly observed during the neuronal development stages of life.[3] DHA and EPA are vital to a number of other physiological processes in the body, where they are often incorporated into phospholipid membranes and play a role in signal transduction from cell membranes.

Free DHA can be found throughout the body and has been shown to bind to cytoplasmic receptors and regulate gene expression. It is important that sufficient n-3 PUFAs are obtained from the diet. This can be a problem when animal feeds are low in n-3 fatty acids, and even when it is present, the animal cannot desaturate ALA efficiently. In humans it has been demonstrated that ingesting n-3 fatty acids regularly can decrease very low-density lipoprotein (VLDL), cholesterol and triglyceride levels in the blood,[6] which may also decrease the risk of cardiovascular disease.[4] There is also some evidence to support a drop in blood pressure in cats when their diet was supplemented with fish oils.[7]

Sudden cardiac death and polyunsaturated fatty acids

n-3 PUFAs prevent fatal cardiac ventricular ischaemia-induced arrhythmias in dogs, rats and primates. In one study, the effect of giving dogs 1–5 mL of concentrated, free n-3 fatty acids from fish oils before an exercise-ischaemia-stress test was investigated, and any ventricular fibrillations recorded.[8] An antiarrhythmic property was observed in 77% of the test animals. In order to identify the component of the fish oil that was responsible for preventing fatal arrhythmias, further investigations were performed on DHA, EPA and ALA (found in many vegetable oils). All components were found to be equally as efficient at preventing fatal cardiac death in dogs.[8] These fatty acids prevent arrhythmias by partitioning into phospholipids of the membranes of the myocytes in the heart, and making them resistant to arrhythmias by modifying ion channels. Supplementation with *n*-3 PUFAs builds up stored fatty acids within cells, making them readily available for use when required, providing protection against exercise-induced ischaemia and sudden death in rodents, canines and primates.[8] As the prevalence of ventricular fibrillations increases as the animal ages, supplementation may be of particular benefit to elderly animals.[9]

Coenzyme Q10

Coenzyme Q10 (Co Q10) has attracted much interest in the veterinary world. It has been extensively studied for its antioxidant properties, and its ability to boost the immune response to bacteria and viruses.[10] Co Q10 is a naturally occurring lipid-soluble benzoquinine that can be synthesised by cells *de novo*, and is found in both humans and animals at high concentrations, particularly in the young.[11] Its levels decrease with age and seem to correspond to the decreasing immune response seen in old age.[12] A large number of Co Q-dependent enzymes exist in the mitochondria of most mammals. These include succinate dehydrogenase-CoQ reductase, succinic-cytochrome *c* reductase and NADH-cytochrome *c* reductase, which all use Co Q10 in the production of ATP, which is vital for energy production within eukaryotic cells.[13]

Protection of ischaemic myocardium with Co Q10

A myocardial infarction occurs when cardiac demand for oxygen exceeds supply. This is often caused by thrombus formation in one of the coronary vessels, which stops oxygenated blood reaching the myocardium in sufficient quantities. As a result there may be myocardial necrosis and thus irreversible damage to the heart muscle.[14] There is evidence to support the use of Co Q10 in dogs as a supplement to protect the heart against necrosis caused by a myocardial infarction. A study carried out in dogs has shown that the protective effect on the myocardium of Co Q10 is not caused by a haemodynamic change.[15] The dose was given as an intravenous infusion containing 20 mg/kg of Co Q10 in a polyethylene hydrogenated castor oil, and myocardial tissue ATP levels were used as a marker for the degree of myocardial ischaemia observed. The study showed that the preservation of myocardial ATP was directly linked to maintaining myocardial contraction during ischaemia. Furthermore, Co Q10 was observed to minimise the disturbance in ATP production and mitochondrial deformity occurring as a result of ischaemia.[15] Although the evidence is minimal, Co Q10 would appear to protect against the high level of necrosis seen in the heart muscle following a myocardial infarction in dogs. This evidence may also be applicable to other small vertebrates.

Coenzyme Q10 and the treatment of hypertension

Long-term oral administration of Co Q10 was found to produce an antihypertensive effect in dogs.[16] Significantly, it had a pathological effect on some of the changes observed in animals suffering from hypertension. A detailed study on the effect of chronic administration in both rats and dogs was seen to produce a raised blood pressure. Oral doses of 1 or 10 mg/kg for four weeks produced no change in blood pressure after one week of dosing. The drop in systolic blood pressure was observed after two weeks of dosing and there appeared to be a significant decrease. From the evidence it was concluded that the antihypertensive effect of Co Q10 appeared after repeated dosing and that the effect was to prevent the onset of hypertension or to reduce advancing hypertension in long-term sufferers. The effect was long lasting and present in both dogs and rats. The mechanism of action in hypertension is not fully understood, although it is thought to be as a result of increased levels of Co Q10 present within the body having an influence on aldosterone production and secretion.[16]

Other uses for Co Q10 in veterinary medicine include periodontal disease, decreased physical performance and immune dysfunction.[12] The use of Co Q10 as a nutraceutical is particularly significant in elderly animals, where intrinsic levels are decreased. There is also a potential for greater exercise tolerance in older horses where symptoms of increased lactic acid production and increased muscle enzymes such as creatine phosphokinase are reduced after supplementation.

There are a number of other situations where using Co Q10 as a nutraceutical may be useful, including sprains and strains, wounds, longhaul shipping, infections and exercise. Co Q10 can be beneficial to any animal in all stages of life. General supplementation in horses should be given at doses of 180–300+ mg/day.[10]

L-Carnitine

L-Carnitine is found mainly in the heart and the skeletal muscles. A high proportion of is secreted in the bile and can undergo enterohepatic recirculation. Acyl-carnitine can help with removal of fatty acids from the liver and these complexes are then eliminated from the body by glomerular filtration.[11] If the concentration of L-carnitine in the body decreases, an animal can become deficient and susceptible to raised levels of triglycerides in the blood, decreased tolerance of exercise and myocardial disease.[12]

Carnitine can also be obtained from the diet. Meat and dairy products provide the best sources, although the concentrations of carnitine can vary greatly after processing.[11] Oral bioavailability can be influenced by the quantity present and the metabolic status of the animal ingesting it. This has led to difficulties in determining optimal dosing requirements, and no cross-species doses have been identified.

Carnitine plays a vital role in the metabolism of fatty acids, acting as a cofactor for the transport of long-chain fatty acids across the mitochondrial membrane. It also has an effect on mitochondrial enzymes and assists in the transport of shortened long-chain fatty acids from peroxisomes to mitochondria.[11] L-Carnitine is vital to the conversion of fatty acids into energy via both the citric acid cycle and beta-oxidation.[12]

The heart obtains much of its energy from the breakdown of fatty acids. This makes L-carnitine essential as a transporter of long-chain fatty acids into the myocardial mitochondria in order for enough energy to be produced. Supplementation of animals with L-carnitine has been shown to be beneficial in cardiovascular disease.[12] A decreased level of L-carnitine in the myocardium of Labrador dogs suffering from dilated cardiomyopathy was observed.[17] One dog was fed 50 mg/kg three times a day for two months and showed a substantial clinical improvement. Confirmatory evidence may be obtained from studies on larger subject numbers. The study also produced evidence of increased exercise tolerance and appetite. This may have applications in the treatment of endocardiosis, ischaemic heart disease and congestive heart failure. Increased energy production from fatty acids has also been observed in cats.[11] This has led to interest in its potential to help cats recover from hepatic lipidosis (a condition in which fat is deposited in the liver).

Joint disease

Glycoaminoglycans

The use of supplements to treat chronic diseases such as osteoarthritis (OA) can be beneficial in areas frequently not addressed by conventional therapy such as the slowing of joint degeneration, the improvement of joint health and the general improvement of an animal's quality of life.[18] Most animals are affected by OA at some point in their lives, with 20% of canines over one year of age affected.[19] This fact highlights the importance of reducing the symptoms and degeneration of the condition in the long term.

Initial symptoms of OA in an animal, which may be minimal, include behavioural changes, stiffness, difficulty getting up and unwillingness to exercise.[20] Secondary OA is commonly seen in pets and is brought on by other joint damage such as anterior cruciate ligament rupture, osteochondritis dissecans, fragmented coronoid process and hip displasia.[19]

The aim of treatment is to improve pain relief and decrease inflammation, improve mobility, and increase cartilage repair. Oral nutraceuticals act as chondroprotectants and have maximal effects when used in conjunction with exercise and conventional therapies.[20]

Glycoaminoglycans (GAGs) are essential for the production of cartilage in the joints of most animals. They are large sugar–protein complexes, which are negatively charged. As a result they can attract water molecules, to help improve bone cushioning and act as shock absorbers.[18] Nutraceutical supplementation with GAGs can increase their availability in the joint where they are required and hence help to decrease inflammation and pain, and to increase cartilage repair by the chondrocytes in OA. GAGs may also decrease the activity of proteolytic enzymes in the joint and delay disease progression.[21]

Glucosamine

A large number of clinical trials have been carried out on the effects of glucosamine in humans, and the results may well be applicable to animals. A number of trials in animals have also shown strong evidence for the beneficial effects of glucosamine supplementation. A study in rats to investigate the antiarthritic effects of glucosamine sulfate at a dose of 50–800 mg/kg showed antireactive activity in subacute and chronic inflammation and arthritis.[22] Similar results were found in rabbits dosed with 100 mg glucosamine hydrochloride, producing a partial disease-modifying effect in OA. However, there was no effect seen on the erosion of cellular cartilage in any of the animals studied, and no effects were detected in joint compartments.[23]

The recommended dose of glucosamine in horses is 9 g daily until a benefit is seen. This can then be titrated down to 1–2 g daily as a maintenance dose. Oral bioavailability has been shown to be between 90 and 98%.[10]

Glucosamine sulfate is also useful in the treatment of canine hip displasias, osteochondritis, spondylitis and disc-degeneration conditions. N-Acetylglucosamine has been shown to possess qualities that suggest it could be useful in other inflammatory diseases such as Crohn's disease and colitis.[12] This promising new area of development comes from the ability of N-acetylglucosamine to increase synthesis of glycoproteins that are essential in the mucous membranes of the gastrointestinal, respiratory and genitourinary tracts. These membranes protect the tracts from damage by bacteria and digestive enzymes and it is important that they are maintained efficiently. Previous work on cells from human subjects with inflammatory bowel disease (IBD) reported an increase in the synthesis of glycoproteins when 1–2 nmol of N-acetylglucosamine, but not ^{14}C-glucosamine, was incubated with mucosal cells. This would suggest that the N-acetylation step necessary to produce N-acetylglucosamine is lacking in patients affected by IBD. As a result it was concluded that animals affected with IBD would also benefit from supplementation with N-acetylglucosamine.[12] It may also help to prevent 'leaky-gut' syndrome, which can lead to allergies, malabsorption and infection.[12]

Chondroitin sulfate

Chondroitin sulfate occurs naturally in the extracellular matrix of animal connective tissue/articular cartilage.[20] It is a large molecular weight GAG with a similar action to that of glucosamine. Chondroitin is useful in the treatment of arthritis, tendon and ligament problems, and many disorders associated with old age.[10] It is of particular benefit in horses and larger dogs, where joint degeneration is most marked. It has been found that chondroitin decreases interleukin 1 production, blocks complement activation, inhibits histamine-mediated inflammation, inhibits metalloproteinases and stimulates glycosaminoglycan and collagen synthesis.[24]

Supplementation with chondroitin allows the body to synthesise GAGs, which are used in the building of new cartilage.[25] After joint damage has occurred, chondrocytes use this material to synthesise new cartilage. A vast reservoir of chondroitin is therefore needed in order for complete repair to occur. The body may not naturally contain adequate levels of the necessary material and, as a result, supplementation is often required.

Chondroitin also neutralises destructive enzymes present in joints. It binds the enzyme and thus inactivates it.[25] After joint injury occurs, the level of these enzymes increases and a higher rate of cartilage breakdown occurs. Neutralising these proteins can therefore decrease, or even halt, joint damage when it is most likely to occur. The presence of chondroitin in the body also stimulates production of hyaluronic acid, which increases the viscosity of the synovial fluid, providing extra joint protection.[10]

A placebo-controlled double-blind study on the effect of chondroitin sulfate supplementation in dogs (as perceived by their owners) has been carried out. A dose of 22 mg/kg body weight per day of chondroitin sulfate was administered to dogs for 12 weeks. The results showed a slight improvement in the perceived pain and lameness observed in the animals.[26]

Studies to investigate the bioavailability and pharmacokinetics of chondroitin sulfate have been reported. A number of doses have been tested in horses and it was found that the oral bioavailability is 32% for a low molecular weight chondroitin sulfate (LMWCS).[27] The same experiment was performed in dogs with a dose of 400–1600 mg LMWCS. Accumulation of the drug was observed and this was hypothesised to account for the continued anti-inflammatory effect seen in animals after dosing has ceased.[10]

The recommended dose of chondroitin sulfate in horses is 7.5 g/day until symptoms start to improve.[12] The dose can then be slowly reduced to 3.5 g/day.

Fish oils

The large number of contraindications for veterinary medicines routinely used to treat OA means that owners are shifting their search for new treatments to alternative therapies such as fish oils. Many investigations have been performed on the use of fish oils to treat OA in humans, but little is known about their effect in animals.

Methylsulfonylmethane

Methylsulfonylmethane (MSM) is a sulfur-containing compound and so is essential for normal functioning of animal cells. In horses, high levels of sulfur are found in the joints, skin and hooves and they require large amounts of sulfur in their diet, which they may not obtain from processed food.[25] It has been suggested that MSM may have the potential to decrease inflammation and pain, and to act as an anti-oxidant, making it useful in the treatment of arthritis.[25] The rationale behind its use in disease is that it can replenish sulfur stores within arthritic joints, allowing collagen molecules to form cross-links and increase the strength and stability of tendons, ligaments and joint tissues. Some evidence also suggests an increase in glucosamine efficacy when co-administered with MSM.[10] Very few clinical trials have been completed on this nutraceutical and the recommendation for its use comes primarily from a manufacturer. MSM is sold as a supplement for humans and is readily available. It is also formulated into tablets and capsules for horses and small animals.[20] The dose recommended in horses is said to be 10 g/day, which can be added to the animal's feed. The toxic dose in rats has also been determined as 20 g/kg, equivalent to 10 kg for a 500 kg horse.[10]

Cetyl myristoleate

One cohort investigation has been carried out by a manufacturer of cetyl myristoleate into the effect of supplementing a dog's regular diet with chews containing a mixture of acetylated fatty acids, at a dose of two chews per day. A benefit was observed in the treatment of musculo-skeletal conditions. Although no clinical changes were observed, the pet owners reported increased mobility and less stiffness in their animals.[28] Very high doses of cetyl myristoleate have been shown to have antiarthritic properties in the rat.[29] It is commonly available as a nutraceutical supplement for the management of pain and inflammation in animals.

A study using pure cetyl myristoleate in mice found evidence that doses of 450 and 900 mg/kg when injected intraperitoneally decreased the incidence and severity of arthritis. Oral dosage of 20 mg/kg was also tested, and modest but statistically significant reductions in clinical symptoms of arthritis were seen.[29] The mechanism of action of this fatty acid ester may be through hydrolysis to form the 14-carbon fatty acid myristoleic acid. This fatty acid may work in a similar manner to *n*-6 and *n*-3 fatty acids, which are already known to be effective against arthritis. Further investigation is required on this product in order to discover the minimum effective dose and investigate its pharmacokinetics.

Periodontal disease

According to the American Veterinary Dental Society, 80% of dogs and 70% of cats above the age of three are affected by oral disease. Other animals, including ferrets, rabbits, other small pets and frequently older horses, can also be affected.[10] Periodontal disease is caused by a build-up of bacteria and food around the gum line in the mouth, which causes plaque and can lead to inflammation if not removed. Tartar forms if the plaque combines with saliva and this adheres strongly to the tooth, making it harder to remove. Gingivitis can occur if tartar starts to irritate the gums surrounding the tooth and the gum may become separated from the tooth, causing 'pockets' to form and encouraging the growth of harmful bacteria. This irreversible damage is called periodontal disease, which can cause an animal to lose teeth and may lead to frequent infections and pain. Periodontal disease commonly affects cats and dogs although the wide range in risk factors means that they are not all affected. Age, diet, environment and breed all play key roles in the development of the disease. The common signs and symptoms include persistent bad breath, bleeding and inflamed gums, loose or missing teeth, drooling and difficulty chewing.[20]

Coenzyme Q10

Supplementation with Co Q10 has been shown to suppress advanced gingival disease in cats and dogs and is therefore beneficial in these animals. It is vital to the production of energy by most cells in the mammalian body and is essential to the bioenergetics of the gingiva. Both gingival and leukocytic deficiencies in Co Q10 occur in humans,[13] which implies that a diet deficient in Co Q10 could lead to the development of gingival disease, and therefore that supplementation may restore the balance and decrease inflammation.

Co Q10 has been shown to decrease the gingival inflammation and 'pocket' depth in dogs with periodontal disease when administered orally to dogs for four weeks. This investigation used a dose of 1.5 mg/kg daily and confirms that Co Q10 can decrease inflammation in advanced periodontal disease.[13] It should be noted, however, that there does not appear to be any benefit when Co Q10 is administered to dogs with healthy gingiva.

Cognitive dysfunction

Many studies have been performed on canine species to investigate the effects of certain nutraceuticals on cognitive decline associated with ageing. Older dogs commonly experience behavioural and cognitive defects, and early prevention with dietary interventions may reduce the occurrence. Signs of this advancing cognitive decline, associated with cognitive dysfunction syndrome (CDS), include decreased social interaction, sleep disturbances, disorientation, loss of prior housetraining and reduced activity.[30] CDS is a degenerative disease and ageing may increase the number of symptoms evident to the owner.

The biology of cognitive dysfunction is analogous to the decline seen in humans. Cortical atrophy, ventricular widening and protein deposition occur in both the human and canine brain.[30] These effects can be toxic to neurons and result in cognitive decline. The generation of free radicals in the body becomes a particular problem in the ageing nervous system as there is a large decrease in oxidative defences and high oxidative metabolism as the brain becomes older.[31] Radicals are produced by the body in processes such as energy production, especially in the mitochondria, and the immune response, and their concentrations increase in older canines. As a result, neurons can become irreversibly damaged when radicals try to regain neutral charge and stabilise. They attack proteins, lipids and nucleotides, which leads to irreversible damage to neurons. In young animals there are a number of systems in place to protect cells from free radical damage (e.g. superoxide dimutase, which converts superoxide ions to hydrogen peroxide and hence detoxifies it). However, as the animal ages it has been shown that these systems can fail, allowing free radical damage to prevail and oxidative damage to accumulate.[30] Antioxidants can be supplemented into an animal's diet to 'mop up' these excess charges and protect cells.[30]

Supplements containing L-carnitine and lipoic acid (mitochondrial cofactors) can improve mitrochondrial function and decrease the production of free radicals during respiration. This will prevent damage to the RNA in brain cells and may decrease cognitive decline.[30] In a study using aged rats it was found that a combination of both L-carnitine and lipoic acid was the most beneficial in reducing the extent of RNA oxidisation.[30] An improvement in cognitive functioning was seen when aged dogs were fed lipoic acid, L-carnitine, DHA and EPA along with their regular diet. The effect on sleep and housetraining was rapid, and it was concluded that supplementation could offer an improvement or simply decrease the rate of age-related cognitive decline in many species.[30]

Antioxidants and mitochondrial cofactors have been shown to work in synergy to produce a slight improvement in cognitive functioning or a delay in the progression of age-related cognitive decline.[32] The effect was observed when using a pre-prepared diet containing L-carnitine, α-lipoic acid and vitamin C, fed to Beagle dogs over a period of six months. (R)-α-Lipoic acid is found naturally in mitochondria throughout the mammalian body and acts as a coenzyme for pyruvate dehydrogenase and α-ketoglutarate dehydrogenase, which is a mitochondrial cofactor. It is also reduced by lipoamide dehydrogenase to form dihydrolipoic acid (DHLA), which is a potent antioxidant. Lipoic acid therefore combines both antioxidant properties and acts as a mitochondrial cofactor. It can improve energy metabolism and reduce oxidative damage. Mitochondrial function and metabolic rate were studied in aged rats and it was concluded that the reduction in oxidative stress might be due to a direct increase in the concentration of unbound DHLA within the rat.[33] Therefore supplementing the diet with vitamin C and E along with L-carnitine or D,L-alpha-lipoic acid may be beneficial as an animal ages.

Cancer

The diagnosis of cancer in a pet can be distressing to the owner, but it may be appropriate to educate people about the use of alternative therapies with functional foods that can decrease the disease progression and maybe even reverse the process of tumour growth. Research has been completed on dogs with cancer in order to develop the optimal nutritional diet for their treatment. These findings may also be relevant for cats.[34] Major nutritional components have been identified as helpful in this context, including fibre, insoluble carbohydrates, arginine, fat and n-3 fatty acids.[2] Tea polyphenols may also be useful and green tea extracts are present in a number of commercially prepared pet foods. Although their use has not been verified in clinical trials in animals, there is a body of clinical evidence in humans.[30]

Fats and polyunsaturated fatty acids

Although lipids are oxidised by normal cells in the body to produce energy, some tumour cells find it hard to utilise this process. This has led to the proposal that a diet relatively high in fats may provide a benefit to cancer sufferers when compared with a high carbohydrate diet.[34] As most pet foods contain a large percentage of carbohydrate (25–60%) and a low percentage of fat (7–25%), they are not very suitable for animals suffering from cancer.

Fish oils containing the *n*-3 fatty acids DHA and EPA are important dietary supplements for animals with cancer. Evidence for their use in animals comes from *in vitro* cell culture, rodent, human and canine studies. Supplementation with EPA helps to reverse some of the catabolic changes associated with cancer. It limits muscle protein degradation[34] and tumour-induced lipolysis in rodents.[1] This can significantly reverse cachexia (wasting away of lean mass), which is often characteristic of advanced disease, especially pancreatic cancer. Catabolic changes have also been linked to decreased response to therapy and increased mortality, so it is essential to reverse these changes in order to give an animal the best chance of recovery. Other studies on the use of DHA/EPA in cancer therapy have been shown to have an effect on tumour growth, metastasis and tumorigenesis in animals.[34]

The mechanism of action by which *n*-3 fatty acids are effective in cancer treatment is complex. A number of possible mechanisms have been proposed, but it is likely that the efficacy does not come from a single action on tumour cells, but from a combination of many processes. One known mechanism is the ability of *n*-3 fatty acids to stop angiogenesis in solid tumour. They produce this effect mainly by altering prostaglandin production and inhibiting protein kinase C, processes which have been observed in the mouse during trials.[2]

A number of studies have been completed on the use of a low-carbohydrate, medium fat and high *n*-3 fatty acid-supplemented diet in canines. In all cases, elevated levels of DHA and EPA were observed in plasma samples taken from the animals within one week, and levels continued to be raised for several weeks after stopping the supplements.[35] Cats have shown increased bleeding times and decreased platelet aggregation when fed a diet high in *n*-3 fatty acids.[36] Their dietary intake should therefore be reduced.

Conclusions

Nutraceuticals may provide a number of new leads on possible new drug therapies for future use in veterinary medicine.

The use of nutraceuticals in animals is still in its infancy, with very few clinical trials showing conclusive evidence for their efficacy.

However, an increasing range of nutraceutical formulations, often combination products, are now available for domestic pets, particularly dogs and cats, with applications promoted for joint health, coat and skin wellbeing, and even obesity.

Before using any of the products outlined in this paper, a veterinarian should be consulted so that the animal can be assessed and the evidence for use of available nutraceuticals evaluated.

References

1. Boothe D M. Balancing fact and fiction of novel ingredients: definitions, regulations and evaluation. *Vet Clin North Am Small Anim Pract* 2004; 34: 7–38.
2. Hardman W E. *n*-3 Fatty acids and cancer therapy. *J Nutr* 2004; 134: 3427S–3430S.
3. Filburn C R D, Griffin D. Effects of supplementation with a docosahexaenoic acid-enriched salmon oil on total plasma and plasma phospholipid fatty acid composition in the cat. *Int J Appl Res Vet Med* 2005; 3: 116–123.
4. DeFilippis A P, Sperling L S. Understanding omega-3s. *Am Heart J* 2006; 151: 564–570.
5. Morris J G. Do cats need arachidonic acid in the diet for reproduction? *J Anim Physiol Anim Nutr* 2004; 88: 131–137.
6. Sanders T A, Sullivan D R, Reeve J, Thompson G R. Triglyceride-lowering effect of marine polyunsaturates in patients with hypertriglyceridemia. *Arteriosclerosis* 1985; 5: 459–465.
7. Chen H W, Lii C K, Chen W T *et al.* Blood pressure-lowering effect of fish oil is independent of thromboxane A2 level in spontaneously hypertensive rats. *Prostaglandins Leukotr Essent Fatty Acids* 1996; 54: 147–154.
8. Billman G E, Kang J X, Leaf A. Prevention of sudden cardiac death by dietary pure omega-3 polyunsaturated fatty acids in dogs. *Circulation* 1999; 99: 2452–2457.
9. Brouwer I A, Heeringa J, Geleijnse J M *et al.* Intake of very long-chain n-3 fatty acids from fish and incidence of atrial fibrillation. The Rotterdam Study. *Am Heart J* 2006; 151: 857–862.
10. Kellon E M. *Equine Supplements and Nutraceuticals*. New York: Break Through Publications, 1998.
11. Center S A. Metabolic, antioxidant, nutraceutical, probiotic, and herbal therapies relating to the management of hepatobiliary disorders. *Vet Clin North Am Small Anim Pract* 2004; 34: 67–172, vi.
12. Kendall R.V. Therapeutic nutrition for the cat, dog, and horse. In: Schoen A M, Wynn S G, eds. *Complementary and Alternative Veterinary Medicine*. St Louis: Mosby, 1998.
13. Shizukuishi S, Inoshita E, Tsunemitsu A *et al.* Therapy by coenzyme Q10 of experimental peridontitis in a dog model supports results of human peridontitis study. *Biomed Clin Asp Coenzyme Q* 1984, 4: 153–162.

14. Fenton D E. Myocardial infarction. http://www.emedicine.com/EMERG/topic327.htm (accessed 1 May 2006).
15. Nakamura Y, Takahashi M, Hayashi J et al. Protection of ischaemic myocardium with coenzyme Q10. *Cardiovasc Res* 1982; 16: 132–137.
16. Igarashi T, Nakajima Y, Tanaka M, Otake S. Effect of coenzyme Q10 on experimental hypertension in rats and dogs. *J Pharmacol Exp Ther* 1974; 189: 149–156.
17. McEntee K, Clercx C, Snaps F, Henroteaux M. Clinical electrocardiographic and echocardiographic improvements after L-carnitine supplementation in a cardimyopathic Labrador. *Canine Pract* 1995; 20: 12.
18. Hawks D. Alternative medicine: musculoskeletal system. *Clin Tech Small Anim Pract* 2002; 17: 41–49.
19. Hegemann N, Kohn B, Brunnberg L, Schmidt M F. Biomarkers of joint tissue metabolism in canine osteoarthritic and arthritic joint disorders. *Osteoarthritis Cartilage* 2002; 10: 714–721.
20. Beale B S. Use of nutraceuticals and chondroprotectants in osteoarthritic dogs and cats. *Vet Clin North Am Small Anim Pract* 2004; 34: 271–289.
21. Lipiello M J, Ioduraine A, McNamara P S. Cartilage stimulatory and antiproteolytic activity is present in sera of dogs treated with a chondroprotectant agent. *Canine Pract* 1998; 23: 10–14.
22. Setnikar I, Pacini M A, Revel L. Antiarthritic effects of glucosamine sulfate studied in animal models. *Arzneimittel-Forschung* 1991; 41: 542–545.
23. Tiraloche G, Girard C, Chouinard L et al. Effect of oral glucosamine on cartilage degradation in a rabbit model of osteoarthritis. *Arthritis Rheum* 2005; 52: 1118–1128.
24. McNamara P S, Johnston S A, Todhunter R J. Slow-acting, disease-modifying osteoarthritis agents. *Vet Clin North Am Small Anim Pract* 1997; 27: 863–881.
25. Brennan M. *Complete Holistic Care and Healing for Horses*. Addington: Kenilworth Press, 2001.
26. Dobenecker B, Beetz Y, Kienzle E. A placebo-controlled double-blind study on the effect of nutraceuticals (chondroitin sulfate and mussel extract) in dogs with joint diseases as perceived by their owners. *J Nutr* 2002; 132: 1690S–1691S.
27. Du J, White N, Eddington N D. The bioavailability and pharmacokinetics of glucosamine hydrochloride and chondroitin sulfate after oral and intravenous single dose administration in the horse. *Biopharm Drug Disp* 2004; 25: 109–116.
28. Hesslink R, Emens-Hesslink K, Sprouse S. The effects of a cetylated fatty-acid for improving quality of life in canines. http://www.celadrin.com/studies/EfficacyCanine.pdf (accessed 27 June 2006).
29. Hunter K W Jr, Gault R A, Stehouwer J S, Tam-Chang S-W. Synthesis of cetyl myristoleate and evaluation of its therapeutic efficacy in a murine model of collagen-induced arthritis. *Pharmacol Res* 2003; 47: 43–47.
30. Head E, Zicker S C. Nutraceuticals, aging, and cognitive dysfunction. *Vet Clin North Am Small Anim Pract* 2004; 34: 217–228.
31. Halliwell B. Reactive oxygen species and the central nervous system. *J Neurochem* 1992; 59: 1609–1623.

32. Milgram N W, Zicker S C, Head E *et al.* Dietary enrichment counteracts age-associated cognitive dysfunction in canines. *Neurobiol Aging* 2002; 23: 737–745.

33. Hagen T M, Ingersoll R T, Lykkesfeldt J *et al.* (R)-Alpha-lipoic acid-supplemented old rats have improved mitochondrial function, decreased oxidative damage, and increased metabolic rate. *FASEB J* 1999; 13: 411–418.

34. Roudebush P, Davenport D J, Novotny B J. The use of nutraceuticals in cancer therapy. *Vet Clin North Am Small Anim Pract* 2004; 34: 249–269.

35. Hansen R A, Ogilvie G K, Davenport D J *et al.* Duration of effects of dietary fish oil supplementation on serum eicosapentaenoic acid and docosahexaenoic acid concentrations in dogs. *Am J Vet Res* 1998; 59: 864–868.

36. Bright J M, Sullivan P S, Melton S L *et al.* The effects of n-3 fatty acid supplementation on bleeding time, plasma fatty acid composition, and in vitro platelet aggregation in cats. *J Vet Intern Med* 1994; 8: 247–252.

19

Meta-analyses and systematic reviews of nutraceutical clinical trials

Researchers are increasingly carrying out meta-analyses of published clinical trials of nutraceuticals in order to generate data involving larger patient numbers, and over 70 have been published to date. Such analyses have been carried out on many of the major nutraceuticals, and sometimes for more than one application. Table 19.1 outlines the results found to date. The numbers of analyses of nutraceuticals for particular applications are summarised in Table 19.2.

The results from meta-analyses appear to show possible improvement in symptoms by glucosamine, chondroitin and S-adenosyl methionine (SAMe) treatment of arthritis, coenzyme Q10 treatment of congestive heart failure, acetyl-L-carnitine in cognitive impairment, SAMe as an antidepressant, melatonin for jet lag, evening primrose oil for atopic eczema, fish oil (docosahexaenoic acid) for reduction in blood pressure, creatine in lean mass interventions, and soy products for reduced low-density lipoprotein–cholesterol (LDL-C), but contradictory evidence for melatonin in sleep improvement, and soy and phytoestrogens in treatment of menopausal symptoms. However, the Cochrane Library of systematic reviews of research on effectiveness of a number of nutraceuticals are less optimistic. This is due to the quality of data analysed by the Cochrane Library, which only takes into account randomised, blinded trials, noting dropouts, and the use of intention-to-treat trials. Bias is also removed by their sponsoring neither the trials nor the meta-analyses of specific manufacturers' products.

Although meta-analyses have been carried out on the use of dehydroepiandrosterone (DHEA) and green tea, no positive associations between these nutraceutical supplementations and disease states has been shown. There is also a noticeable absence of meta-analyses on carnitine, conjugated linoleic acid (CLA), flaxseed and its lignans, Pycnogenol, resveratrol, grape seed proanthocyanidin extract (GSPE) and lipoic acid. To date, there are limited data of any type on methyl-sulfonylmethane (MSM).

Table 19.1 Published outcomes from a number of meta-analyses of nutraceuticals

Nutraceutical	Outcome
Glucosamine[1]	Moderate to large effects on osteoarthritis
Glucosamine[2]	Significant efficacy in knee osteoarthritis
Glucosamine[3]	Moderate help in arthritis joint pain
Glucosamine[4]	Safe and effective, further research for treatment of osteoarthritis required[a]
Glucosamine[5]	May be effective in delaying progression and improving symptoms of knee osteoarthritis
Chondroitin[1]	Moderate to large effects on osteoarthritis
Chondroitin[6]	May be useful in osteoarthritis
Chondroitin[2]	Effective in knee osteoarthritis
Glucosamine/chondroitin[7]	Significant improvement of symptoms in patients with moderate to severe pain
Coenzyme Q10[8]	Useful adjunctive treatment for congestive heart failure
Coenzyme Q10[9]	Significant improvement in cardiac parameters in congestive heart failure
Coenzyme Q10[10]	Variable benefit in physical exercise, reduction in hypertension, insufficient patient numbers for conclusions in heart failure
Coenzyme Q10[11]	Inconclusive results on efficacy of coenzyme Q10 for improved tolerability of cancer treatments
Acetyl-L-carnitine[12]	Significant advantage over placebo in cognitive impairment and Alzheimer's disease
Acetyl-L-carnitine[13]	Further research required for use in dementia[a]
Lipoic acid[14]	Improves diabetic polyneuropathy
Lipoic acid[15]	No evidence for improvement in dementia until randomised controlled trials available[a]
S-Adenosyl methionine[16]	Symptomatic improvement in intrahepatic cholestasis
S-Adenosyl methionine[17]	Significant advantage compared with placebo in depression
S-Adenosyl methionine[18]	Significant improvement in depression, pain in osteoarthritis and pruritus, compared with placebo, but not conventional treatment.
S-Adenosyl methionine[19]	As effective as NSAIDs in reducing pain and improving functional limitations on osteoarthritis
S-Adenosyl methionine[20]	Role in the treatment of major depression in adults
Melatonin[21]	0.5–6 mg melatonin improves initial sleep quality in selected elderly insomniacs
Melatonin[22]	Insufficient data for resetting of circadian acrophase
Melatonin[23]	8 out of 10 trials show reduction in jet lag symptoms[a]

continued

Table 19.1 Continued

Nutraceutical	Outcome
Melatonin[24]	Marked efficacy in animal models of focal cerebral ischaemia
Melatonin[25]	Little evidence to suggest that melatonin is effective in primary insomnia
Melatonin[26]	Reduction in sleep onset latency, increased sleep efficiency, and increased total sleep duration
Melatonin[27]	Reduction in risk of death at one year, irrespective of cancer type
Melatonin[28]	Some evidence for efficacy in treating delayed sleep phase syndrome
Melatonin[29]	No evidence for efficacy in treating sleep disorders
Lycopene/tomato products[30]	May prevent prostate cancer
β-Cryptoxanthin[31]	May modestly reduce risk of lung cancer in smokers
α-Linolenic acid[32]	Reduced risk of congestive heart failure, but increased risk of prostate cancer
α-Linolenic acid[33]	Most cardiovascular risk markers unaffected
γ-Linolenic acid[34]	Potential anti-inflammatory benefits
γ-Linolenic acid[35]	Potential benefits in rheumatoid arthritis[a]
Evening primrose oil[36]	Marked improvement in symptoms of atopic eczma, changes correlated to plasma levels of dihomo gamma-linolenic and arachidonic acids
Evening primrose oil[37]	Marked improvement in symptoms of atopic eczma
Evening primrose oil[38]	Little benefit for premenstrual syndrome
Docosahexaenoic acid[39]	Higher performance in visual resolution acuity tasks at two, and possibly four months of age
Eicosapentaenoic acid/docosahexaenoic acid (EPA/DHA)[40]	Further research needed before use in schizophrenia[a]
Fish oil[41]	Restenosis after coronary angioplasty is reduced by fish oil supplementation, in a dose-dependent manner
Fish oil[42]	Fish oil causes a dose-dependent reduction in blood pressure
Fish oil[43]	3 g/day reduces blood pressure in untreated hypertension
Fish oil[44]	Number of tender joints and duration of morning stiffness at three months, reduced
Fish oil[45]	Reduction in overall mortality, mortality due to myocardial infarction, and sudden death in coronary heart disease patients
Fish oil[46]	Ratio of total cholesterol to HDL-C decreased

continued

Table 19.1 Continued

Nutraceutical	Outcome
Fish oil[47]	Daily intake over 37 months decreased all causes of mortality by 16% and incidence of death due to MI by 24%. However, suboptimal quality of studies in meta-analysis do not justify use!
Fish oil[48]	Reduction in heart rate
Fish oil[49]	Fish oil (eicosapentaenoic acid/docosahexaenoic acid) has demonstrated a significant reduction in total mortality, coronary heart disease death, and sudden death
n-3 Fatty acids[50]	No significant association between n-3 fatty acids and cancer
n-3 Fatty acids[51]	Possible association between n-3 fatty acids and reduced risk of dementia
n-3 Fatty acids[52]	No clear effect on total mortality, combined cardiovascular events, or cancer
Dehydroepiandrosterone[53]	No lean mass or strength gains
Dehydroepiandrosterone[54]	No support for increased cognitive function[a]
Tea[55]	Increased risk of cornoary heart disease in UK, and stroke in Australia. Reduction in continental Europe
Green tea[56]	No evidence it helps prevent stomach/intestinal cancer
Green tea[57]	Non-significant effect on breast cancer development
Creatine[58]	Combined with resistance training, increased maximal weight lifted in young men, not older individuals/women
Creatine[53]	Increased lean mass, minimal increase in strength
Creatine[59]	Increased lean body mass, lab-based exercise and upper body exercise
Soy isoflavones[60]	Reduced plasma cholesterol levels
Soy isoflavones[61]	Consumption not related to changes in LDL-C or HDL–C
Phytoestrogens[62]	Shows promise of treatment of menopausal symptoms
Phytoestrogens[63]	High concentrations associated with reduction in breast cancer
Phytoestrogens[64]	Hot flush frequency decreased by 5%
Phytoestrogens[65]	Some evidence for efficacy in menopausal symptoms
Phytoestrogens[66]	No improvement in hot flushes or other menopausal symptoms
Soy protein/isoflavones[67]	Reduced total and LDL-C may be due to other factors
Soy protein/isoflavones[68]	Use of products containing up to 150 mg isoflavones/day show no benefits on serum lipids

continued

Table 19.1 Continued

Nutraceutical	Outcome
Soy protein/isoflavones[69]	Significant decrease in LDL-C
Soy protein/isoflavones[70]	Significant reduction in total cholesterol, LDL-C and increased HDL-C
Soy isoflavones[71]	Contradictory results for hot flushes
Soy protein[72]	Significant reduction in total and LDL-C
Soy food[73]	Reduced risk of prostate cancer in men
Soy food[74]	Intake may be associated with a small reduction in breast cancer risk
Stanols/sterols[75]	Lowered LDL-C
Policosanol[76]	Reduction of LDL-C, more effective than plant sterols and stanols

[a]Cochrane review.

NSAIDs, non-steroidal anti-inflammatory drugs; LDL-C, low-density lipoprotein–cholesterol; HDL-C, high-density lipoprotein–cholesterol; MI, myocardial infarction.

In many meta-analyses the conclusion is that 'Further investigations in larger cohorts for longer time periods are needed to prove usefulness'.[6] Sometimes meta-analyses include confirmation of a good safety profile, such as that reported for glucosamine and chondroitin, although limited data may be available on 'structural efficacy for an accurate disease-modifying characterisation'.[2]

In a number of instances there are still questions to be resolved relating to the mechanism of action, bioavailability and absorption of nutraceuticals, for instance in the case of SAMe.[20] Other studies have reported dose-dependent effects, for example with soy supplementation, in which beneficial effects in total cholesterol, LDL-C and HDL-C were noted.[70] In some instances the causes and effects are not clearly understood, as, for example, in the case of α-linolenic acid (ALA) and coronary heart disease,[32] and sometimes incomplete treatment has been reported, such as functional limitations to the disease state without any pain relief, as noted with the use of SAMe in osteoarthritis.[19]

A recent large-scale analysis of data using nearly 37 000 pooled participants in a survey of the data on *n*-3 fatty acid use in cardiovascular disease and cancer has provided no positive evidence to substantiate its use.[52] Similar lack of evidence for the use of melatonin in a number of sleep disorders has also recently been published. Interestingly, this latter analysis was also the subject of a forceful accompanying editorial extolling the virtues of melatonin in jet lag, and also questioning the methods used in the analysis.[77]

Table 19.2 Summary of results from meta-analyses listed in Table 19.1

Nutraceutical	Disease state	Number
Glucosamine	Osteoarthritis	4
Glucosamine	Joint pain	1
Chondroitin	Osteoarthritis	3
Coenzyme Q10	Various cardiac parameters	3
Acetyl-L-carnitine	Alzheimer's/dementia	2
S-Adenosyl methionine	Depression	3
S-Adenosyl methionine	Osteoarthritis	2
Melatonin	Beneficial sleep modification	5
Melatonin	Reduction of mortality in cancer	1
Lycopene	Prostate cancer	1
γ-Linolenic acid	Anti-inflammatory	2
γ-Linolenic acid	Atopic eczema improvement	1
n-3 fatty acids/fish oil (DHA/EPA)	Visual acuity	1
n-3 fatty acids/fish oil (DHA/EPA)	Reduction in blood pressure	2
n-3 fatty acids/fish oil (DHA/EPA)	Reduced mortality in heart disease	2
Creatine	Increased weight-lifting ability	1
Creatine	Reduced lean body mass	2
Soy	Reduced serum lipids	5
Soy	Reduced cancers	2
Phytoestrogens	Contradictory evidence in menopausal symptoms	3
Policosanol	Reduced LDL-C	1

DHA, docosahexaenoic acid; EPA, eicosapentaenoic acid; LDL-C, low-density lipoprotein–cholesterol.

Many meta-analyses and critical reviews of published clinical trials of a number of nutraceuticals have now been published, and more original data and reviews are still being published. In general, data from meta-analyses is more meaningful, but the overall conclusions often do not provide clear corroboration of particular trials claiming beneficial effects.

References

1. McAlindon T E, LaValley M P, Gulin J P, Felson D T. Glucosamine and chondroitin for treatment of osteoarthritis: a systematic quality assessment and meta-analysis. *JAMA* 2000; 283: 1469–1475.
2. Richy F, Bruyere O, Ethgen O *et al.* Structural and symptomatic efficacy of glucosamine and chondroitin in knee osteoarthritis: a comprehensive meta-analysis. *Arch Intern Med* 2003; 163: 1514–1522.

3. Miller D C, Richardson J. Does glucosamine relieve arthritis joint pain? *J Fam Pract* 2003; 52: 645–647.

4. Towheed T E, Anastassiades T P, Shea B *et al.* Glucosamine therapy for treating osteoarthritis (Cochrane Review). In: *The Cochrane Library*, Issue 2. Chichester: John Wiley & Sons, 2004.

5. Poolsup N, Suthisisang C, Channark P, Kittikulsuth W. Glucosamine long-term treatment and the progression of knee osteoarthritis: systematic review of randomized controlled trials. *Ann Pharmacother* 2005; 39: 1080–1087.

6. Leeb B F, Schweitzer H, Montag K, Smolen J S. A metaanalysis of chondroitin sulfate in the treatment of osteoarthritis. *J Rheumatol* 2000; 27: 205–211.

7. Clegg DO, Reda DJ, Harris CL *et al.* Glucosamine, chondroitin sulfate and the two in combination for painful knee ostearthritis. *N Engl J Med.* 2006; 354: 795–808.

8. Soja A M, Mortensen S A. Treatment of congestive heart failure with coenzyme Q10 illuminated by meta-analyses of clinical trials. *Mol Aspect Med* 1997; 18: s159–s168.

9. Soja A M, Mortensen S A. Treatment of chronic cardiac insufficiency with coenzyme Q10 , results of meta-analysis in controlled clinical trials. *Ugeskrift Laeger* 1997; 159: 7302–7308.

10. Rosenfeldt F, Hilton D, Pepe S, Krum H. Systematic review of effect of coenzyme Q10 in physical exercise, hypertension and heart failure. *BioFactors* 2003; 18: 91–100.

11. Roffe L, Schmidt K, Ernst E. Efficacy of coenzyme Q10 for improved tolerability of cancer treatments: a systematic review. *J Clin Oncol* 2004; 22: 4418–4424.

12. Montgomery S A, Thal L J, Amrein R. Meta-analysis of double blind randomized controlled clinical trials of acetyl-L-carnitine versus placebo in the treatment of mild cognitive impairment and mild Alzheimer's disease. *Int Clin Psychopharmacol* 2003; 18: 61–71.

13. Hudson S, Tabet N. Acetyl-L-carnitine for dementia (Cochrane Review). In: *The Cochrane Library*, Issue 2. Chichester: John Wiley & Sons, 2004.

14. Ziegler D, Nowak H, Kempler P *et al.* Treatment of symptomatic diabetic polyneuropathy with the antioxidant α-lipoic acid: a meta-analysis. *Diabetic Med* 2004; 21: 114–121.

15. Sauer J, Tabet N, Howard R. Alpha lipoic acid for dementia (Cochrane Review). In: *The Cochrane Library*, Issue 2. Chichester: John Wiley & Sons, 2004.

16. Frezza M. A meta-analysis of therapeutic trials with ademetionine in the treatment of intrahepatic cholestasis. *Ann Ital Med Intern* 1993; 8: 48S–51S.

17. Bressa G M. S-adenosyl-L-methionine (SAMe) as antidepressant: meta-analysis of clinical studies. *Acta Neurol Scand Suppl* 1994; 154: 7–14.

18. Agency for Healthcare Research and Quality. S-Adenosyl-L-methionine for treatment of depression, osteoarthritis, and liver disease. 2002: 1–3. http://www.ahrq.gov/clinic/epcsums/samesum.pdf (accessed 16 June 2006).

19. Soeken K L, Lee W-L, Bausell R B *et al.* Safety and efficacy of S-adenosylmethionine (SAMe) for osteoarthritis. *J Fam Pract* 2002; 51: 425–430.

20. Williams A-L, Girard C, Jui D *et al.* S-Adenosylmethionine (SAMe) as

treatment for depression: a systematic review. *Clin Invest Med* 2005; 28: 132–139.

21. Olde Rikkert M G, Rigaud A S. Melatonin in elderly patients with insomnia. A systematic review. *Z Gerontol Geriat* 2001; 34: 491–497.

22. Cornelissen G, Halberg F, Tarquini R *et al.* Point and interval estimations of circadian melatonin ecphasia in Smith-Magenis syndrome. *Biomed Pharmacother* 2003; 57: 31s–34s.

23. Herxheimer A, Petrie K J. Melatonin for the prevention and treatment of jet lag (Cochrane Review). In: *The Cochrane Library*, Issue 2. Chichester: John Wiley & Sons, 2004.

24. Macleod M R, O'Collins T, Horky L L *et al.* Systematic review and meta-analysis of the efficacy of melatonin in experimental stroke. *J Pineal Res* 2005; 38: 35–41.

25. MacMahon K M A, Broomfield N M, Espie C A. A systematic review of the effectiveness of oral melatonin for adults (18 to 65 years) with delayed sleep phase syndrome and adults (18 to 65 years) with primary insomnia. *Curr Psychiat Rev* 2005; 1: 103–113.

26. Brzezinski A, Vangel M G, Wurtman R J *et al.* Effects of exogenous melatonin on sleep : a meta-analysis. *Sleep Med Rev* 2005; 9: 41–50.

27. Mills E, W P, Seely D, Guyatt G. Melatonin in the treatment of cancer: a systematic review of randomized controlled trials and meta-analysis. *J Pineal Res* 2005; 39: 360–366.

28. Buscemi N, Vandermeer B, Hooton N *et al.* The efficacy and safety of exogenous melatonin for primary sleep disorders. A meta-analysis. *J Gen Intern Med* 2005; 20: 1151–1158.

29. Buscemi N, Vandermeer B, Hooton N *et al.* Efficacy and safety of exogenous melatonin for secondary sleep disorders and sleep disorders accompanying sleep restriction: meta-analysis. *BMJ* 2006; 332: 385–388.

30. Etminan M, Takkouche B, Caamano-Isorna F. The role of tomato products and lycopene in the prevention of prostate cancer: a meta-analysis of observational studies. *Cancer Epidemiol Biomarkers Prev* 2004; 13: 340–345.

31. Mannisto S, Smith-Warner S A, Spiegelman D *et al.* Dietary carotenoids and risk of lung cancer in a pooled analysis of seven cohort studies. *Cancer Epidemiol Biomarkers Prev* 2004; 13: 40–48.

32. Brouwer I A, Katan M B, Zock P L. Dietary α-linolenic acid is associated with reduced risk of fatal coronary heart disease, but increased prostate cancer risk: a meta-analysis. *J Nutr* 2004; 134: 919–922.

33. Wendland E, Farmer A, Glasziou P, Neil A. Effect of α-linolenic acid on cardiovascular risk markers: a systematic review. *Heart* 2006; 92: 166–169.

34. Zilberberg M D, Levine C, Komaroff E, *et al.* Clinical uses of γ-linolenic acid: a systematic review of the literature. In: *γ-Linolenic Acid: Recent Advances in Biotechnology and Clinical Applications*. International Symposium on γ-Linolenic Acid, San Diego, CA, USA, April 25–28, 2000. Champaign, IL: AOCS Press, 2001: 90–104.

35. Little C, Parsons T. Herbal therapy for treating rheumatoid arthritis (Cochrane Review). In: *The Cochrane Library*, Issue 2. Chichester: John Wiley & Sons, 2004.

36. Morse P F, Horrobin D F, Manku M S *et al.* Meta-analysis of placebo-

controlled studies of the efficacy of Epogam in the treatment of atopic eczema. Relationship between plasma essential fatty acid changes and clinical response. *Br J Dermatol* 1989; 121: 75–90.

37. Kerscher M J, Korting H C. Treatment of atopic eczema with evening primrose oil: rationale and clinical results. *Clin Invest* 1992; 70: 167–171.

38. Budeiri D, Li Wan Po A, Dornan J C. Is evening primrose oil of value in the treatment of premenstrual syndrome? *Controlled Clin Trial* 1996; 17: 60–68.

39. SanGiovanni J P, Berkey C S, Dwyer J T, Colditz G A. Dietary essential fatty acids , long-chain polyunsaturated fatty acids , and visual resolution acuity in healthy fullterm infants: a systematic review. *Early Human Dev* 2000; 57: 165–188.

40. Joy C B, Mumby-Croft R, Joy L A. Polyunsaturated fatty acid supplementation for schizophrenia (Cochrane Review). In: *The Cochrane Library*, Issue 2. Chichester: John Wiley & Sons, 2004.

41. Gapinski J P, VanRuiswyk J V, Heudebert G R, Schectman G S. Preventing restenosis with fish oils following coronary angioplasty. A meta-analysis. *Arch Intern Med* 1993; 153: 1595–1601.

42. Morris M C, Sacks F, Rosner B. Does fish oil lower blood pressure ? A meta-analysis of controlled trials. *Circulation* 1993; 88: 523–533.

43. Appel L J, Miller E R III, Seidler A J, Whelton P K. Does supplementation of diet with 'fish oil' reduce blood pressure? A meta-analysis of controlled clinical trials. *Arch Intern Med* 1993; 153: 1429–1438.

44. Fortin P R, Lew R A, Liang M H *et al*. Validation of a meta-analysis: the effects of fish oil in rheumatoid arthritis. *J Clin Epidemiol* 1995; 48: 1379–1390.

45. Bucher H C, Hengstler P, Schindler C, Meier G. N-3 Polyunsaturated fatty acids in coronary heart disease: a meta-analysis of randomized controlled trials. *Am J Med* 2002; 112: 298–304.

46. Mensink R P, Zock P L, Kester A D M, Katan M B. Effects of dietary fatty acids and carbohydrates on the ratio of serum total to HDL cholesterol and on serum lipids and apolipoproteins: a meta-analysis of 60 controlled trials. *Am J Clin Nutr* 2003; 77: 1146–1155.

47. Yzebe D, Lievre M. Fish oils in the care of coronary heart disease patients: a meta-analysis of randomized controlled trials. *Fundam Clin Pharmacol* 2004; 18: 581–592.

48. Mozaffarian D, Geelen A, Brouwer I A *et al*. Effect of fish oil on heart rate in humans: a meta-analysis of randomized controlled trials. *Circulation* 2005; 112: 1945–1952.

49. Harper C R, Jacobson T A. Usefulness of omega-3 fatty acids and the prevention of coronary heart disease. *Am J Cardiol* 2005; 96: 1521–1529.

50. MacLean C H, Newberry S J, Mojica W A *et al*. Effects of omega-3 fatty acids on cancer risk. A systematic review. *JAMA* 2006; 295: 403–415.

51. Issa A M, Mojica W A, Morton S C *et al*. The efficacy of omega-3 fatty acids on cognitive function in aging and dementia: a systematic review. *Dement Geriatr Cogn Disord* 2006; 21: 88–96.

52. Hooper L, Thompson R , Harrison R A *et al*. Risks and benefits of omega 3 fats for mortality, cardiovascular disease, and cancer: systematic review. *BMJ* 2006; 332: 752–760.

53. Nissen S L, Sharp R L. Effect of dietary supplements on lean mass and strength gains with resistance exercise: a meta-analysis. *J Appl Physiol* 2003; 94: 651–659.

54. Huppert F A, Van Niekerk J K. Dehydroepiandrosterone (DHEA) supplementation for cognitive function (Cochrane Review). In: *The Cochrane Library*, Issue 2. Chichester: John Wiley & Sons, 2004.

55. Peters U, Poole C, Arab L. Does tea affect cardiovascular disease? A meta-analysis. *Am J Epidemiol* 2001; 154: 495–503.

56. Borrelli F, Capasso R, Russo A, Ernst E. Systematic review: green tea and gastrointestinal cancer risk. *Aliment Pharmacol Ther* 2004; 19: 497–510.

57. Seely D, Mills E J, Wu P *et al.* The effects of green tea consumption on incidence of breast cancer and recurrence of breast cancer: a systematic review and meta-analysis. *Integr Cancer Ther* 2005; 4: 144–155.

58. Dempsey R L, Mazzone M F, Meurer L N. Does oral creatine supplementation improve strength? A meta-analysis. *J Fam Pract* 2002; 51: 945–951.

59. Branch J D. Effect of creatine supplementation on body composition and performance: a meta-analysis. *Int J Sport Nutr Exercise Metab* 2003; 13: 198–226.

60. Tikkanen M J, Adlercreutz H. Dietary soy-derived isoflavone phytoestrogens. Could they have a role in coronary heart disease prevention? *Biochem Pharmacol* 2000; 60: 1–5.

61. Weggemans R M, Trautwein E A. Relation between soy-associated isoflavones and LDL and HDL cholesterol concentrations in humans: a meta-analysis. *Eur J Clin Nutr* 2003; 57: 940–946.

62. Kronenberg F, Fugh-Berman A. Complementary and alternative medicine for menopausal symptoms: a review of randomized, controlled trials. *Ann Intern Med* 2002; 137: 805–813.

63. Dodin S, Blanchet C, Marc I. Phytoestrogens in menopausal women: a review of recent findings. *Med Sci* 2003; 19: 1030–1037.

64. Messina M, Hughes C. Efficacy of soyfoods and soybean isoflavone supplements for alleviating menopausal symptoms is positively related to initial hot flush frequency. *J Med Food* 2003; 6: 1–11.

65. Huntley A L, Ernst E. Soy for the treatment of perimenopausal symptoms – a systematic review. *Maturitas* 2004; 47: 1–9.

66. Krebs E E, Ensrud K E, MacDonald R, Wilt T J. Phytoestrogens for treatment of menopausal symptoms: a systematic review. *Obstet Gynecol* 2004; 104: 824–836.

67. Gardner C D, Newell K A, Cherin R, Haskell W L. The effect of soy protein with or without isoflavones relative to milk protein on plasma lipids in hyper-cholesterolemic postmenopausal women. *Am J Clin Nutr* 2001; 73: 728–735.

68. Yeung J, Yu T-F. Effects of isoflavones (soy phyto-estrogens) on serum lipids: a meta-analysis of randomized controlled trials. *Nutr J* 2003; 2: 15.

69. Zhuo X-G, Melby M K, Watanabe S. Soy isoflavone intake lowers serum LDL cholesterol: a meta-analysis of 8 randomized controlled trials in humans. *J Nutr* 2004; 134: 2395–2400.

70. Zhan S, Ho S C. Meta-analysis of the effects of soy protein containing isoflavones on the lipid profile. *Am J Clin Nutr* 2005; 81: 397–408.

71. Nelson H D, Vesco K K, Haney E *et al.* Nonhormonal therapies for

menopausal hot flashes. Systematic review and meta-analysis. *JAMA* 2006; 295: 2057–2071.

72. Anderson J W, Johnstone B M, Cook-Newell M. Meta-analysis of the effects of soy protein intake on serum lipids. *N Engl J Med* 1995; 333: 276–282.

73. Yan L, Spitznagel E L. Meta-analysis of soy food and risk of prostate cancer in men. *Int J Cancer* 2005; 117: 667–669.

74. Trock B J, Hilakivi-Clarke L, Clarke R. Meta-analysis of soy intake and breast cancer risk. *J Natl Cancer Inst* 2006; 98: 459–471.

75. Katan M B, Grundy S M, Jones P *et al.* Efficacy and safety of plant stanols and sterols in the management of blood cholesterol levels. *Mayo Clin Proc* 2003; 78: 965–978.

76. Chen J T, Wesley R, Shamburek R D, Pucino F, Csako G. Meta-analysis of natural therapies for hyperlipidemia: plant sterols and stanols versus policosanol. *Pharmacotherapy* 2005; 25: 171–183.

77. Herxheimer A. Does melatonin help people sleep? *BMJ* 2006; 332: 373–374.

20

Synergism, beneficial interactions and combination products

As more and more combination products becoming available, some involving more than one nutraceutical, some including other entities with claimed biological activity, the identification and study of synergistic and additive effects becomes more important. Synergy is the interaction between two or more constituents, resulting in potentiation of the therapeutic effects and a quantitative increase in the particular effect, above and beyond that expected simply by adding the effects seen by the individual constituents. Synergistic interactions may result from events taking place at many possible loci: absorption, distribution, metabolism, site of action or excretion. Any or all of these can vary with route of administration, age, gender, health, nutritional status etc. Additive effects, on the other hand, require independent mechanisms and that any rate- or effect-limiting steps in the process are not saturated by any of the individual components acting alone.[1]

Synergism has been reported to occur between conventional medicines, herbal medicines and biologically active food constituents. The major benefits of synergistic reactions between two or more active constituents include reduced dosing levels required to obtain the same response, concomitant reduction of adverse effects, and avoidance of use of potentially toxic medicines. Consumption of plant foods such as fruit and vegetables, as well as grains, has been strongly associated with reduced risk of many disease states, including cardiovascular disease, cancer, diabetes, Alzheimer's disease and age-related disorders. Plant foods contain a wide range of pharmacologically and physiologically active constituents, including antioxidants. It is now thought that a number of these constituents may act synergistically, and increasingly those examples are being used as nutraceutical supplementation to our diets.

Data are emerging concerning a number of both additive and synergistic interactions between nutraceuticals and other biologically active constituents. A number of patents have been filed concerning these

Table 20.1 Examples of claimed synergistic effects between nutraceuticals and medicines, other nutraceuticals and biologically active natural products in filed patents

Medical application	Nutraceutical	Nutraceutical/medicine
Analgesic[2]	Glucosamine	NSAID/opioid
Articular cartilage repair[3]	Chondroitin/MSM	Four glucosamine derivatives
Anti-inflammatory[4]	Glucosamine	Green-lipped mussel extract
Growth hormone release[5]	Acetyl-L-carnitine	L-Ornithine
Antioxidant effect[6]	Astaxanthin	Mixed tocotrienols
	Carotenoid	Tocotrienol
	Melatonin	Astaxanthin
Treatment of vascular disease[7]	Propionyl carnitine	Chitosan plus derivatives

NSAID, non-steroidal anti-inflammatory drug.

synergistic interactions with nutraceuticals. Some examples are listed in Table 20.1.

The synergistic effects claimed in patents are usually not corroborated by parallel publications in the medical/scientific literature concerning their *in vitro* activity, whole animal *in vivo* results, or randomised clinical trials in either patients or human volunteers. An increasing number of research papers are now being published in the area of synergistic and beneficial interactions of the nutraceuticals.

Glycoaminoglycan supplementation in arthritis, liver injury and pain

The glycoaminoglycans (GAGs) are arguably the most widely used nutraceuticals, mainly being taken for symptom reduction and correction of the underlying pathophysiology in osteoarthritis and rheumatic arthritis. In a review of the use of GAGs for preservation of cartilage in arthritic pain, it was argued that supplementation with GAGs, particularly glucosamine, caused an increase in synovial hyaluronic acid synthesis, whilst certain sulfated GAGs such as chondroitin actually stimulated synovial hyaluronic acid synthesis, apparently due to a hormone-like effect triggered by its binding to membrane proteins of synovial cells.[8] One synergistic effect has been reported from an *in vitro* study on the incorporation of ^{35}S into GAGs, in which a combination of glucosamine and chondroitin demonstrated an effect of the order of 50% greater than the combined effects of the individual entities.[9] The feeding of a glucosamine/chondroitin dietary bar to rats has been shown to produce a more pronounced effect on arthritic disease than chondroitin alone.[10]

It has been suggested that a combination of glucosamine, methyl-sulfonylmethane (MSM), carnitine, coenzyme Q10 (Co Q10) and Pycnogenol, plus vitamins C and K and silica may be a useful treatment for Ehlers–Danlos syndrome, which is characterised by a combination of symptoms including musculoskeletal problems plus a susceptibility to arthritis. This proposal is based upon evidence of the individual entities being used for the treatment of separate symptoms of the disease.[11]

More recently, Japanese workers claimed a synergistic effect between water-soluble collagen and glucosamine in rabbit cartilage. Enzymically degraded collagen (10 000 Da) was rapidly absorbed from the digestive tract and induced cartilage repair with an acceleration of cartilage matrix synthesis. Simultaneous supplementation with glucosamine and collagen showed a synergistic effect on regeneration of hyaline cartilage.[12] The same group later investigated co-supplementation with glucosamine and collagen after surgical removal of cartilage, and reported cartilage to have been rebuilt by proliferating chondroblasts after only 2–3 weeks. In addition, cartilage proteoglycan and GAG content of cartilage was increased.[13] Green-lipped mussel extract has been claimed to amplify the potency of salicylates, prednisone and mefenamic acid for treating chronic inflammation in arthritis, and was shown to have abolished non-steroidal anti-inflammatory drug (NSAID) gastropathy in some combinations.[14]

The antioxidant activities of chondroitin sulfate and hyaluronic acid were investigated in carbon tetrachloride-induced injury in the liver of rats. Supplementation with 12.5 mg/kg of each reversed all the enzymatic indicators associated with liver injury, whilst supplementation with 25 mg/kg failed to exert any beneficial effect. It was postulated that the beneficial effects were due to the different modes of antioxidant activity of the two GAGs.[15]

The combination of glucosamine and NSAIDs for the treatment of pain in mice was investigated, and significant antinociceptive synergism was elicited by fixed combinations of glucosamine with either ibuprofen or ketoprofen. Glucosamine/ibuprofen in ratios of 2/1 to 19/1 showed synergistic effect on pain levels in the mouse abdominal irritant test.[16]

Effects with antioxidants

Many nutraceuticals have free radical or antioxidant activity, which may contribute to a wide range of biological activities, including anti-inflammatory effects. The carotenoids are probably the most widely investigated antioxidants in the area of synergism. The synergistic antioxidant effects of β-carotene and quercetrin (quercetin rhamnoside) on lipid radical chain reactions were investigated, and the inhibitory effect of 150 μmol/L of both was found to be stronger than 300 μmol/L of either during peroxidation of the methyl ester of linoleic acid. A further peroxidation experiment using rabbit red cell ghosts with 150 μmol/L of both showed greater inhibitory effect than 600 μmol/L of either alone.[17] Both *in vivo* and *in vitro* cellular protection against the nitric oxide metabolites NO_2· and $OONO^-$ was demonstrated for β-carotene in the presence of vitamins E and C. Synergistic protection was observed, and it was postulated that depleted β-carotene radical was repaired by vitamin C.[18] Synergistic involvement of β-carotene with the cytotoxic activity of mitomycin was reported, and again an electron transfer process was postulated to be involved.[19]

In healthy human subjects the antioxidant lycopene was shown to synergistically inhibit low-density lipoprotein (LDL) oxidation when in combination with vitamin E, rosmarinic acid or carnosine. The 30 mg dose of lycopene from tomato oleoresin decreased LDL oxidation by 21%, 5 hours after dosing.[20] Ferulic acid, also claimed to work as an antioxidant, was investigated in its role of inhibiting lipid oxidation. Although it was more powerful than α-tocopherol, β-carotene or vitamin C, combination with either of these was still more powerful.[21] Recent research into the beneficial effects of supplementation with cranberry extract highlighted the possible actions of antioxidants present. It was found that both additive and synergistic antiproliferative activities against human tumour cell lines were evident, presumably caused by the anthocyanins proanthocyanin and flavonol glycoside.[22]

To date, many carotenoids have been shown to protect the skin against photo-oxidative damage, and mixtures have been shown to be more effective than single compounds. Recently it has been postulated that carotenoids are active due to their ability to filter blue light, as most have an absorption maximum at about 450 nm.[23]

Melatonin synergism in miscellaneous therapeutic areas

Melatonin (12.5 mg/kg) has been shown to act synergistically with monoamine oxidase (MAO)-A inhibitors (clorgyline, 2.5 mg/kg, and moclobemide, 50 mg/kg) but not MAO-B inhibitors (e.g. selegiline, 25 mg/kg) in suppression of the frog righting reflex, which none of these individual compounds affected on their own.[24] Antioxidants are widely used in topical products for reducing the signs of ageing in the skin, and work combining glycolic acid with α-tocopherol and melatonin demonstrated high levels of synergy *in vitro* either in a biomimetic liposomal system or in human skin homogenates. Combinations of α-tocopherol or melatonin with glycolic acid in a 1:5 to 1:200 molar ratio resulted in a clear synergistic protection of liposomes at levels of 250% for α-tocopherol and 80% for melatonin. The rate of breakdown of α-tocopherol during liposome peroxidation in the absence or presence of glycolic acid suggested that α-tocopherol regeneration may be partly responsible for the observed effect. Synergistic antioxidant activity between α-tocopherol and glycolic acid was also demonstrated in skin homogenates, whereas only additive activity was seen with melatonin and glycolic acid.[25]

Investigation into the potential of melatonin to synergise with the antitumour activity of 9-*cis*-retinoic acid in a model for mammary carcinogenesis demonstrated both additive and synergistic effects. In fact, a single low dose of 9-*cis*-retinoic acid had no effect on the breast cancer cell cultures used, unless in combination with melatonin. The consequence of this is that significantly lowered doses of 9-*cis*-retinoic acid are required, greatly reducing the risks of toxicity.[26]

Miscellaneous nutraceutical interactions

Two synergistic interactions of lipoic acid have been reported. In one, lipoic acid and γ-linolenic acid improved NO-mediated neurogenic and endothelium-dependent relaxation of corpus cavernosum in experimental diabetes,[27] and in another, lipoic acid (16 mg/kg) and doxorubicin (5 mg/kg) were reported to be synergistic in cytotoxic and antitumor effects on L1210 mouse leukaemia cells. Its mechanism of action was considered to be improved scavenging of free radicals and metal ions. The usual most serious side-effects of doxorubicin are associated with its cardiotoxicity, but lipoic acid shows a cardioprotective effect.[28]

Docosahexaenoic acid (DHA) and tea catechin have been reported to show synergistic activity on blood plasma and liver lipids in mice. Total plasma cholesterol was the lowest when a combination of DHA ethyl ester (1%) and catechin (0.3%) was included in the diet.[29] Two further interactions have been reported with DHA: First, when used in combination with eicosapentaenoic acid (EPA) in the ratio in which the two are present in fish oils, DHA showed a synergistic inhibition of proliferation of smooth muscle cells, used as an indicator of the risk of developing cardiovascular disease.[30] Second, a synergistic interaction between DHA and two neutrophil agonists, methionine-leucine-phenylalanine and a phorbol ester, was reported when their ability to stimulate an oxygen-dependent respiratory burst was investigated.[31]

In a study involving phytoestrogens, the antioxidant activities of genistein, daidzein and equol were measured in terms of LDL oxidative susceptibility. Increasing levels inhibited the oxidation, and this effect was further enhanced with ascorbic acid. This particular synergistic effect is of clinical importance as the phytoestrogen antioxidant activity is evident at concentrations well within the range found in plasma of individuals consuming soy products.[32] Another interaction observed with soy and a tea constituent, epigallocatechin gallate, was the synergistic suppression of superoxide and nitric oxide generation from inflammatory cells.[33] A synergistic antioxidative effect of green tea extract containing epigallocatechin gallate and either butylated hydroxytoluene (0.5 mg) or α-tocopherol (2 mg) has been reported. Butylated hydroxytoluene was more potent, and it was postulated that the synergistic antioxidant activity was due to inhibition of peroxidation, free radical scavenging and binding action of ferric ions, mainly by tea polyphenol constituents.[34] Another tea constituent, this time caffeine (1.67 and 16.7 mg/kg), has been reported to exhibit an enhanced analgesic effect in combination with clomipramine (3 mg/kg).[35]

Policosanol (25 mg/kg), whose major component is octacosanol, and aspirin (30 mg/kg) are individually ineffective in protecting Mongolian gerbils against cerebral ischaemia induced by unilateral ligation of their common carotid artery. In combination, however, protection was observed.[36]

The synergistic interactions of a large number of natural products with anticancer activity have recently been reviewed. Polyphenols from tea and soy have been reported to be involved in synergistic activities both with nutraceuticals and with conventional pharmaceuticals. The antitumour activity of (—)-epigallocatechin gallate (EGCG) was found to be synergistically increased by the NSAID sulindac in two animal cancers, and thearubigins were found to inhibit the growth of tumour cells when in combination with genistein, but not when alone. Genistein has also been shown to act synergistically with EPA in the inhibition of human breast carcinoma cells, and showed significant synergy with tamoxifen in breast cancer cells.[37]

Table 20.2 Examples of claimed beneficial interactions between nutraceuticals and other biologically active natural products in filed patents

Medical application	Nutraceutical	Nutraceutical/medicine
Vascular disease treatment[38]	Coenzyme Q10	Propionyl-L-carnitine
Anti-inflammatory[39]	Glucosamine	Capsaicinoids
Arthritis treatment[40]	Glucosamine	Chinese herbs
CNS injuries[41]	Lipoic acid	Lipoic acid derivatives
Ophthalmic antimicrobial[42]	Grape seed extract, pine bark extract	Resveratrol and Pycnogenol

Beneficial interactions between nutraceuticals and medicines

A similar number of filed patents claim beneficial interactions between nutraceuticals, and medicines, again mainly in the areas of GAG supplementation for use in arthritis, and also in antioxidant combinations. Table 20.2 summarises a number of examples of documented beneficial interactions reported with nutraceuticals.

A wide range of published scientific and medical papers have detailed the extent to which research has been conducted in this area. The overwhelming activity is seen in the area of interactions with conventional medicines (Table 20.3).

One clinical trial was carried out on athletes undergoing progressive training, in which creatine (20 g/day for 7 days, 10 g/day for 14 days) and hydroxymethylbutyrate (3 g/day) were taken. This combination was shown to produce additive increases in lean body mass and muscle strength.[64]

Novel actions and interactions of piperine

The alkaloid piperine, responsible for much of the smell and taste of black pepper, *Piper longum*, displays a range of interesting effects. In mice with experimentally induced diarrhoea it showed antidiarrhoeal activity when given orally at doses of 8 and 32 mg/kg.[67] It also inhibited gastric emptying and gastrointestinal transit in rats and mice at levels of 1 mg/kg and 1.3 mg/kg.[68] Piperine has also been found to exhibit novel interactions, and is in fact a long-standing synergist for insecticides.[69] Two of the first publications in the area of drug potentiation showed a potentiating action for piperine on hexobarbital hypnosis[70] and pentobarbital-induced hypnosis in rats.[71] Later, rats treated with

Table 20.3 Beneficial interactions reported between a range of nutraceuticals, medicines and other natural products

Medical application	Nutraceutical	Nutraceutical/medicine
Body fat reduction[43]	Hydroxycitrate/carnitine	Metformin
Prevention of migraine[44]	Fish oil	Magnesium taurate
Increased antibacterial effect[45]	Epicatechin gallate	Oxacillin/other β-lactam antibiotics
Enhanced antitumour activity[46]	Theanine	Doxorubicin
Increased antifungal activity[47]	Green tea catechin	Amphotericin B
Microcirculatory function in diabetes[48]	Coenzyme Q10	Fenofibrate
Treat left ventricular disfunction[49]	Carnitine/coenzyme Q10/taurine, 'MyoVive'	
Hypotensive effect[50]	Coenzyme Q10	Enalapril/nitrendipine
Repairs gastric lesions[51]	Policosanol	Cimetidine
Antioxidant combination[52]	Lipoic acid	Ascorbic acid, tocopherol
Lipid-lowering diet[53]	Soy	Oats
Lipid-lowering[54]	Carnitine	Simvastatin
Thrombosis prevention[55]	Carnitine	Prostacycline
Tuberculosis and leprosy treatment[56]	Piperine	Isoniazid, rifampicin
Hepatic fatty acid oxidation[57]	Carnitine	Propionate
Breast cancer cell inhibition[58]	Melatonin	Vitamin D3
Cytoprotective[59]	Melatonin	Chalcones
Cytotoxic[60]	Melatonin	Tamoxifen
Ischaemic stroke protection[61]	Melatonin	Meloxicam
Anxiolytic activity[62]	Melatonin	Diazepam
Alzheimer's disease[63]	Lipoic acid	Acety-L-carnitine
Improvement in muscle mass and lean body mass[64]	Creatine	Hydroxymethylbutyrate
Topical penetration enhancement of NSAIDs[65]	DHA/EPA	Ibuprofen/ketoprofen
Topical penetration enhancement of tamoxifen[66]	GLA	Tamoxifen

NSAID, non-steroidal anti-inflammatory drug; DHA, docosahexaenoic acid; EPA, eicosapentaenoic acid; GLA, γ-linolenic acid.

radiolabelled vascine and sparteine at the same time as *Piper longum*, the major source of piperine, were shown to exhibit an increase in blood levels of vascine by nearly 233% and sparteine by more than 100%. It was proposed that piperine increased bioavailability either by promoting rapid absorption from the gastrointestinal tract, or by protecting the drugs from being metabolised or oxidised in the first passage through the liver after being absorbed, or by a combination of these two mechanisms.[72]

In 1993 a patent was filed claiming enhanced activity of anti-tuberculosis or antileprosy drugs when administered in combination with 20 mg of piperine. Pharmacokinetics were compared in humans with those of the formulations containing no piperine.[56]

Perhaps the most interesting activity of piperine involves inhibition of hepatic and intestinal glucuronidation of certain medicinal agents. Work carried out on both animals and humans showed a significant decrease in the metabolism of curcumin 2 g/kg when given in combination with 20 mg piperine.[73] Work using mice showed piperine 10 mg/kg significantly increased the analgesic activity of nimesulide administered at the submaximal dose of 10 mg/kg. Plasma concentrations of nimesulide increased 15% in this combination.[74]

One clinical trial evaluated piperine for its ability to improve the serum response of beta-carotene during oral supplementation in a double-blind crossover study. Subjects ingested 15 mg of beta-carotene with 5 mg of piperine daily for 14 days, and this resulted in 60% higher beta-carotene serum levels compared with beta-carotene plus placebo. The authors suggested that this was caused by a non-specific thermogenic property of piperine, although similar thermogenic effects of capsaicin did not have the same ability.[75] A further clinical trial using 90 and 120 mg of Co Q10 in combination with 5 mg piperine daily for 21 days produced 30% greater plasma levels than in the absence of piperine.[76]

Later research in 2002 suggested that piperine's bioavailability-enhancing properties may be attributed to increased absorption, which be due to an alteration in membrane lipid dynamics and a change in the conformation of enzymes in the intestine. It was further thought that piperine was able to modify permeation characteristics along with induction of the synthesis of proteins associated with cytoskeletal function, resulting in an increase in the small intestinal absorptive surface, thus increasing permeation of xenobiotics through the epithelial barrier.[77]

As stated earlier, piperine is an example of a methylenedioxyphenyl insecticide synergist, and these compounds are known to act as both inhibitors and inducers of CYP 450 monoxygenase activity. In fact their activity is biphasic, since following a single dose, the time courses for inhibition and induction differ: initially there is a decrease in activity, followed by an increase, with levels ultimately returning to those of the control.[1]

In addition to potentiation of the effect of medicines and nutraceuticals, piperine has been reported to potentiate the toxicity of both benzopyrene[78] and carbon tetrachloride.[79] Its use should therefore be considered carefully due to the possibility of potentiation of side-effects.

Combination products

Increasingly, combination nutraceutical formulations are becoming available. Some of these are based upon scientific and medical evidence, others perhaps are designed to aid patient compliance or possibly to give a marketing edge over competitors. Most fall within the area of treatments for joint pain and include glucosamine amongst their component nutraceuticals, but there is also a wide range of antioxidant combinations available.

Combination products for joint pain

In addition to single-entity glucosamine products, there are two other nutraceuticals that are widely sold in combination with glucosamine. The most common of these is the GAG chondroitin. One trial using a combination of glucosamine and chondroitin showed significant improvement of knee symptoms, but not low back symptoms in navy personnel.[80] In another trial, only those with mild to moderate osteoarthritis showed significant improvement.[81] The other common nutraceutical offered in combination with glucosamine is MSM. This has recently been subjected to clinical trials both on its own and in combination. When 500 mg of both glucosamine and MSM in combination was administered three times daily to patients with osteoarthritis, a statistically significant reduction in mean pain index at the knee joint was seen, compared with the individual entities. In addition, there was a reduction in the swelling index and significant decrease in the Lequesne Index. There was no suggestion that these improvements were synergistic.[82]

Recently, a range of combination products containing mainly herbal ingredients (e.g. turmeric, bromelain, boswellia, yucca and even aromatherapy oils) have appeared on the market, probably adding to the confusion of patients. Some of these adjuncts may have anti-inflammatory activity, but no clinical trials of these combinations have been carried out.

Combination of α-lipoic acid and acetyl-L-carnitine

In a study designed to investigate the effect of acetyl-L-carnitine and α-lipoic acid on memory loss, tasks testing spatial and temporal memory in rats were undertaken[83] and these were shown to improve during combination supplementation. Oxidative damage to nucleic acids is also reduced and mitochondrial structural decay is reversed. The rats involved in another study were reported to show increased energy.[84] The two compounds act synergistically to improve both fatty acid and glucose catabolism and also to improve energy production. These reactions occur along with the amelioration of oxidative stress, loss of metabolic function and mild cognitive impairment.[84]

Oxidative damage is associated with cognitive deficits in both spatial and temporal memory. Both types of memory rely on the hippocampus, but temporal memory also relies on the striatum and cerebellum. Spatial memory decreases with age but this study on rats[83] showed that supplementation with the combination of acetyl-L-carnitine and α-lipoic acid restored some of this function. Each compound on its own was found to restore this function to a small extent, but the combination use was significantly more effective. The combination product can also reduce mitochondrial dysfunction in peripheral systems such as the sensory systems. The removal of these effects may be linked with a reverse in the age-related decline in nervous, cardiovascular, visual and auditory systems, as well as effects on motivation and physical strength.[83]

Temporal memory affects learning processes, attention and exploratory behaviour. Peak rate is the measurement used to monitor the decline in this function, and it reflects the change in a response learning mechanism. The older rats involved in the study described above showed lower peak rates, suggesting difficulty in learning the relevant response. Use of the combination product showed an improvement in the peak rates.[83]

The use of α-lipoic acid and acetyl-L-carnitine in combination is of primary interest to those engaged in the development of anti-ageing therapies, attempting to prevent the symptoms associated with growing old. However, widely circulated claims are only partially justified, as the majority of the studies performed on this combination of supplements have been carried out on rats. Although combination acetyl-L-carnitine and alpha-lipoic acid appear to improve memory loss, decrease oxidative stress, improve metabolic function and decrease mitochondrial decay in rats, further study is required to be able to be more specific on the precise benefits and long-term side-effects.[63]

Combinations of plant sterols and sterolins

The possibility of lowering LDL–cholesterol levels through consumption of products enriched with plant sterols and stanols may be beneficial for mildly and hypercholesteraemic patients, and is now a widely accepted approach.[85] β-Sitosterol, the most widely occurring plant sterol, is one of the most widely used sterols in this role, but is increasingly available in combination with its glycoside, β-sitosterolin. Naturally occurring mixtures of these two exist in many plants, and as such may be responsible for some of the activity elicited by a number of plant medicines.

Interest has been shown in the anti-inflammatory activity of a combination product consisting of β-sitosterol and β-sitosterolin in a ratio of 100:1 capable of reducing the secretion of proinflammatory cytokines and tumour necrosis factor-alpha.[86] Clinical studies have also been carried out to investigate its use as an adjuvant in the treatment of pulmonary tuberculosis; it resulted in faster recovery from infection, less inflammation and improved weight gain of patients. It has also been shown to inhibit immune stress in marathon runners, and was used in the management of HIV-infected patients, where it demonstrated viral control and inhibition of CD4+ cell loss in the absence of antiretroviral drugs. The combination formulation has also shown promise in treating rheumatoid arthritis, where the response to treatment was twice that of the placebo-treated patients, and in another inflammatory disease, allergic rhinitis.[86]

Combination products of ornithine and arginine

Products containing ornithine and arginine have become popular recently, although there is no reported scientific or medical evidence of disease prevention or treatment to support their combined use. About half of ingested arginine is rapidly converted to ornithine in the body, and ornithine is metabolised to putrescine and polyamines.[87] It is in the area of exercise enhancement that this combination (1–2 g of each) is used, based on one report of higher gains in strength and enhancement of lean body mass when compared with placebo. Subjects involved in this trial also had significantly lower urinary hydroxyproline, a marker of tissue breakdown.[88]

Combinations for cognitive enhancements

This is an area where there is little published work to date, but it is thought that different nutraceuticals may affect different memory processes, and therefore combinations may be beneficial. It is possible, for example, that agents thought to have effects on the structural integrity of neurons, such as phosphatidylserine, may have greater effects on storage processes, whereas compounds that boost the energy production of neurons, such as acetyl-L-carnitine, may have greater effects on more laborious memory processes such as tasks requiring deep processing or self-initiated retrieval.[89]

Commercially available combinations

The commercial availability of a few combination products such as lipoic acid and acetyl-L-carnitine have been discussed, but a number of proprietary products are also available, with little if any published evidence to substantiate their applications. Phototrop, containing acetyl-L-carnitine, *n*-3 fatty acids and Co Q10, has been proposed for use in macular degeneration. One trial has been reported in a conference proceeding, showing its effect in restoring mitochondrial and retinal functions in age-related macular degeneration (AMD) patients.[90] LifePak is a much more complex supplement, containing around 30 components such as vitamins, carotenoids, grape seed proanthocyanidin extract (GSPE), soy isoflavones, lipoic acid, lycopene and lutein. This product claims to have anti-ageing properties.[91]

Examples of other combination products becoming available for treatment of joint problems include combinations of polyunsaturated fatty acids (PUFAs) and GAGs plus MSM. A few of the combinations used are listed in Table 20.4.

A number of possible synergistic effects of components in complex components have been cited in this text, such as green tea and soy. Commercial samples of soy in particular are more complex than previously believed, and a range of soy products have been found to contain levels of plant lignans normally associated with flaxseed. Although these levels are lower than those in flax, their presence may be responsible for modified or improved activity.[92]

Table 20.4 Examples of available combination products

Nutraceutical A	Nutraceutical B	Nutraceutical C
Fish oil	Evening primrose oil	
Glucosamine	n-3 PUFAs	
Glucosamine	Fish oil	
Glucosamine	Cetyl myristoleate	
Glucosamine	Chondroitin	MSM
Lutein	Zeaxanthin	
Coenzyme Q10	Policosanol	
Lipoic acid	Acetyl-L-carnitine	

PUFA, polyunsaturated fatty acid; MSM, methylsulfonylmethane.

Miscellaneous combinations

A number of other combinations for which there is no documentary evidence have been suggested as possible treatments for particular ailments. Combinations of chitosan with chromium picolinate or chitosan with carnitine, for example, are claimed to aid weight loss.[93] Two further examples available for sale are acetyl-L-carnitine and resveratrol for ageing and cerebral disorders, and soy protein with grape seed extract for skin health; possibly these combinations appeal to users with exotic tastes.

Conclusions

Common synergistic effects appear between antioxidant and anti-inflammatory nutraceuticals, but many others have been patented and often published. There also appears to be a wide range of other therapeutic synergies reported between nutraceuticals and conventional medicines. Recently a review on the potential for synergistic activity between tea and soy entities and prescription medicines used in cancer treatment has been published; this is evidence of the increased interest in this area.[94] It is also becoming better understood that the health benefits of a wide range of fruits and vegetables containing nutraceuticals are often due to additive and synergistic interactions.[95]

References

1. Hodgson E, Ryu D, Adams N, Levi P E. Biphasic responses in synergistic interactions. *Toxicology* 1995; 105: 211–216.

2. Raffa R, Cowan A, Tallarida R. Analgesic and glucosamine compositions. PCT International Applications, 2002: 1–24.

3. Madere S P. Compositions of orally administered nutritional supplements to repair articular cartilage. PCT International Applications, 2001: 1–29.

4. Croft J E. A synergistic composition comprising mussel protein extract and glycosaminoglycan suitable for treatment of arthritis. British UK Patent Application, 2000: 1–10.

5. Parr T B. Dietary supplement containing two bioactive components acting synergistically to elevate growth hormone release in vertebrates. US Patent Application Publication, 2002: 1–8.

6. Babish J G, Howell T. Compositions containing carotenoids and tocotrienols and having synergistic antioxidant effect. PCT International Application, 2002: 1–30.

7. Cavazza C. Composition for the prevention and/or treatment of disorders due to abnormal lipid metabolism, comprising propionyl L-carnitine and chitosan. PCT International Application, 2001: 1–12.

8. McCarty M F, Russell A L, Seed M P. Sulfated glycosaminoglycans and glucosamine may synergize in promoting synovial hyaluronic acid synthesis. *Med Hypotheses* 2000; 54: 798–802.

9. Lippiello L, Woodward J, Karpman R, Hammad T A. In vivo chondro-protection and metabolic synergy of glucosamine and chondroitin sulfate. *Clin Orthop Relat Res* 2000; 381: 229–240.

10. Chou M M, Vergnolle N, McDougall J J et al. Effects of chondroitin and glucosamine sulfate in a dietary bar formulation on inflammation, interleukin-1β, matrix metalloprotease-9, and cartilage damage in arthritis. *Exp Biol Med* 2005; 230: 255–262.

11. Mantle D, Wilkins R M, Preedy V. A novel therapeutic strategy for Ehlers–Danlos syndrome based on nutritional supplements. *Med Hypotheses* 2005; 64: 279–283.

12. Minami S, Hashida M, Miyatake K et al. Synergistic effect of water soluble collagen and D-glucosamine on injured cartilage. *Adv Chitin Sci* 2002; 6: 191–194.

13. Hashida M, Miyatake K, Okamoto Y et al. Synergistic effects of D-glucosamine and collagen peptides on healing experimental cartilage injury. *Macromol Biosci* 2003; 3: 596–603.

14. Whitehouse M W, Butters D E. Combination anti-inflammatory therapy: synergism in rats of NSAIDs/corticosteroids with some herbal/animal products. *Inflammopharmacology* 2003; 11: 453–464.

15. Campo G M, Avenoso A, Campo S et al. Hyaluronic acid and chondroitin-4-sulphate treatment reduces damage in carbon tetrachloride-induced acute rat liver injury. *Life Sci* 2004; 74: 1289–1305.

16. Tallarida R J, Cowan A, Raffa R B. Antinociceptive synergy, additivity, and subadditivity with combinations of oral glucosamine plus nonopioid analgesics in mice. *J Pharmacol Exp Ther* 2003; 307: 699–704.

17. Maoka T, Ito Y. Synergistic antioxidant effect of β-carotene and quercitrin. *Igaku to Seibutsugaku* 1994; 129: 69–73.

18. Bohm F, Edge R, McGarvey D J. Truscott T G. β-Carotene with vitamins E

and C offers synergistic cell protection against NOx. *FEBS Lett* 1998; 436: 387–389.

19. Kammerer C, Czermak I, Getoff N, Kodym R. Enhancement of mitomycin C efficiency by vitamin C, E-acetate and β-carotene under irradiation. A study in vitro. *Anticancer Res* 1999; 19: 5319–5321.

20. Fuhrman B, Volkova N, Rosenblat M, Aviram M. Lycopene synergistically inhibits LDL oxidation in combination with vitamin E, glabridin, rosmarinic acid, carnosic acid, or garlic. *Antiox Redox Signal* 2000; 2: 491–506.

21. Trombino S, Serini S, Di Nicuolo F *et al*. Antioxidant effect of ferulic acid in isolated membranes and intact cells: synergistic interactions with α-tocopherol, β-carotene, and ascorbic acid. *J Agric Food Chem* 2004; 52: 2411–2420.

22. Seeram N P, Adams L S, Hardy M L, Heber D. Total cranberry extract versus its phytochemical constituents: antiproliferative and synergistic effects against human tumor cell lines. *J Agric Food Chem* 2004; 52: 2512–2517.

23. Stahl W, Sies H. Antioxidant activity of carotenoids. *Mol Aspects Med* 2003; 24: 345–351.

24. Requintina P J, Oxenkrug G F, Yuwiler A, Oxenkrug A G. Synergistic sedative effect of selective MAO-A, but not MAO-B, inhibitors and melatonin in frogs. *J Neural Transm* 1994; 41: 141–144.

25. Morreale M, Livrea M A. Synergistic effect of glycolic acid on the antioxidant activity of α-tocopherol and melatonin in lipid bilayers and in human skin homogenates. *Biochem Mol Biol Int* 1997; 42: 1093–1102.

26. Nowfar S, Teplitzky S R, Melancon K *et al*. Tumor prevention by 9-cis-retinoic acid in the N-nitroso-N-methylurea model of mammary carcinogenesis is potentiated by the pineal hormone melatonin. *Breast Cancer Res Treat* 2002; 72: 33–43.

27. Keegan A, Cotter M A, Cameron N E. Corpus cavernosum dysfunction in diabetic rats: effects of combined alpha-lipoic acid and gamma-linolenic acid treatment. *Diabetes/Metab Res Rev* 2001; 17: 380–386.

28. Dovinova I, Novotny L, Rauko P, Kvasnicka P. Combined effect of lipoic acid and doxorubicin in murine leukemia. *Neoplasma* 1999; 46: 237–241.

29. Shirai N, Suzuki H. Effects of simultaneous docosahexaenoic acid and catechin intakes on the plasma and liver lipids in low- and high-fat diet fed mice. *Nutr Res* 2003; 23: 959–969.

30. Pakala R. Vascular smooth muscle cells preloaded with eicosapentaenoic acid and docosahexaenoic acid fail to respond to serotonin stimulation. *Atherosclerosis* 2000; 153: 47–57.

31. Poulos A, Robinson B S, Ferrante A *et al*. Effect of 22–32 carbon n-3 polyunsaturated fatty acids on superoxide production in human neutrophils: synergism of docosahexaenoic acid with f-Met-Leu-Phe and phorbol ester. *Immunology* 1991; 73: 102–108.

32. Hwang J, Sevanian A, Hodis H N, Ursini F. Synergistic inhibition of LDL oxidation by phytoestrogens and ascorbic acid. *Free Radic Biol Med* 2000; 29: 79–89.

33. Murakami A, Takahashi D, Koshimizu K, Ohigashi H. Synergistic suppression of superoxide and nitric oxide generation from inflammatory cells by combined food factors. *Mutat Res* 2003; 523–524: 151–161.

34. Yeo S-G, Ahn C-W, Lee Y-W *et al.* Antioxidative effect of tea extracts from green tea, oolong tea and black tea. *Han'guk Yongyang Siklyong Hakhoechi* 1995; 24: 299–304.

35. Bach-Rojecky L. Analgesic effect of caffeine and clomipramine: a possible interaction between adenosine and serotonon systems. *Acta Pharm* 2003; 53: 33–39.

36. Arruzazabala M L, Molina V, Carbajal D *et al.* Effect of policosanol on cerebral ischemia in Mongolian gerbils: role of prostacyclin and thromboxane A2. *Prostaglandins Leukot Essent Fatty Acids* 1993; 49: 695–697.

37. Hemalswarya S, Doble M. Potential synergism of natural products in the treatment of cancer. *Phytother Res* 2006; 20: 239–249.

38. Cavazza C. Composition for the prevention and/or treatment of vascular diseases, comprising propionyl L-carnitine and coenzyme Q10. PCT International Application, 2001: 1–19.

39. Dickson J R. Transdermal delivery of an anti-inflammatory composition of a capsaicinoids in combination with a primary amine. US Patent, 2004: 1–8.

40. Zhong S, Yu H, Babish J G. Combination of glucosamine with herbal extracts of Tripterygium, Ligustrum and Erycibe. PCT International Application, 2000: 1–20.

41. Meyerhoff J L, Yoorick D L, Koenig M L. Lipoic acid-containing pharmaceutical compositions for treatment, prevention or inhibition of central nervous system injuries and diseases. PCT International Application, 2001: 1–47.

42. De Bruijn C, Christ F, Dziabo A J, Vigh J. Ophthalmic, pharmaceutical and other health care preparations with naturally occurring plant compounds, extracts and derivatives. US Patent Application Publication, 2003: 1–17.

43. McCarty M F. Utility of metformin as an adjunct to hydroxycitrate/carnitine for reducing body fat in diabetics. *Med Hypotheses* 1998; 51: 399–403.

44. McCarty M F. Magnesium taurate and fish oil for prevention of migraine. *Med Hypotheses* 1996; 47: 461–466.

45. Shiota S, Shimizu M, Mizushima T *et al.* Marked reduction in the minimum inhibitory concentration (MIC) of β-lactams in methicillin-resistant *Staphylococcus aureus* produced by epicatechin gallate, an ingredient of green tea (*Camellia sinensis*). *Biol Pharm Bull* 1999; 22: 1388–1390.

46. Sugiyama T, Sadzuka Y. Enhancing effects of green tea components on the antitumor activity of adriamycin against M5076 ovarian sarcoma. *Cancer Lett* 1998; 133: 19–26.

47. Hirasawa M, Takada K. Multiple effects of green tea catechin on the antifungal activity of antimycotics against *Candida albicans*. *J Antimicrob Chemother* 2004; 53: 225–229.

48. Playford D A, Watts G F, Croft K D, Burke V. Combined effect of coenzyme Q10 and fenofibrate on forearm microcirculatory function in type 2 diabetes. *Atherosclerosis* 2003; 168: 169–179.

49. Jeejeebhoy F, Keith M, Freeman M *et al.* Nutritional supplementation with MyoVive repletes essential cardiac myocyte nutrients and reduces left ventricular size in patients with left ventricular dysfunction. *Am Heart J* 2002; 143: 1092–1100.

50. Danysz A, Oledzka K, Bukowska-Kiliszek M. Influence of coenzyme Q-10 on

the hypotensive effects of enalapril and nitrendipine in spontaneously hypertensive rats. *Pol J Pharmacol* 1994; 46: 457–461.

51. Valdes S, Carbajal D, Molina V *et al*. Interaction of D-002 and cimetidine in gastric lesions induced experimentally. *Rev CENIC, Ciencias Biol* 2000; 31: 185–188.

52. Lu C, Liu Y. Interactions of lipoic acid radical cations with vitamins C and E analogues and hydroxycinnamic acid derivatives. *Arch Biochem Biophys* 2002; 406: 78–84.

53. Van Horn L, Liu K, Gerber J *et al*. Oats and soy in lipid-lowering diets for women with hypercholesterolemia: is there synergy? *J Am Diet Assoc* 2001; 101: 1319–1325.

54. Brescia F, Balestra E, Iasella M G, Damato A B. Effects of combined treatment with simvastatin and L-carnitine on triglyceride levels in diabetic patients with hyperlipidemia. *Clin Drug Invest* 2002; 22: 23–28.

55. Bertelli A, Bertelli A A E, Giovannini L. The potentiating effect of propionyl carnitine on prostacycline prevention of thrombosis induced by endothelin (ET-1) and K-carrageenin. *Drugs Exp Clin Res* 1994; 20: 7–11.

56. Johri R K, Dhar S K, Kaul J L *et al*. A process for preparation of pharmaceutical composition for treatment of tuberculosis and leprosy having increased therapeutic efficacy. Indian Patent No. 172689, 1993: 1–22.

57. Brass E P, Beyerinck R A. Effects of propionate and carnitine on the hepatic oxidation of short- and medium-chain-length fatty acids. *Biochem J* 1988; 250: 819–825.

58. Bizzarri M, Cucina A, Valente M G *et al*. Melatonin and vitamin D3 increase TGF-β1 release and induce growth inhibition in breast cancer cell cultures. *J Surg Res* 2003; 110: 332–337.

59. de la Rocha N, Maria A O M, Gianello J C, Pelzer L. Cytoprotective effects of chalcones from Zuccagnia punctata and melatonin on the gastroduodenal tract in rats. *Pharmacol Res* 2003; 48: 97–99.

60. Hermann R, Podhaisky S, Jungnickel S, Lerchl A. Potentiation of antiproliferative effects of tamoxifen and ethanol on mouse hepatoma cells by melatonin: possible involvement of mitogen-activated protein kinase and induction of apoptosis. *J Pineal Res* 2002; 33: 8–13.

61. Gupta Y K, Chaudhary G, Sinha K. Enhanced protection by melatonin and meloxicam combination in a middle cerebral artery occlusion model of acute ischemic stroke in rat. *Can J Physiol Pharmacol* 2002; 80: 210–217.

62. Guardiola-Lemaitre B, Lenegre A, Porsolt R D. Combined effects of diazepam and melatonin in two tests for anxiolytic activity in the mouse. *Pharmacol Biochem Behav* 1992; 41: 405–408.

63. Wadsworth F, Lockwood G B. Combined alpha-lipoic acid and acetyl-L-carnitine supplementation. *Pharm J* 2003; 270: 587–589.

64. Jowko E, Ostaszewski P, Jank M *et al*. Creatine and beta-hydroxy-beta-methylbutyrate (HMB) additively increase lean body mass and muscle strength during a weight-training program. *Nutrition* 2001; 17: 558–566.

65. Heard C M, Gallagher S J, Harwood J, Maguire P B. The in vitro delivery of NSAIDs across skin was in proportion to the delivery of essential fatty acids in the vehicle-evidence that solutes permeate skin associated with their solvation cages? *Int J Pharmac* 2003; 261: 165–169.

66. Heard C M, Gallagher S J, Congiatu C, *et al.* Preferential π–π complexation between tamoxifen and borage oil/gamma linolenic acid: Transcutaneous delivery and NMR spectral modulation. *Int J Pharmac* 2005; 302: 47–55.

67. Bajad S, Bedi K L, Singla A K, Johri R K. Antidiarrhoeal activity of piperine in mice. *Planta Med* 2001; 67: 284–286.

68. Bajad S, Bedi K L, Singla A K, Johri R K. Piperine inhibits gastric emptying and gastrointestinal transit in rats and mice. *Planta Med* 2001; 67: 176–179.

69. Matsubara H, Tanimura R. Synergist for insecticides. XXIV. Utilization of constituents of pepper as an insecticide and as a synergist for pyrethrins or allethrin. *Bochu Kagaku* 1966; 31: 162–167.

70. Woo W S, Shin K H, Kim Y S. Investigation of the synergistic effects of *Piper nigrum* on hexobarbital. *Soul Taehakkyo Saengyak Yonguso Opjukjip* 1979; 18: 12–16.

71. Mujumdar A M, Dhuley J N, Deshmukh V K *et al.* Effect of piperine on pentobarbitone induced hypnosis in rats. *Indian J Exp Biol* 1990; 28: 486–487.

72. Atal C K, Zutshi U, Rao P G. Scientific evidence on the role of Ayurvedic herbals on bioavailability of drugs. *J Ethnopharmacol* 1981; 4: 229–232.

73. Shoba G, Joy D, Thangam J *et al.* Influence of piperine on the pharmacokinetics of curcumin in animals and human volunteers. *Planta Med* 1998; 64: 353–356.

74. Gupta S K, Velpandian T, Sengupta S *et al.* Influence of piperine on nimesulide-induced antinociception. *Phytother Res* 1998; 12: 266–269.

75. Badmaev V, Majeed M, Norkus E P. Piperine, an alkaloid derived from black pepper increases serum response of beta-carotene during 14-days of oral beta-carotene supplementation. *Nutr Res* 1999; 19: 381–388.

76. Badmaev V, Majeed M, Lakshmi P. Piperine derived from black pepper increases the plasma levels of coenzyme Q10 following oral supplementation. *J Nutr Biochem* 2000; 11: 109–113.

77. Khajuria A, Thusu N, Zutshi U. Piperine modulates permeability characteristics of intestine by inducing alterations in membrane dynamics: influence on brush border membrane fluidity, ultrastructure and enzyme kinetics. *Phytomedicine* 2002; 9: 224–231.

78. Chu C Y, Chang J P, Wang C J. Modulatory effect of piperine on benzo[a]pyrene cytotoxicity and DNA adduct formation in V-79 lung fibroblast cells. *Food Chem Toxicol* 1994; 32: 373–377.

79. Piyachaturawat P, Kingkaeohoi S, Toskulkao C. Potentiation of carbon tetrachloride hepatotoxicity by piperine. *Drug Chem Toxicol* 1995; 18: 333–344.

80. Leffler C T, Philippi A F, Leffler S G *et al.* Glucosamine, chondroitin, and manganese ascorbate for degenerative joint disease of the knee or low back: a randomized, double-blind, placebo-controlled pilot study. *Mil Med* 1999; 164: 85–91.

81. Das A, Hammond T A. Efficacy of a combination of FCHG49 glucosamine hydrochloride, TRH122 low molecular weight sodium chondroitin sulfate and manganese ascorbate in the management of knee osteoarthritis. *Osteoarthritis Cartilage* 2000; 8: 343–350.

82. Usha P R, Naidu M U R. Randomised, double-blind, parallel, placebo-controlled study of oral glucosamine, methylsulfonylmethane and their combination in osteoarthritis. *Clin Drug Invest* 2004; 24: 353–363.

83. Liu J, Head E, Gharib A M *et al.* Memory loss in old rats is associated with brain mitochondrial decay and RNA/DNA oxidation: partial reversal by feeding acetyl-L-carnitine and/or R-α-lipoic acid. *Proc Natl Acad Sci USA* 2002; 99: 2356–2361.

84. Hagen T M, Liu J, Lykkesfeldt J *et al.* Feeding acetyl-L-carnitine and lipoic acid to old rats significantly improves metabolic function while decreasing oxidative stress. *Proc Nat Acad Sci USA* 2002; 99: 1870–1875.

85. De Jong A, Plat J, Mensink R P. Metabolic effects of plant sterols and stanols. *J Nutr Biochem* 2003; 14: 362–369.

86. Bouic P J D. Sterols and sterolins: new drugs for the immune system? *Drug Discov Today* 2002; 7: 775–778.

87. Appleton J. Arginine: clinical potential of a semi-essential amino acid. *Altern Med Rev* 2002; 7: 512–522.

88. Elam E P, Hardin D H, Sutton R A, Hagen L. Effect of arginine and ornithine on strength, lean body mass, and urinary hydroxyproline in adult males. *J Sport Nutr* 1989; 9: 52–56.

89. McDaniel M A, Maier S F, Einstein G O. 'Brain specific' nutrients: a memory cure? *Nutrition* 2003; 19: 957–975.

90. MD Support (2006). www.mdsupport.org (accessed 13 April 2006).

91. Pharmanex (2006). www.Pharmanex.com (accessed 13 April 2006).

92. Penalvo J L, Heinonen S-M, Nurmi T *et al.* Plant lignans in soy -based health supplements. *J Agric Food Chem* 2004; 52: 4133–4138.

93. Candlish T K. What you need to know: over the counter slimming products – their rationality and legality. *Singapore Med J* 1999; 40: 550–552.

94. HemaIswarya S, Doble M. Potential synergism of natural products in the treatment of cancer. *Phytother Res* 2006; 20: 239–249.

95. Liu R H. Health benefits of fruit and vegetables are from additive and synergistic combinations of phytochemicals. *Am J Clin Nutr* 2003; 78: 517S–520S.

21

Minor nutraceuticals and their therapeutic applications

This chapter is included to allow coverage of nutraceuticals about which there is, as yet, little published scientific data although they are widely available in the form of commercial products. Examples of human metabolites such as superoxide dismutase (SOD) and ribonucleic acid (RNA) are being touted as treatments for a number of ailments with virtually no therapeutic evidence, while others such as theanine, cetyl myristoleate (CMO), the reduced form of nicotinamide adenine dinucleotide (NADH), polyamines and caprylic acid have very limited published evidence to substantiate their use. Table 21.1 lists a number of these entities. The data on theanine, CMO, NADH, SOD, polyamines, plant sterols and stanols and RNA are discussed below. Evidence on phosphatidylserine, phosphatidylcholine and carnosine has been discussed previously in the chapter on mental health (Chapter 8).

Theanine

Theanine is a non-protein amino acid present in tea and in the leaves of other species of the genus *Camellia*. It is the major amino acid in tea, and constitutes 1–2% of the dry weight of tea.[1] Theanine has been shown to possess three potentially useful activities: as a relaxant, an ability to lower blood pressure and an ability to improve learning ability.

An oral dose of 50–200 mg theanine once weekly, in water, was reported to cause generation of α-brain waves, which is considered to be an index of relaxation. The incidence of α-waves (30–60 minutes after theanine ingestion) in the occipital and parietal regions of the brains of volunteers was dose-dependent and did not apparently cause drowsiness, presumably because θ-waves, which are known to promote drowsiness, were not increased.

It has been demonstrated that after administration theanine was absorbed and reduced levels of serotonin were recorded. A reduction in blood pressure was noted after 60 minutes, which again appeared to be dose-related. It has been postulated that the reduction in blood pressure

Table 21.1 Structures, sources and applications of minor nutraceuticals

Nutraceutical	Structure	Source	Applications
Theanine [1]		*Camellia sinensis*	Relaxation, lowering blood pressure, mental ability
Cetyl myristoleate [7]		Experimental mice	Osteoarthritis
NADH [9]		Yeast	Chronic fatigue syndrome

Table 21.1 Continued

Nutraceutical	Structure	Source	Applications
Superoxide dismutase (SOD)[14,15]	——	Brain, kidney, liver	Heart disease, cancer, ageing, osteoarthritis
Polyamines, e.g. spermidine[17]		Soy, tea, mushrooms	Hair growth
Plant sterols/stanols,[25] e.g. β-sitosterol		Food seeds/oils	Reduction of cholesterol absorption/LDL
sitostanol			
RNA[20]	Polynucleotide containing adenosine, guanosine, cytidine and uridine	Yeast	Anticoagulant?

Table 21.1 Continued

Nutraceutical	Structure	Source	Applications
Phosphatidylserine		Brain	Memory loss, depression
Phosphatidylcholine (lecithin)	Mixture of fatty acid triglycerides linked to choline ester of phosphoric acid	Nervous tissue, brain	Memory loss
Carnosine		Brain, Muscle	Memory loss

NADH, reduced form of nicotinamide adenine dinucleotide.

is responsible for mental calming.[1] The reduction in serotonin, and also dopamine, may have an effect on memory and learning ability. Administration of 180 mg/day of theanine to rats showed increased ability in the Operant Test, and long-term administration of 1 g/100 mL in drinking water showed improvement in learning ability, as demonstrated by laboratory tests.[1]

Long-term social tea drinking appears to have no side-effects apart from the effects of the caffeine content, therefore it may be assumed that realistic levels of theanine consumption comparable with those obtained from tea drinking should be safe.

In vitro research on the neuroprotective effects of theanine has shown that destruction of rat cortical neurons by glutamic acid was suppressed, and that the mechanism of action was related not only to the glutamate receptor, but also to other mechanisms such as the glutamate transporter.[2] Theanine and other glutamate transporter inhibitors have been shown to enhance the antitumour activity of doxorubicin in mice, partially by increasing the doxorubicin concentration in the tumours.[3] Theanine has been shown to be a precursor of the non-peptide antigen ethylamine, and it has been suggested that this may prime human γδT cells, which may then provide natural resistance to microbial infections and even tumours.[4]

In addition to being available in tablets and capsule formulations, theanine is increasingly being formulated into foods such as confectionery, chewing gum and chocolates. Confectionery containing 72 mg was reported to cause relaxation, as indicated by increased generation of α-waves. Theanine is also used as a flavour enhancer, and concentrations of 0.002–0.2% have been shown to suppress bitterness in products such as grapefruit juice and beer.[5]

Cetyl myristoleate

CMO was first isolated from an NIH Swiss albino mouse strain that was resistant to adjuvant-induced arthritis.[6] It was first shown to give protection against adjuvant-induced arthritis states in rats at doses of about 400 mg/kg;[7] later on, both oral (20 mg/kg) and intraperitoneal (450–900 mg/kg) doses were shown to reduce the incidence and severity of arthritis in mice.[6] One clinical trial investigated a proprietary product (Celadrin) containing lecithin in combination with CMO and other cetylated fatty acids and claimed improvement in knee range of motion and overall function in osteoarthritis patients (see Chapter 5).[8]

No guidance on human dosage is available for CMO, but it has been used at levels of 400–500 mg daily for 30 days.

Reduced form of nicotinamide adenine dinucleotide

NADH is a coenzyme found in mitochondria and cellular cytosol, and is synthesised in the body. It triggers energy production through ATP generation, which has been postulated as the rationale for NADH supplementation in chronic fatigue syndrome (CFS), allowing replenishment of depleted cellular stores of ATP. One pilot study on the use of NADH in CFS has been carried out involving 26 patients taking 10 mg daily. The results showed a mild benefit to patients.[9] NADH has also been used to treat a number of neurological diseases, such as depression, Alzheimer's disease and Parkinson's disease, as it affects the metabolism of neurotransmitters. In one study patients with dementia associated with Alzheimer's disease were treated with intramuscular NADH for 8–12 weeks and improvement in their condition was reported.[10] The rationale for use in Parkinson's disease is that NADH may boost dopamine production, since it has been shown to increase tyrosinase hydroxylase and dopamine biosynthesis.[11] A number of trials with both oral and intravenous NADH have been published, one comparing two different routes of administration (5 mg capsules on alternate days for 14 days versus 12.5 mg by intravenous administration), and have reported similar outcomes. In 80% of the patients a beneficial clinical effect was seen, 19% showed a very good improvement of disability and 22% showed no response to treatment. Most improvement was seen in younger patients and those in the early stages of the disease.[12]

An investigation into the effect of NADH on cardiovascular disease showed that oral supplementation in animals resulted in a reduced systolic blood pressure after the first month of treatment. In addition, total cholesterol and low-density lipoprotein–cholesterol (LDL-C) levels were reduced, but no effect was noted in high-density lipoprotein–cholesterol (HDL-C) or triglyceride levels.[13]

Superoxide dismutase

The rationale for the use of SOD, which scavenges free radicals, in inflammatory joint disease is that this is frequently caused by reactive oxygen species (ROS) which aggravate and perpetuate inflammation and contribute to the degeneration of connective tissue. Intrarticular injection of SOD has been shown to be effective in symptom reduction in arthritis, and is approved for medical treatment in a number of countries.[14] The main problem with the use of intrarticular SOD is the non-human source of the enzyme, which has been found to cause immunological problems. The development of low molecular weight SOD mimetics may overcome these problems.[15]

Polyamines

Polyamines such as spermine and spermidine are ubiquitous in living cells. Spermine occurs particularly in blood, saliva, milk, sperm and urine, and is involved in cellular growth, including hair growth. Spermidine 0.5 mg daily was found to significantly reduce the clinical symptoms of telogen effluvium, demonstrating the possibility of an effect against hair loss.[16] Another study showed that spermidine partially overcame growth depression in hair follicles, suggesting a role in hair growth.[17]

Other candidates

Plant sterols/stanols have been the subject of animal and human research into their ability to reduce total cholesterol and LDL-C for over 40 years.[18] Most work has focused on plant sterol/stanol enrichment of the diet and has shown a positive association. Typical research has studied a plant sterol-enriched reduced fat spread, such as that used in the National Cholesterol Education Program Step 1 diet in the USA. This study investigated the effects of both 1.1 and 2.2 g daily of sterol and a 40% reduced fat spread, and subjects were monitored over five weeks. Total cholesterol and LDL-C values were reduced by 5.2% and 6.6%, and 7.6% and 8.1% respectively for the two dosage level groups.[18]

A later comparison of trials using a range of foods containing sterols and stanols found that effective doses ranged from 1.5 to 3.0 g daily, and LDL-C reductions were between 8% and 15%. The principle mechanism of action was considered to interference with the solubilisation of cholesterol in intestinal micelles, consequently reducing cholesterol absorption.[19] Formulated nutraceuticals in tablet and capsule form are widely available, but no evidence exists for their efficacy, the majority of published work having been carried out using fat spreads.

RNA is a crucial component of 'life on earth', having both a passive role as an information store and an active role as an enzyme that propagates the information. It has also been investigated for its potential as an anticlotting agent that avoids the possibility of excess bleeding due to production of its own aptamer antidote.[20] Despite the fact that there is no evidence to substantiate the theory that supranormal supplementation with RNA improves any health state, the molecule is widely commercially available as a nutraceutical.

Applications of phosphatidylserine, phosphatidylcholine and carnosine have been previously discussed in Chapter 8.

References

1. Juneja L R, Chu D-C, Okubo T *et al*. L-Theanine – a unique amino acid of green tea and its relaxation effect in humans. *Trends Food Sci Technol* 1999; 10: 199–204.

2. Kakuda T. Neuroprotective effects of the green tea components theanine and catechins. *Biol Pharm Bull* 2002; 25: 1513–1518.

3. Sugiyama T, Sadzuka Y. Theanine and glutamate transporter inhibitors enhance the antitumor efficacy of chemotherapeutic agents. *Biochim Biophys Acta Rev Cancer* 2003; 1653: 47–59.

4. Kamath A B, Wang L, Das H *et al*. Antigens in tea-beverage prime human gamma/delta T cells in vitro and in vivo for memory and nonmemory antibacterial cytokine responses. *Proc Natl Acad Sci USA* 2003; 100: 6009–6014.

5. Okubo T, Juneja L R. Characteristics and food uses of L-theanine. *Japan Fudo Saiensu* 2001; 40: 33–36.

6. Hunter K W Jr, Gault R A, Stehouwer J S, Tam-Chang S-W. Synthesis of cetyl myristoleate and evaluation of its therapeutic efficacy in a murine model of collagen-induced arthritis. *Pharmacol Res* 2003; 47: 43–47.

7. Diehl H W, May E L. Cetyl myristoleate isolated from Swiss albino mice: an apparent protective agent against adjuvant arthritis in rats. *J Pharm Sci* 1994; 83: 296–299.

8. Hesslink R Jr, Armstrong D III, Nagendran M V *et al*. Cetylated fatty acids improve knee function in patients with osteoarthritis. *J Rheumatol* 2002; 29: 1708–1712.

9. Forsyth L M, Preuss H G, MacDowell A L *et al*. Therapeutic effects of oral NADH on the symptoms of patients with chronic fatigue syndrome. *Ann Allergy Asthma Immunol* 1999; 82: 185–191.

10. Birkmayer J G. Coenzyme nicotinamide adenine dinucleotide: new therapeutic approach for improving dementia of the Alzheimer type. *Ann Clin Lab Sci* 1996; 26: 1–9.

11. Swerdlow R H. Is NADH effective in the treatment of Parkinson's disease? *Drugs Aging* 1998; 13: 263–268.

12. Birkmayer J G, Vrecko C, Volc D, Birkmayer W. Nicotinamide adenine dinucleotide (NADH) – a new therapeutic approach to Parkinson's disease. Comparison of oral and parenteral application. *Acta Neurol Scand Suppl* 1993; 146: 32–35.

13. Bushehri N, Jarrell S T, Lieberman S *et al*. Oral reduced B-nicotinamide

adenine dinucleotide (NADH) affects blood pressure, lipid peroxidation, and lipid profile in hypertensive rats (SHR). *Geriatr Nephrol Urol* 1998; 8: 95–100.

14. Puhl W, Flohe L, Biehl G *et al.* SOD treatment in osteoarthritis of the knee joint. *Proceedings of the 3rd International Conference on Oxygen Radicals Chemistry and Biology, 1983.* Berlin: De Gruyter, 1984: 813–820.

15. Salvemini D, Cuzzocrea S. Therapeutic potential of superoxide dismutase mimetics as therapeutic agents in critical care medicine. *Crit Care Med* 2003; 31: S29–S38.

16. Rinaldi F, Sorbellini E, Bezzola P, Marchioretto D I. Biogenina-based dietary additives. Stimulation of hair shaft growth. *Cosm Technol* 2002; 5: 9–15.

17. Hynd P I, Nancarrow M J. Inhibition of polyamine synthesis alters hair follicle function and fiber composition. *J Invest Dermatol* 1996; 106: 249–253.

18. Maki K C, Davidson M H, Umporowicz D M *et al.* Lipid responses to plant-sterol-enriched reduced-fat spreads incorporated into a National Cholesterol Education Program Step I diet. *Am J Clin Nutr* 2001; 74: 33–43.

19. Quilez J, Garcia-Lorda P, Salas-Salvado J. Potential uses and benefits of phytosterols in diet : present situation and future directions. *Clin Nutr* 2003; 22: 343–351.

20. Tuddenham E. RNA as drug and antidote. *Nature* 2002; 419: 23–24.

22

Safety, adverse effects and interactions of nutraceuticals

Although many of the nutraceuticals discussed in this book are natural components of body tissues and dietary constituents, evidence is starting to appear concerning adverse effects and interactions. This chapter will discuss examples of published safety data on nutraceuticals, general adverse effects and drug interactions, examining in particular, carnitine, acetyl-L-carnitine, soy isoflavones, tea catechins and wine polyphenols, melatonin and glucosamine, and studies of specific adverse effects and toxicity of these products. Compared with pharmaceuticals there is still little evidence available, although information is slowly increasing, due partly to increasing usage, but also due to interest from clinicians and nutraceutical manufacturers.

Safety data

Safety data derived from animal studies after single-dose treatment with a number of nutraceuticals has been collated.[1] LD_{50} values and safe doses are available for glucosamine,[2] chondroitin,[3] carnitine,[4] melatonin,[5] Pycnogenol,[6] grape seed proanthocyanidin extract (GSPE),[7] methylsulfonylmethane (MSM),[8] lutein,[9] policosanol,[10] lycopene[11] and daidzein.[12] These examples of nutraceuticals would appear to be very safe at therapeutic levels, but long-term usage may show further adverse effects than these data shown for single-dose treatment.

General adverse effects

Since 1999, the Natural Standard Research Collaboration has graded complementary medicines, including nutraceuticals, according to their efficacy. Importantly, they also collate data on adverse effects and interactions with medicines, which until recently were only sporadically reported. A number of their data-retrieval protocols have uncovered possibly serious associations, a few of which are documented in this chapter.[13] US Poison Control Centers have also reported problems with

Table 22.1 Incidence of adverse effects of a number of nutraceuticals

Symptom	Nutraceutical	Incidence cases (single ingredients)
Drowsiness/lethargy	Melatonin	26 (22)
Headache	Creatine	35 (16)
Peripheral numbness or weakness, possible neuropathy or ischaemia	Glucosamine/chondroitin	1
Coma	Melatonin	1 (1)
Ataxia	Melatonin	1 (1)
Tachycardia	Melatonin	2 (2)
Hypertension	Melatonin	1 (1)
Conduction disturbances and dysrhythmias	DHEA	1
Anaemia	Glucosamine/chondroitin	1
Anaemia with bleeding	Melatonin	1
Anaemia with hepatotoxicity	Melatonin	1
Electrolyte abnormalities	Creatine	1
Dyspnoea/shortness of breath	Melatonin	1 (1)
Urinary retention	Creatine	1 (1)

Data collated from Palmer M E, Haller C, McKinney P E *et al.* Adverse events associated with dietary supplements: an observational study. *Lancet* 2003; 361: 101–106, with permission of Elsevier.

the increasing use of nutraceuticals. The most commonly cited adverse effects were drowsiness, lethargy and headaches. Symptoms from moderate to severe were seen in a number of entities and the authors warned that it was difficult to identify the cause in multicomponent formulations or if the product was incompletely labelled. Table 22.1 summarises the incidence of life-threatening or potentially serious adverse effects of nutraceuticals found in the survey.[14] Melatonin accounted for 4% of the total adverse effects reported (also included were herbal remedies). These results were perhaps unexpected, but may be a reflection of the popularity of supplementing with melatonin and creatine in the population surveyed.

Nutraceuticals are frequently involved in basic metabolic pathways in the body, and the presence and levels of a particular nutrient may impair or enhance the action of another. This interaction has been reported for nutrients such as dietary fatty acids and vitamin A,[15] other examples being depression of glucose levels by coenzyme Q10 (Co Q10) and levels of thyroid hormone depressed by carnitine or soy products.[16] Nine oral prescription medicines have been shown to have reduced absorption after administration with flaxseed products.[17] However, most adverse effects are mild and experienced by a small proportion of consumers.

Some patients have experienced mild gastrointestinal effects after taking Pycnogenol,[6] S-adenosyl methionine (SAMe),[18] carnitine,[4] chondroitin[19] or glucosamine.[20] In addition, it has been claimed that there is a possible risk of significant psychiatric and cardiovascular adverse effects with SAMe; this is unsurprising with such an important endogenous metabolite.[18] The incidence of hypomania caused by SAMe in a number of studies has been reviewed.[21] α-Lipoic acid has been found to cause allergic skin reactions and possible hypoglycaemia in diabetic patients as a consequence of improved glucose utilisation.[21]

Daily intakes of carotenoids greater than 30 mg per day have been found to cause hypercarotenaemia (yellowing skin).[19] Slightly more serious effects have been reported with creatine, and include weight gain, typically 1–2 kg, muscle cramps, and isolated cases of renal dysfunction, and also the possibility of cytotoxicity.[23] Chronic creatine supplementation has been reported to increase the bodily production of potentially dangerous formaldehyde, which is known to cross-link proteins and DNAs.[24] There is also now mounting evidence that both creatine and creatinine are precursors of mutagenic amino-imidazoazaarenes. This is of significance in the light of the increasing prevalence of diet supplementation with several hundred times the levels of creatine naturally present in food.[25]

Dehydroepiandrosterone (DHEA) has been postulated to have a number of potential side-effects including hair loss and menstrual irregularities in women, and increased risk of prostate cancer in men.[19] As DHEA is a hormone, masculinisation may occur in women, and gynaecomastia and breast tenderness in men may become evident.[13] DHEA may also be responsible for causing an increase in blood sugar levels.[13] An increased risk of prostate cancer is reported in individuals being treated with α-linolenic acid to reduce the risk of heart disease,[26] and increased cell damage during intense exercise has been reported after use of Co Q10.[27]

Potential adverse effects of conjugated linoleic acid (CLA) have been reported, based mainly on evidence obtained from animals. Rats given 1% CLA in their diets showed decreased mineral apposition rate and bone formation in the tibia. The authors also questioned the wisdom of using CLA isomers that do not exist in foods in commercial preparations.[28] There is increasing evidence from both animal and human work that the CLA isomer *trans*-10, *cis*-12 may produce liver hypertrophy and insulin resistance, using a mechanism resembling lipodystrophy that redistributes fat.[29] Both black and green teas contain caffeine, from which multiple adverse effects have been reported, mainly due to its activity as a CNS stimulant.[13]

Drug interactions

A number of interactions have been reported both between nutraceuticals and with prescribed medicines.

Work in rats has shown policosanol to increase the anti-ulcer effects of cimetidine.[30] Interactions between the two antidepressants SAMe and clomipramine have been reported,[31] and it is possible that there are interactions between SAMe and tyramine and other centrally acting pharmaceuticals. Prostaglandin excretion has been shown to be lowered after supplementation with n-3 fatty acids and α-linolenic acid, in combination with indometacin.[32] The anticoagulant activity of warfarin is decreased after Co Q10 administration,[33] but raised when taken in conjunction with policosanol.[16] Increased anticoagulant effects have been reported with nicoumalone taken in combination with carnitine, and gastrointestinal bleeding was also noted.[34]

Many of the effects of CLA in the hepatic activity of lipogenic enzymes and gene expression have been reported to be reversed by fish oil containing docosahexaenoic acid (DHA) and eicosapentaenoic acid (EPA).[35] γ-linolenic acid (GLA) is known to inhibit *in vitro* the activity of a number of CYP enzymes, suggesting a clinical interaction with phenothiazines, and theoretical considerations suggest a possible interaction with tamoxifen.[36] There have been multiple reports of seizures occurring in patients taking evening primrose oil in combination with phenothiazine neuroleptics such as chlorpromazine, trifluoperazine and thioridazine. n-3 Fatty acids may reduce blood pressure and enhance the effects of medications used for this purpose, and flaxseed, but not the oil, may reduce the absorption of oral medication. To prevent this latter problem, medication should be taken 2 hours after flaxseed consumption. The use of creatine with diuretics such as furosemide should be avoided due to the risks of dehydration, and kidney damage may be greater when creatine is used with medicines that may damage kidneys, such as anti-inflammatories (e.g. ibuprofen) or cimetidine. Finally, the caffeine content of teas has been documented as causing severe cardiovascular events when used in conjunction with ephedrine, and it is also thought to be synergistic in combination with other stimulants.[13]

A number of reports have highlighted the possibility of prescription medicines depressing levels of nutraceuticals. Acetohexamide, propranolol, phenothiazine and tricyclic antidepressants have lowered levels of Co Q10, and valproic acid has been shown to lower levels of carnitine and acetyl-ʟ-carnitine. It has been recommended that increased Co Q10 supplementation is required when taking statins.[1] This advice is particularly important as statins are available without prescriptions in the UK, and consequently require pharmaceutical intervention for safe use. Although Co Q10 depletion may be tolerated by young patients in the short term, higher doses over longer periods of time and to elderly patients with chronic conditions may be dangerous.[37]

Carnitine and acetyl-ʟ-carnitine

Carnitine and acetylcarnitine are endogenous constituents in human metabolism, but only the ʟ-carnitine and acetyl-ʟ-carnitine occur naturally; the synthetic ᴅ-isomers show more serious adverse effects.

Drug interactions

Sodium valproate, pivampicillin and isotretinoin have been reported to induce carnitine deficiency.[38] Sodium valproate interferes with carnitine uptake by forming valproyl-CoA and valproyl carnitine, which results in direct competitive inhibition of carnitine uptake at the transport site, and reduction in efficiency of carnitine transporters.[1] Valproate-induced hepatotoxicity, overdose and other acute metabolic crises linked with carnitine deficiency require intravenous supplementation, while non-emergency situations (e.g. infants and young children taking valproate) may need oral supplementation.[39]

Pivampicillin has been found to lower carnitine levels, suggesting the need for carnitine supplementation, and zidovudine has been reported to be less effective when administered with carnitine.[38]

A positive effect has been reported in cystic acne patients on iso-tretinoin therapy concurrently taking ʟ-carnitine. Isotretinoin elicits some of the adverse effects associated with carnitine deficiency, but patients taking ʟ-carnitine along with isotretinoin found that the adverse effects disappeared without the need to discontinue or reduce the isotretinoin.[40]

Adverse effects and toxicity

Both ʟ-carnitine and acetyl-ʟ-carnitine have been shown to have very low toxicity with rare and generally minor side-effects.[1]

The adverse effects have recently been reviewed. They include sporadic reports with the use of carnitine, such as pungent skin odour and a fishy body or urine odour following administration. Nausea and vomiting, as well as diarrhoea and muscle cramping have been reported with both carnitine and acetyl-L-carnitine supplementation. Aggression and agitation have been reported in some patients following administration of acetyl-L-carnitine.[1]

D-Carnitine

Most dietary supplements contain L-carnitine or a DL-carnitine mixture, which is a result of chemical synthesis. D-Carnitine is a competitive inhibitor of L-carnitine uptake, and this delays mitochondrial fatty acid oxidation and energy formation. D-Carnitine administration results in a depletion in L-carnitine in cardiac and skeletal muscle, which can cause cardiac arrhythmias and muscle weakness. Toxicity has been seen following administration of DL-carnitine, and D-carnitine has been classed as not safe for human consumption in the USA.[41]

Soy isoflavones

A few isolated adverse effects have been reported with soy isoflavones. An epidemiological study revealed a relationship between soy intake and an increased risk of bladder cancer.[42] Work carried out in animals has demonstrated the possibility of reproductive problems, but no human data have been published. Healthy postmenopausal women were administered 150 mg soy isoflavones daily for 5 years, and they exhibited an increased occurrence of endometrial hyperplasia.[43] One report has found that low-dose genistein stimulates proliferation of breast cancer cells *in vitro*, and high tofu consumption in men has been claimed to be responsible for lower brain weights and reduced scores on cognitive tests.[44] Asthma has been reported in young adults after drinking soy beverages.[45]

Toxicity

Studies in animals have revealed potentially mutagenic, carcinogenic and teratogenic properties of phytoestrogens,[46] and an influence on reproductive physiology has been associated with production of equol from daidzein. Equol is thought to be responsible for permanent histological damage to the reproductive organs of the ewe.[47]

Possible toxic effects of genistein related to its ability to inhibit tyrosine kinase and topoisomerase have been reported in animal studies.[1] The relevance of these findings has yet to be reported in humans. Genistein and daidzein have been investigated to examine their ability to induce chromosomal aberrations in cultured human peripheral blood lymphocytes, and chromatid aberrations have been observed, but *in vivo* data have not been reported.[1]

Adverse effects

A study into the effects of individual soy isoflavones in women found cases of loss of appetite, pedal oedema, nausea and breast tenderness, possibly caused by the isoflavones. Reductions of blood pressure and neutrophil count have also been reported.[48] Genistein administration causes hypophosphataemia, and may affect phosphorous deposition in the bone, leading to inhibition of bone formation over an extended period of time.[49]

Caution should be taken with excessive consumption of the isoflavones. At present although there is little evidence on the effects of chronic or high dosage on toxicity in humans, high mid-life tofu consumption has been linked to cognitive impairment and brain atrophy in late life.[50] Soy allergy has also been documented from skin tests, and is reported to occur in up to 6% of all children.[13]

Catechins

Catechins, which are a class of proanthocyanidins, are present in many plant food products, particularly wine and tea, and are generally thought to be safe.[1]

Toxicity and adverse effects

High levels of antioxidants such as catechins may cause pro-oxidation in some individuals, potentially worsening cardiovascular damage and atherosclerosis.[38]

A range of adverse effects have been reported with teas, and some with specified tea constituents. The first rather unexpected effect is the erosive effect of black tea on dental enamel, even though the effect is only 20% of that recorded for a number of herbal teas.[51] One case report detailed the inhibition of efficacy of oral iron treatment in iron-deficiency anaemia with excessive tea consumption, and it has been recommended that oral iron medications should not be taken with tea.[52] However, work carried out on the inhibitory action of (—)-epigallocatechin gallate (EGCG) at doses up to 300 mg on non-haem iron absorption was found to be much lower than that for black tea itself.[53] The possible pro-oxidant effects of tea catechins have been considered, and it is known that they can be both pro- and antioxidant, being capable of causing damage to biological molecules and tissues.[54] Allergies have also been reported with teas, for example the widely quoted induction of asthma in workers in a green tea factory, probably caused by airborne inhalation,[55] which is probably irrelevant to tea drinkers. Another symptom is activation of hypoxia-inducible factor 1, which can be a serious effect in cases of consumption of high doses of tea catechins.[56]

A recent review discussed adverse effects of catechin derivatives, and reported them to inhibit most digestive enzymes, including pectinase, amylase, lipase and proteolytic enzymes. They are said to interfere with the digestion and absorption of carbohydrates, and also to interfere with iron metabolism. Despite being investigated for anticarcinogenic effects, catechins have also been suspected to cause cancers, although it is thought that this carcinogenic activity may be due to the irritation and cellular damage that they cause rather than direct mutation of DNA. *In vitro*, epicatechin-(4β-8)-catechin and catechin have been shown to possess a strong inhibitory effect on sperm motility, showing a dose–response relationship. However, it is not known whether these effects are exerted *in vivo*.[1]

Melatonin

During the chemical synthesis of melatonin L-kynurenine is produced, which has been reported to have a convulsant effect. Another side-product, quinolinic acid, has been reported to be neurotoxic.[57]

Adverse effects

Side-effects of melatonin that have been demonstrated include inhibition of reproductive function, delayed timing of puberty and influence (when taken during pregnancy and lactation) on the circadian status of the fetus and neonate and on future development.[58]

Melatonin administration has been reported to cause residual drowsiness the following morning, sleep disturbance and excitement after wakening and before going to sleep.[59] It has also been reported that asynchronous supplementation disrupts sleep and alters the circadian rhythm.[60]

A large number of wide-ranging adverse effects have been noted, and it is obviously safer to take the minimum effective dose on the minimum of occasions.[1] One report of the formation of secondary oxidation products, such as the endoperoxides, has been published, which may explain the pro-oxidant property of melatonin.[61]

Few studies have been carried out to determine the effect of melatonin on the human reproductive system, although in one interesting experiment in young women a large dose of 300 mg daily for four months was found to suppress the midcycle surge in luteinising hormone and to partially inhibit ovulation. This effect was increased by the addition of a progestin mini-pill. Side-effects with this contraceptive use of melatonin included abnormal bleeding and headaches, but interestingly, no effect on sleep was reported.[62,63] Most studies on reproduction and melatonin have been carried out in animals, as many animals have a seasonal reproduction cycle, which may be affected by melatonin levels. The role of melatonin in non-seasonal breeders, such as humans, has not been defined but should be considered when starting melatonin therapy.[64]

Toxic effects and drug interactions

Melatonin has been reported to interact with a number of prescription drugs, for example, serum melatonin levels have been shown to increase after taking fluvoxamine due to fluvoxamine reducing the metabolism of melatonin by inhibiting P450CYP enzymes. Certain sedative medications may have a similar effect, which could lead to exaggerated enhancement of their sedative effects.[65] Melatonin interacts with nifedipine, increasing the blood pressure and heart rate of patients taking the two products concurrently.[66] It should not be given to children or pregnant or lactating women, as it crosses the placenta and has been responsible for rhythmic variations in milk in both humans and goats. Furthermore, it has been shown that melatonin interferes with glucose metabolism.[67]

Glucosamine

Glucosamine is generally safe, but gastrointestinal side-effects occur in up to 12% of consumers. These effects included upset stomach, nausea, heartburn and diarrhoea.[20]

Adverse effects

Glucosamine has been reported to produce an immediate-hypersensitivity reaction (urticaria) in one case study,[68] and asthma exacerbation[69] and renal toxicity[70] have been reported when used in combination with chondroitin. Animal studies have shown that high levels of glucosamine administration can raise plasma glucose levels, and this may also happen in humans.[71] This is of particular significance in elderly populations where there is an high risk of both type 2 diabetes and rheumatoid arthritis occurring, the latter often being treated with glucosamine. It has been claimed that glucosamine affects insulin secretion and/or action in humans due to its involvement in the hexosamine pathway.[72] However, in a recent study it was reported that oral glucosamine did not cause significant alterations in glucose metabolism in patients with type 2 diabetes.[71]

One report has suggested that a number of glycosaminoglycans, including chondroitin (but glucosamine has not been investigated) provoke autoimmune dysfunction, thereby promoting inflammation. These data were obtained both in a murine model and in patients with rheumatoid arthritis.[73] A recent publication by the Committee on Safety of Medicines (CSM) and the Medicines and Healthcare products Regulatory Agency (MHRA) in the UK has highlighted an interaction with warfarin. Seven incidences of increased prothrombin times in patients with previously stable levels have been reported.[74]

Conclusions

Carnitine, soy isoflavones, teas and proanthocyanidins are safely consumed routinely by many populations in their habitual diets, however, as they are increasingly being used as nutraceuticals, further investigations must be made concerning their possible toxicity, as supra-normal levels may be consumed. Melatonin and glucosamine are normal components of human metabolism, but in unusual dosages and with chronic administration they may show side-effects.

Nutraceuticals show fewer adverse effects and interactions with medicines than prescription medicines and herbal remedies; however, the absence of documented effects does not indicate that these products are necessarily safe. In the interests of patient safety all use of nutraceuticals should be made available to healthcare prescribers to ensure that precautions are explained and acted upon.

Although many nutraceuticals are present as components of food or as molecules in human metabolism, a number of adverse effects and toxicities have been reported. Increasing use of these compounds by consumers at higher doses and chronic administration may reveal further adverse effects in the future.[1]

References

1. Davies E, Greenacre D, Lockwood G B. Adverse effects and toxicity of nutraceuticals. *Rev Food Nutr Toxicol* 2005; 3: 165–195.
2. Lenga R E. *The Sigma-Aldrich Library of Chemical Safety Data*, 2nd edn. Milwaukee: Sigma-Aldrich, 1988.
3. Takeuchi M, Edanaga M. Antiatherosclerotic agents. 8. Toxicological studies of sodium chondroitin polysulfate. 1. *Oyo Yakuri* 1972; 6: 573–587.
4. Kelly G S. L-Carnitine: therapeutic applications of a conditionally-essential amino acid. *Altern Med Rev* 1998; 3: 345–360.
5. Sugden D. Psychopharmacological effects of melatonin in mouse and rat. *J Pharmacol Exp Ther* 1983; 227: 587–591.
6. Rohdewald P. A review of the French maritime pine bark extract (Pycnogenol), a herbal medication with a diverse clinical pharmacology. *Int J Clin Pharmacol Ther* 2002; 40: 158–168.
7. Yamakoshi J, Saito M, Kataoka S, Kikuchi M. Safety evaluation of proanthocyanidin-rich extract from grape seeds. *Food Chem Toxicol* 2002; 40: 599–607.
8. Horvath K, Noker P E, Somfai-Relle S *et al.* Toxicity of methylsulfonylmethane in rats. *Food Chem Toxicol* 2002; 40: 1459–1462.
9. Kruger C L, Murphy M, DeFreitas Z *et al.* An innovative approach to the determination of safety for a dietary ingredient derived from a new source: case study using a crystalline lutein product. *Food Chem Toxicol* 2002; 40: 1535–1549.
10. Aleman C, Rodeiro I, Noa M *et al.* One-year dog toxicity study of D-002, a mixture of aliphatic alcohols. *J Appl Toxicol* 2001; 21: 179–184.
11. Mellert W, Deckardt K, Gembardt C *et al.* Thirteen-week oral toxicity study of synthetic lycopene products in rats. *Food Chem Toxicol* 2002; 40: 1581–1588.
12. Munro I C, Harwood M, Hlywka J J *et al.* Soy isoflavones: a safety review. *Nutr Rev* 2003; 61: 1–33.
13. Ulbricht C E, Basch E M. *Natural Standard Herb and Supplement Reference.* St Louis: Elsevier/Mosby, 2005.
14. Palmer M E, Haller C, McKinney P E *et al.* Adverse events associated with dietary supplements: an observational study. *Lancet* 2003; 361: 101–106.
15. Dillard C J, German J B. Phytochemicals: nutraceuticals and human health. *J Sci Food Agric* 2000; 80: 1744–1756.
16. Harkness R, Bratman S. *Handbook of Drug-Herb and Drug-Supplement Interactions.* St Louis: Mosby, 2003.
17. Ly J, Percy L. Dhanani S. Use of dietary supplements and their interactions with prescription drugs in the elderly. *Am J Health-Syst Pharm* 2002; 59: 1759–1762.
18. Fetrow C W, Avila J R. Efficacy of the dietary supplement S-adenosyl-L-methionine. *Ann Pharmacother* 2001; 35: 1414–1425.

19. Mason P. *Dietary Supplements*, 2nd edn. London; Pharmaceutical Press, 2001.

20. Murray M T. Glucosamine sulphate: effective osteoarthritis treatment. *Am J Nat Med* 1994; 1: 10–14.

21. Friedel H A, Goa K L, Benfield P. *S*-Adenosyl-L-methionine. A review of its pharmacological properties and therapeutic potential in liver dysfunction and affective disorders in relation to its physiological role in cell metabolism. *Drugs* 1989; 38: 389–416.

22. Packer L, Witt E H, Tritschler H J. alpha-Lipoic acid as a biological antioxidant. *Free Radic Biol Med* 1995; 19: 227–250.

23. Persky A M, Brazeau G A. Clinical pharmacology of the dietary supplement creatine monohydrate. *Pharmacol Rev* 2001; 53: 161–176.

24. Yu P H, Deng Y. Potential cytotoxic effect of chronic administration of creatine, a nutrition supplement to augment athletic performance. *Med Hypotheses* 2000; 54: 726–728.

25. Brudnak M A. Creatine: are the benefits worth the risk? *Toxicol Lett* 2004; 150: 123–130.

26. Brouwer I A, Katan M B, Zock P L. Dietary γ-linolenic acid is associated with reduced risk of fatal coronary heart disease, but increased prostate cancer risk: a meta-analysis. *J Nutr* 2004; 134: 919–922.

27. Malm C, Svensson M, Joeberg B *et al.* Supplementation with ubiquinone-10 causes cellular damage during intense exercise. *Acta Physiol Scand* 1996; 157: 511–512.

28. Watkins B A, Li Y. Conjugated linoleic acid: the present state of knowledge. In: Wildman R E C, ed. *Handbook of Nutraceuticals and Functional Foods*. Boca Raton, FL: CRC Press, 2001.

29. Larsen T M, Toubro S, Astrup A. Efficacy and safety of dietary supplements containing CLA for the treatment of obesity: evidence from animal and human studies. *J Lipid Res* 2003; 44: 2234–2241.

30. Valdes S, Molina V, Carbajal D, Arruzazabala L, Mas R. Comparative study of the antiulcer effects of D-002 with sucralfate and omeprazole. *Rev CENIC, Ciencias Biol* 2000; 31: 117–120.

31. Iruela L M, Minguez L, Merino J, Monedero G. Toxic interaction of S-adenosylmethionine and clomipramine. *Am J Psychiatry* 1993; 150: 522.

32. Codde J P, Beilin L J, Croft K D, Vandongen R. Study of diet and drug interactions on prostanoid metabolism. *Prostaglandins* 1985; 29: 895–910.

33. Landbo C, Almdal T P. Interaction between warfarin and coenzyme Q10. *Ugeskrift Laeger* 1998; 160: 3226–3227.

34. Martinez E, Domingo P, Roca-Cusachs A. Potentiation of acenocoumarol action by L-carnitine. *J Intern Med* 1993; 233: 94.

35. Ide T. Interaction of fish oil and conjugated linoleic acid in affecting hepatic activity of lipogenic enzymes and gene expression in liver and adipose tissue. *Diabetes* 2005; 54: 412–423.

36. Williamson E M. Interactions between herbal and conventional medicines. *Exp Opin Drug Safety* 2005; 4: 355–378.

37. Preedy V, Mantle D. Adverse effect on coenzyme Q10 levels. *Pharm J* 2004; 272: 13.

38. Rapport L, Lockwood B. *Nutraceuticals*. London: Pharmaceutical Press, 2002.

39. De Vivo D C, Bohan T P, Coulter D L *et al.* L-Carnitine supplementation in childhood epilepsy: current perspectives. *Epilepsia* 1998; 39: 1216–1225.

40. Georgala S, Schulpis K H, Georgala C, Michas T. L-Carnitine supplementation in patients with cystic acne on isotretinoin therapy. *J Eur Acad Dermatol Venereol* 1999; 13: 205–209.

41. Fuhrmann M. Stereospecific purity of L-carnitine and analytical control of deleterious D-carnitine. *Ann Nutr Metab* 2000; 44: 75–76.

42. Sun C-L, Yuan J-M, Arakawa K *et al.* Dietary soy and increased risk of bladder cancer: the Singapore Chinese Health Study. *Cancer Epidemiol Biomarkers Prev* 2002; 11: 1674–1677.

43. Unfer V, Casini M L, Costabile L *et al.* Endometrial effects of long-term treatment with phytoestrogens: a randomized, double-blind, placebo-controlled study. *Fertil Steril* 2004; 82: 145–148.

44. Sarwar G, L'Abbe M R, Brooks S P J *et al.* *Dietary Phytoestrogens: Safety, Nutritional Quality, and Health Considerations.* ACS Symposium Series 2002, 803 (Quality Management of Nutraceuticals), 241–257.

45. Woods R K, Walters E H, Raven J M *et al.* Food and nutrient intakes and asthma risk in young adults. *Am J Clin Nutr* 2003; 78: 414–421.

46. Sirtori C R. Dubious benefits and potential risk of soy phyto-oestrogens. *Lancet* 2000; 355: 849.

47. Cassidy A. Physiological effects of phyto-oestrogens in relation to cancer and other human health risks. *Proc Nutr Soc* 1996; 55: 399–417.

48. Bloedon L T, Jeffcoat A R, Lopaczynski W *et al.* Safety and pharmacokinetics of purified soy isoflavones: single-dose administration to post menopausal women. *Am J Clin Nutr* 2002; 76: 1126–1137.

49. Busby M G, Jeffcoat R A, Bloedon L T *et al.* Clinical characteristics and pharmacokinetics of purified soy isoflavones: single-dose administration to healthy men. *Am J Clin Nutr* 2002; 75: 126–136.

50. White L R, Petrovitch H, Ross G W *et al.* Brain aging and midlife tofu consumption. *J Am Coll Nutr* 2000; 19: 242–255.

51. Brunton P A, Hussain A. The erosive effect of herbal tea on dental enamel. *J Dent* 2001; 29: 517–520.

52. Gabrielli G B, De Sandre G. Excessive tea consumption can inhibit the efficacy of oral iron treatment in iron-deficiency anemia. *Haematologica* 1995; 80: 518–520.

53. Ullmann U, Haller J, Bakker G C M *et al.* Epigallocatechin gallate (EGCG) (TEAVIGO) does not impair nonhaem-iron absorption in man. *Phytomedicine* 2005: 12: 410–415.

54. DiSilvestro R A. Flavonoids as antioxidants. In: Wildman R E C, ed. *Handbook of Nutraceuticals and Functional Foods.* Boca Raton, FL: CRC Press, 2001: 127–142.

55. Dubick M A, Omaye S T. Modification of atherogenesis and heart disease by grape wine and tea polyphenols. In: Wildman R E C, ed. *Handbook of Nutraceuticals and Functional Foods.* Boca Raton, FL: CRC Press, 2001; 235–260.

56. Zhou Y-D, Kim Y-P, Li X-C *et al.* Hypoxia-inducible factor-1 activation by (—)-epicatechin gallate: potential adverse effects of cancer chemoprevention with high-dose green tea extracts. *J Nat Prod* 2004; 67: 2063–2069.

57. Heyes M P, Saito K, Devinsky O, Nadi N S. Kynurenine pathway metabolites in cerebrospinal fluid and serum in complex partial seizures. *Epilepsia* 1994; 2: 251–257.

58. Arendt J. Safety of melatonin in long term use (?) *J Biol Rhythm* 1997; 12: 673–681.

59. Ishizaki A, Sugama M, Takeuchi N. Usefulness of melatonin for developmental sleep and emotional behavior disorders – studies of melatonin trial on 50 patients with developmental disorders. *No To Hattatsu [Brain and development]* 1999; 31: 428–437.

60. Samel A. Melatonin and jet lag. *Eur J Med Res* 1999; 4: 385–388.

61. Medina-Navarro R, Duran-Reyes G, Hicks J J. Pro-oxidating properties of melatonin in the in vitro interaction with the singlet oxygen. *Endocrine Res* 1999; 25: 263–280.

62. Brzezinski A. Melatonin in humans. *N Engl J Med* 1997; 336: 186–195.

63. Reiter R J, Maestroni G J M. Melatonin in relation to the antioxidative defense and immune systems: possible implications for cell and organ transplantation. *J Mol Med* 1999; 77: 36–39.

64. Birdsall T C. The biological effects and clinical uses of the pineal hormone melatonin. *Altern Med Rev* 1996; 1: 94–101.

65. Hartter S, Grozinger M, Weigmann H. Increased bioavailability of oral melatonin after fluvoxamine coadministration. *Clin Pharmacol Ther* 2000; 67: 1–6.

66. Lusardi P, Piazza E, Fogari R. Cardiovascular effects of melatonin in hypertensive patients well controlled by nifedipine: a 24-hour study. *Br J Clin Pharmacol* 2000; 49: 423–427.

67. Lemaître B. Toxicology of melatonin. *J Biol Rhythm* 1997; 12: 697–706.

68. Matheu V, Gracia Bara M T, Pelta R *et al.* Immediate-hypersensitivity reaction to glucosamine sulfate. *Allergy* 1999; 54: 643.

69. Tallia A F, Cardone D A. Asthma exacerbation associated with glucosamine-chondroitin supplement. *J Am Board Fam Pract* 2002; 15: 481–484.

70. Guillaume M P, Peretz A. Possible association between glucosamine treatment and renal toxicity: comment on the letter by Danao-Camara. *Arthritis Rheum* 2001; 44: 2943–2944.

71. Scroggie D A, Albright A, Harris M D. The effect of glucosamine-chondroitin supplementation on glycosylated hemoglobin levels in patients with type 2 diabetes mellitus: A placebo-controlled, double-blinded, randomized clinical trial. *Arch Intern Med* 2003; 163: 1587–1590.

72. Monauni T, Zenti G M, Cretti A *et al.* Effects of glucosamine infusion on insulin secretion and insulin action in humans. *Diabetes* 2000; 49: 926–935.

73. Wang J Y, Roehrl M H. Glycosaminoglycans are a potential cause of rheumatoid arthritis. *Proc Natl Acad Sci USA* 2002; 99: 14362–14367.

74. Anon. Glucosamin adverse reactions and interactions. *Curr Prob Pharmacovigilance* 2006; 31: 8.

23

Quality of nutraceuticals

The quality of biologically active materials, of whatever genre, is an integral part of their overall effects. Rigorous quality control and quality assurance of pharmaceuticals ensures that they are fit for their purpose, that they contain the stated dose of active constituents and that they have suitable disintegration characteristics, allowing for absorption in the gastrointestinal tract. Complementary medicines are increasingly being evaluated for quality by independent experts and some of them found to be substandard.

Herbal medicines are a case in point, and we have seen many herbal products banned by regulatory authorities because they have misleading label information (inaccurate component description), they contain totally unsuitable components and contaminants, or they have in-accurate statements on the levels of active constituents. Regulatory authorities are addressing these concerns worldwide and a range of quality control monographs are being introduced at the same time as dangerous products are being removed from the marketplace. This type of control is now being seen with food supplements as well, in instances where their use and possible abuse is not in the interest of the general public. In May 2003, the UK Food Standards Agency (FSA) effectively banned a range of chromium picolinate products and issued a warning concerning products containing high levels of beta-carotene and other vitamins.[1]

Monographs are being published describing analytical standards for active constituents, and the US Food and Drug Administration (FDA) and the Office of Dietary Supplements of the National Institutes of Health in the US have plans to publish monographs on up to 20 nutraceuticals.[2] The following text outlines examples of the levels of quality seen in a number of nutraceuticals that have been evaluated to date.

Glucosamine and chondroitin products

Products for joint health, particularly glucosamine and chondroitin, are of particular interest to the general public, independent researchers and consumer organisations. These two products are arguably the most widely used and available in a wide variety of nutraceutical formulations. Specifications for pharmaceuticals normally require 95–105% content of claimed active constituent,[3] and nutraceuticals are now widely assessed to this standard, notably by consumer organisations.

Glucosamine exists in a number of different forms, and it is usually the sulfate, hydrochloride or N-acetyl forms that are available. Because the proportion of the whole molecule that is glucosamine varies depending on the form used, different products will have wide variations in the levels of the glucosamine base. This information may not necessarily be stated clearly on the label. In addition to this complication, either potassium or sodium chloride may be added as a stabilising agent. Again, the presence of this may not be stated on the label, and if the weight of total glucosamine salt plus stabilising agent is quoted on the label, the actual glucosamine content is even further reduced.[4]

A number of values determined for levels of active constituents in samples of formulated glucosamine products have been reported. Wide variations are seen, particularly from one report, where only 1 out of the 15 products tested passed the criteria used. One product with no indication as to the weight of active constituent contained no glucosamine at all![4] Other analyses have reported that most products have unsatisfactory levels of active constituent.[5,6] However, three out of four products passed in another survey,[7] and there were no failures in the ConsumerLab tests.[8]

A study carried out for the American Nutraceutical Association investigated the glucosamine contents of 14 glucosamine or combination glucosamine and chondroitin products; 12 were found to contain at least 90%, one contained less than 40%, one contained about 70%, and overall they had levels ranging from 25% to 115% of the content stated on the label.[9]

In one report, four samples of glucosamine raw material were assayed and found to contain 99% and 102% of the stated content. Intra-batch levels of glucosamine in one capsule product were found to be between 93% and 104% of stated content, with only one individual falling below 95%.[10]

Commercially available chondroitin raw materials often vary in size, with molecular weights ranging widely from 50 000 to below

1000 Da,[11] but this variation has not been confirmed in formulated products.

An additional concern regarding chondroitin is whether the products could be contaminated with the causative agent of "mad cow disease" (bovine spongiform encephalitis, BSE) because they are derived from bovine cartilage. The risk appears to be extremely small, however, because the prion thought to be the causative agent of BSE exists only in very low levels in cartilage; it is most abundant in nervous and glandular tissues, which are not used for extraction of chondroitin. In addition, some manufacturers have stated that the process used to make chondroitin supplements should inactivate the prion – although this has not been shown conclusively. There is no simple way to test for BSE prion contamination in supplements, and no reports of testing have been published.

Levels of active constituents in samples of formulated chondroitin products have been reported. Data in the public domain published on the Internet by ConsumerLab[12] listed one product containing less than 85%, two pet products containing 18%, and one product containing no chondroitin at all. Products containing the correct level of constituent were not listed. The report published in *Consumer Reports*[7] failed all three products tested, while another report[5] showed that two products out of seven passed. More recently, a survey found that six out of 15 products passed.[13] Chondroitin is comparatively expensive because it typically comes from cow cartilage, and it has been suggested that cost may have influenced the amount used in formulations.[12]

The American Nutraceutical Association surveyed 32 chondroitin products. Five were found to contain more than 90%, 17 less than 40%, and overall levels were between 0 and 110%. They also recorded high variability between levels in capsules made by one particular manufacturer, reflecting quality control problems.[9]

The range of values determined for levels of active constituents in samples of formulated combination glucosamine and chondroitin products have also shown great variability. ConsumerLab found that all 13 combination products tested contained between 95 and 105% of the stated glucosamine content, but 7 out of 13 did contain sufficient chondroitin.[8] Two of the four products tested passed,[5] and 3 out of the 12 tested by *Consumer Reports* passed on levels of both components, chondroitin levels being most frequently less than 95% of the stated level.[7]

Other nutraceuticals

Although only few researchers have investigated the quality of glucosamine and chondroitin, a number of reports have been published concerning the quality of other nutraceuticals. The chemical entities of nearly 40 nutraceuticals have now been evaluated by a range of consumer organisations and researchers.

Some nutraceuticals are classed as medicines in certain countries, and as such will be subject to strict regulation. A survey of ten Japanese pharmaceutical-grade coenzyme Q10 (Co Q10) products showed that all passed, as they complied with their labelled contents,[14] but considerable variability has been reported for other nutraceuticals.

Table 23.1 shows constituent levels and passing rates for other nutraceuticals.

Overall, random and realistic numbers of most formulated nutraceutical products have been tested in representative categories, although no examples of acetyl-L-carnitine, lipoic acid, Pycnogenol or resveratrol have been reported. Relatively high-quality products were found for Co Q10, melatonin and methylsulfonylmethane (MSM), but poor quality was found with soy isoflavones, proanthocyanidins and α-tocopherol. Other reports on the quality of nutraceuticals recorded data on lycopene,[30] S-adenosyl methionine (SAMe)[32,33] and dehydro-epiandrosterone (DHEA) products,[34,35] but they show a similar picture of low-quality products available for sale.

Product identity is obviously of help to informed readers wanting to select brands, but a comparatively small proportion of scientific publications identify levels of nutraceuticals in named products; Consumerlab.com specify levels for all products analysed.

Problems relating to the precise chemical form of the named nutraceutical used in a product exist for some materials, namely glycosides, salts and glucosamine. The isoflavones, for example, exist in nature in the form of glycosides, and because the sugar content of the molecule may constitute up to 40–50% of the total, the isoflavone aglycone levels will be much lower than those claimed for the glycoside. ConsumerLab[12] reported varying levels of individual isoflavones in both soy and clover preparations (see above), and Nurmi et al.[36] also found wide variations in 15 products examined. Levels of three individual isoflavonoids – daidzein, genistein and glycitein – ranged from 9.7% to zero, and total isoflavone levels from 20.1% to trace level. Tosylate or butanedisulfonate salt forms, required for stability of SAMe, dramatically reduce the actual level of SAMe.[8]

Table 23.1 Constituent levels and passing rates for a range of nutraceuticals

Nutraceutical	Origin	No. tested	No. passed	No. >90% label claim	Comments
MSM[8]	USA	17	15	15	Levels of 85 and 88% (2)
Co Q10[12]	USA	29	28	28	Level of 17% (1)
Co Q10[15]	USA	X	X	X	All passed
Co Q10[16]	New Zealand	7[b]	1	7	All 100% and over
Melatonin[12]	USA	18	16	16	Level of 83% (1)
Carnitine[17]	3 Czech	3[b]	1	2	
	1 USA	1	0	0	
Policosanol[12]	USA	7	3	3	Levels of 23–78% (6)
Flaxseed oil[12]	USA	9	5	5	Levels of 70–83% linoleic acid (4)
SAMe[12]	USA	11	10	10	Level of 30% (1)
SAMe[12]	USA	13	7	7	Level of 5% (1)
DHA/EPA[12]	USA	20	14	14	Levels of 50–83% (6)
DHA[18]	USA	8[b]	1	4	
EPA[18]	USA	8[b]	0	1	
GLA[19]	Germany	19[b]	5	6	
Proanthocyanidins[20]	Japan health food	4	0	2	Levels of 70–125%
Proanthocyanidins[20]	Japan grape seed oil	2	0	0	ND
Lutein[21]	USA	3	0	3	
Lutein/zeaxanthin[12]	USA	19	18	18	
Lutein/zeaxanthin[22]	7 German	7	0	3	16–136%
	7 USA	7	2	5	11–122%
DHEA[12]	USA	17	14	14	Levels of 19%, 79%, 84%
Soy isoflavones[23]	Australia	10[b]	2	3	One < 1%
Soy isoflavones[24] [a]	Finland	14	2	3	
Soy isoflavones[25] [a]	USA	13	2	3	None above 99%
Phytoestrogens[26]	31 USA 1 UK	32[c]	4	11	1 at 0%, 1 at 383%
Green tea extracts[27]	USA	4	0	0	9–48% catechin content stated on labels
Creatine[12]	USA	1	0	0	Level of >1%
Creatine[12]	USA	X	X/2	X/2	Half no. tested, failed
Creatine[28]	USA	6[b]	4	6	Level of 100% in 4
Creatine[29]	USA	3[b]	1	2	'Serum' formulation, 1.7% of claimed level
α-Tocopherol[30]	Canada	7	0	5	Levels of 59–149%
Branched-chain amino acids[31]	Italy	3	3	3	All passed
Sterol[12]	USA	4	3	3	Level of 77% (1)

[a]Products specifying levels of particular isoflavones, genistein and daidzein all failed to meet claims.
[b]Disclosure of product identity.
[c]Predominantly soy-based formulations. Nine products contained formononetin and/or biochanin A, usually associated with red clover.
NS, not stated; ND, none detected.
MSM, methylsulfonylmethane; Co Q10, coenzyme Q10; SAMe, S-adenosyl methionine; DHA, docosahexaenoic acid; EPA, eicosapentaenoic acid; GLA, γ-linolenic acid; DHEA, dehydroepiandrosterone.

Four commercial conjugated linoleic acid (CLA) products have been analysed, and total CLA contents found to range from 65.1 to 77.9 mg/100 mg, while specific isomers such as the *cis*-9, *trans*-11 CLA isomer were present at levels of 24.3–37.7 mg/100 mg.[37]

Non-formulated products

The problem relating to the precise chemical form of the nutraceutical present also arises with flax, teas and soy.

Flaxseed

The effect of three flaxseed cultivars with differing contents of α-linoleic acid and lignans have been shown to have marked differences in a number of biomarkers for atherosclerosis and mental stress, thus demonstrating the importance of nutraceutical composition on biological activity.[38] Popularisation of the health benefits of flax lignans has stimulated the development of a large number of proprietary breads and breakfast cereals containing flax. In one survey of breads available in Canada, 13 flaxseed-containing breads were stated to contain from 0 to 10.1% flaxseed, and analysis of lignan aglycones resulting from fermentation of the constitutent glycosides revealed a wide range of levels of the metabolites secoisolariciresinol, enterolactone and enterodiol. Total levels ranged from 1 to 32 μmol/100 g of bread, with the metabolite enterolactone appearing as the major product in all samples. Similar investigation of six breakfast cereals revealed a metabolite level ranging from 2 to 48 μmol/100 g, with enterolactone usually present as the predominant metabolite.[39] This report disclosed the identity of the samples, allowing consumers to choose products to purchase, as stated flax contents did not necessarily correspond to levels of lignan metabolites.

Teas

More complex sources of nutraceuticals such as green teas are increasingly popular as a source of antioxidants, but the levels of claimed active compounds are very variable and will depend upon method of preparation of the infusion, as well as choice of tea type. One survey of three teas with two methods of preparation showed differences in theanine levels, and wide variations in catechin derivatives.[40] Another survey of three tea products showed similar wide variations in both catechin constituents and theanine.[41] One hundred and ninety-one specific types of green teas were investigated in one study, and Longjing teas were found to have the highest levels of theanine, gallic acid and certain catechin derivatives.[42] Comparison of a range of tea bags containing green tea also revealed a wide variation in both individual and total catechin contents, the latter ranging from 6.9 to 48.3 mg/g.[27]

Similar wide variations were reported in a survey of 12 named black teas, with total catechin contents varying from 5.6 to 47.5 mg/g,[43] and further evidence of high variability of commercial products found total catechins in canned green tea drinks to vary between 7.5 and 346.1 µg/mL, with extreme differences in levels of the individual catechins (—)-epicatechin (EC), (—)-epicatechin gallate (ECG), (—)-epigallocatechin (EGC) and (—)-epigallocatechin gallate (EGCG).[44] Further variability has been reported in 18 teas and one green tea supplement, with levels of catechins varying from 21.2 to 103.2 mg/g for regular teas, and 4.6–39.0 mg/g for decaffeinated teas. This publication showed further evidence for the importance of the catechin levels by finding a positive correlation between levels and antioxidant activity as measured by oxygen radical absorbance capacity (ORAC) assay.[45]

One final publication on teas reported a variation in catechin levels between 11 different teas and 14 commercial tea drinks ranging from 2.4 to 144.4 mg/g and 2.6 to 341.7 mg/g, respectively. In addition, they investigated the effect of degradation of the catechins under various processing conditions. Although the catechins were stable in water at room temperature, brewing Longjing tea at 98°C for 7 hours caused 20% loss of catechins. Autoclaving at 120°C for 20 minutes was found to cause epimerisation of EGCG to (—)-gallocatechin gallate (GCG), which was found in a number of commercial tea drinks, probably caused by high-temperature treatment. GCG itself is liable to further degradation dependent upon the medium in which it is present, irrespective of a low pH.[46]

Resveratrol

The resveratrol content of grape products have been investigated, and again showed a wide range of levels. Juices from white grapes were found to contain a mean of 0.5 mg/L, while those from red grapes had a mean of 3.1 mg/L, with a maximum level of 15.3 mg/L.[47] The resveratrol levels of grapes were shown to depend on the variety of the plant, and hence different types of wines contained a wide range of levels, from 98 to 1803 µg /100 mL.[48]

Soy-based infant formulas and foods

One of the first reported investigations into the isoflavone content of six commercial soy products revealed that there was variability in the levels in soy-based infant formulas available in the USA. The range of isoflavones found in dry products was 214–285 µg/g, and 25–30 µg/mL in reconstituted products, and it was postulated that this was caused by the use of different amounts of soy isolate used in product formulation. Individual isoflavone contents within particular products showed even greater variability, with genistin levels ranging from 75 to 134 µg/g and daidzin levels from 31 to 76 µg/g.[49] Later work by the same team on the isoflavone levels in 65 commercially available soy-based foods and those available in certain US institutions showed further variations both between different and within the product types.

Levels of glycosides and aglycones were estimated for seven soymilk products, 12 tofu products, six fermented soy food products, including soy sauce, miso and tempeh, and 13 meat analogue/hamburger products, and variations in individual isoflavone levels were found to vary by factors up to 150%.[50] More recent work has also shown wide variation in total isoflavone content in particular commercial products over a 3-year period, with up to 200% variation between products and up to 150% variation in values in one specific brand. Large variations are evident in both isoflavone content and individual isoflavones in near identical food sources, using similar processing conditions, as was found from the analysis of 85 soymilks.[51]

Another interesting finding reported in one analysis of formulated soy products was that in addition to the variability of isoflavone constituents in the 14 formulations, there was also up to six lignans present, including secoisolariciresinol, albeit at much lower levels.[24] This concomitant occurrence of two nutraceuticals in the raw material and in the formulated products suggests the possibility of similar 'contamination' in grape products with the presence of both resveratrol and grape seed proanthocyanidin extract (GSPE).

Possible contaminants in nutraceuticals

A range of breakdown products, synthetic intermediates and co-occurring related constituents in nutraceuticals are possible contaminants. A number of evaluations of the levels of some of these possible contaminants have been published. Table 23.2 lists examples found in the literature.

Table 23.2 Investigation of contaminants in a range of individual products

Nutraceutical	Contaminant	Level
Glucosamine[8]	Manganese	> 11 mg/day[a]
Policosanol[52]	Alkanol esters	None quantified
MSM[12]	DMSO	None
MSM[12]	DMSO	0.05%
Creatine[12]	Creatinine	> Creatine
Creatine[53]	Creatinine	9 × Creatine level
DHA/EPA[12]	Magnesium	None
Melatonin[8]	Lead (1 in 18 products)	0.5 µg/daily dose[a]
DHEA[12]	Other steroids	None

[a]When taken at recommended dose.
MSM, methylsulfonylmethane; DMSO, dimethyl sulfoxide; DHA, docosahexaenoic acid; EPA, eicosapentaenoic acid.

Overall, levels of contaminants reported in isolated formulations are low. These figures show single examples of failed products, and many ranges contain no contaminants. The possible presence of dioxins and polychlorinated biphenyls (PCBs) in fish oil supplements available in the UK was investigated by the FSA, and 2 out of 33 named branded liquid and capsule products were withdrawn from sale due to levels which could lead to ingestion of twice the tolerable daily intake.[54]

Often there is no information concerning the identity and quantity of the contaminant, as it is simply not investigated. Contaminants have been quantified in one report, in which up to 40% contaminant levels were recorded in a range of soy isoflavone formulations.[25]

Creatinine, a metabolite of creatine, also appears in impure creatine supplements as a result of improper manufacturing or breakdown of the creatine, as could another manufacturing by-product, dicyandiamide. It has been speculated that creatine sold in liquid forms, particularly products for sporting enhancement, is more liable to breakdown within the product into creatinine. Although creatinine and dicyandiamide in small amounts may not pose a safety risk, they are not useful, and should not be present. Purity has become an issue with creatine because dosages are relatively large – often as much as 20 g/day.[12]

Three commercial melatonin preparations have been analysed using high-performance liqiud chromatography/UV and liquid chromatography electrospray ionisation tandem mass spectrometry (LC/ESI-MS) and a number of contaminants have been found at levels up to

0.5%. Six of these contaminants were related to impurities which had been previously discovered in a sample of L-tryptophan,[55] associated with an eosinophilia-myalgia syndrome.[56]

A recent survey by the Cologne doping laboratory of nutraceutical supplements used by athletes found a risk of 25% contamination with prohibited substances, including contamination of carnitine.[57]

The events of 11 September 2001 have stimulated wide ranging interest into safety of medicines, foods and nutraceuticals, not only in the areas of quality control and assurance, but also in the covert introduction of chemical and microbiological toxins as agents of terrorism or counterfeiting.[58] Traceability is now being considered using a combination of global positioning and bar/chip coding, and hazard analysis critical control point management, coupled with nanotechnology marker assays.

Analytical issues

One important requirement to ensure quality control of raw and formulated products is the provision of detailed monographs about the routine analysis of nutraceuticals. This is particularly important if the material can be analysed by a range of methods, giving different results, hence making comparison between workers and products impossible. One example of this situation is in the analysis of carnitine, for which four different electrophoretic methods are available. Levels of carnitine in various products have been shown to be 19.3–25.3 g/100 g dependent on method, demonstrating the importance of establishing and using standard analytical techniques.[17] A range of melatonin tablets has been tested against the USP General Tests and Assays for Nutritional Supplements, which outlines standard quantitative test parameters, including disintegration, dissolution, weight variation, friability and hardness, for tablet formulations. Eleven products available in the Baltimore-Washington area were tested, and the results are outlined in Table 23.3.

Individual samples of one of the products revealed a threefold difference in hardness; one controlled-release product released 90% of the melatonin in 4 hours in the dissolution test, while another released 90% of its content in 12 hours. This example of poor quality control should be of concern to both consumers and healthcare providers.

Overall, the data give evidence of poor formulation, and the intra-batch variation of hardness in one product demonstrates lack of attention to quality control. One benefit of this report is that the brands

Table 23.3 Comparison of melatonin products with USP standards

Parameter	Results
Disintegration	4/9 immediate-release products failed
Dissolution	4/9 immediate-release products failed
Weight variation	All passed
Friability	2/11 products had excessive friability due to capping
Hardness	Range from 55.6–154.0 N[a]

[a]Standard deviation of 30.2% in one product.

of melatonin were identified, allowing consumers to select the best-performing products, but unfortunately the results did not include the content of active ingredient![59]

Similar parameters for one policosanol tablet product have been investigated, revealing minimum variability between batches and uniform content of active ingredient. Stability at elevated temperatures and humidity allowed realistic expiry dates of 3–9 years to be claimed.[52]

Other quality issues

As with pharmaceuticals and other alternative medicines, it is essential that tablets and capsules disintegrate after ingestion and that other formulations release their components to make the active constituents bioavailable. The vast majority of products tested have been found to have satisfactory disintegration rates.[8,12] Ten Japanese coenzyme Q10 products were all found to be satisfactory,[14] but one in four sterol products was found to be unsatisfactory.[12] To date very few publications have appeared which contain disintegration values for nutraceuticals.

The stability of active constituents and microbiological control have also rarely been reported. Policosanol tablets have been tested for stability at climatic conditions of both zones 2 ($25 \pm 2°C$, relative humidity $60 \pm 5\%$) and 4 ($30 \pm 2°C$, relative humidity $70 \pm 5\%$), and USP standard microbiological assays carried out. Excellent stability was reported from these tests.[60]

One further problem which has been reported is that some manufacturers use instruction labels advising the use of doses below those used in clinical trials. For example, 5 out of 12 combination glucosamine and chondroitin products, 2 out of 4 glucosamine products, and 3 out of 3 chondroitin products were labelled with low recommended doses.[7] Suggested daily doses of lutein have been reported to range from 0.25

to 22.5 mg, a 90-fold difference.[12] Manufacturers have not yet followed the route of pharmaceutical companies who usually include detailed patient information leaflets with their products, enabling patients to look out for side-effects and possible interactions with prescription medicines.

The range of formulations in use for delivery of nutraceuticals is increasing. For example, glucosamine is now available as a gel rub, gel patch, effervescent and new liquid, as well as tablets. Other formulations of nutraceuticals now available include caplets, capsules, controlled-release preparations and softgels. No investigation into the levels of active constituents has yet studied liquid formulations, which would be expected to be affected by stability problems to a greater extent than solid formulations.

ConsumerLab.com testing

ConsumerLab.com is an independent consumer association concerned with evaluating the quality of vitamins and supplements. They have a detailed website supplying, on a subscription basis, analytical results on a large number of commercially available examples of 13 supplements and herbal remedies available in the USA. Limited analytical data are available for free concerning the general levels of constituents, and sometimes pertinent contaminants present in the ranges of products. General data has also been made available in a published book,[61] the main feature of which is the lists of named products passing their testing procedures. Confusingly, ConsumerLab apply different levels of nutraceutical contents for different products to rate a 'passing' score.

Table 23.4 outlines the levels of active components and contaminant limits required in particular products for a pass score for different nutraceuticals, and the proportion of products that pass.

These published data are particularly useful to consumers in the USA because all products are sourced there, but also to consumers outside, because a number of the branded products are available outside the USA and also on the Internet. However, it is difficult to see how products are selected for testing, and we do not know whether products of manufacturers with wide product ranges have had their individual products tested or failed! Reading the data, it is not possible to detect any trends in successful manufacturers, and therefore individual products have to be selected on the basis of whether or not they 'pass' in that particular category.

Table 23.4 Active constituent levels, contaminant limits, and pass levels for the seven nutraceuticals evaluated

Nutraceutical	Active constituent level required for passing (%)	Other criteria	Proportion passing
Coenzyme Q10	100–150		28/29
Creatine	Minimum 99.9	Maximum 0.1% dicyanamide	11/13
n-3 Fatty acids	100–150	Maximum 10 meq/kg peroxide	14/20
Glucosamine	95–105		10/10
Chondroitin	95–105		0/2
Glucosamine/chondroitin combination products	95–105		7/13
MSM	100–125	Maximum 100 ppb Mg	15/17
SAMe	100–110		7/13
Soy and red clover isoflavones	100	100% of claimed individual isoflavones	13/18

MSM, methylsulfonylmethane; SAMe, S-adenosyl methionine.

Cost comparisons of different products

A quick look at any range of commercial nutraceuticals will show that there is a marked difference in prices (Table 23.5).

The price variations for these nutraceuticals are particularly wide for formulated soy isoflavones, which vary by a factor of nearly 22 times! This difference may possibly be explained in marketing terms: the product is priced differently for different markets, but there is no evidence that quality is responsible for these variations.

Conclusions

Surveys about the quality of nutraceuticals are increasingly being reported by both individual researchers and consumer organisations, and it is hoped that the stigma of published information concerning unsatisfactory product quality will stimulate manufacturers to improve standards of quality control. Interested consumers are able to view detailed results for

Table 23.5 The spread of costs in four nutraceuticals

Nutraceutical	Minimum cost	Maximum cost
Glucosamine[7]	$0.30	$0.70
Glucosamine[62]	£0.11	£0.61
Chondroitin[7]	$0.85	$1.35
Soy isoflavones[25]	$0.10	$2.19

named US nutraceuticals for a subscription at ConsumerLab.com, and recently another website, www.supplementchoice.com also offer information on independent product evaluations for a subscription fee. Official monographs outlining analytical standards will surely help to improve the situation.[63]

References

1. Food Standards Agency. Expert Group on Vitamins and Minerals. *Safer Upper Limits for Vitamins and Minerals*. London: FSA, 2003.
2. Wechsler J. Standards for supplements. *Pharm Technol Eur* 2003; 18–20.
3. Anon. Commission Directive 2003/63/EC. *Official Journal of the European Union* 2003; L159/46.
4. Russell A S, Aghazadeh-Habashi A, Jamali F. Active ingredient consistency of commercially available glucosamine sulfate products. *J Rheumatol* 2002; 29: 2407–2409.
5. Adebowale A, Liang Z, Eddington N D. Nutraceuticals, a call for quality control of delivery systems: A case study with chondroitin sulfate and glucosamine. *J Nutraceuticals Funct Med Food* 1999; 2: 15–30.
6. Sullivan C, Sherma J. Development and validation of an HPTLC-densitometry method for assay of glucosamine of different forms in dietary supplement tablets and capsules. *Acta Chromatogr* 2005; 15: 119–130.
7. Anon. Joint remedies. *Consumer Reports* (2002) 18–21.
8. ConsumerLab. www.ConsumerLab.com (accessed 27 October 2003).
9. American Nutraceutical Association (2000) Obtained via Cupp M J (ed.) *Dietary Supplements. Toxicology and Clinical Pharmacology*. Totowa, NJ: Humana Press, 2003.
10. Liang Z, Leslie J, Adebowale A *et al*. Determination of the nutraceutical, glucosamine hydrochloride, in raw materials, dosage forms and plasma using pre-column derivatization with ultraviolet HPLC. *J Pharm Biomed Anal* 1999; 20: 807–814.
11. Green R. The laboratory notebook. *Nutraceuticals World* 2004; 24–25.
12. ConsumerLab. www.ConsumerLab.com (accessed 30 April 2004).
13. Sim J-S, Jun G, Toida T *et al*. Quantitative analysis of chondroitin sulfate in raw materials, ophthalmic solutions, soft capsules, and liquid preparations. *J Chromatogr* 2005; 818: 133–139.

14. Nishii S, Wada M, Maruta E *et al.* Quality test of commercial ubidecarenone tablets. *Byoin Yakugaku* 1983; 9: 14–18.
15. Johnson C, Spradley N, SubbaRao L *et al.* Analysis of CoQ10 in nutraceuticals. *Abstracts of papers, 229th ACS National Meeting, San Diego, CA, USA, March 13–17, 2005.* CHED-193. Washington DC: American Chemical Society, 2005.
16. Molyneux S, Florkowski C, Lever M, George P. The bioavailability of coenzyme Q10 supplements available in New Zealand differs markedly. *N Z Med J* 2004; 117: U1108.
17. Prokoratova V, Kvasnicka F, Sevcik R, Voldrich M. Capillary electrophoresis determination of carnitine in food supplements. *J Chromatogr A* 2005; 1081: 60–64.
18. Chee K M, Gong J X, Rees D M *et al.* Fatty acid content of marine oil capsules. *Lipids* 1990; 25: 523–528.
19. Ihrig M , Blume H. Preparations of evening primrose oil: a quality comparison. *Pharmaz Z* 1994; 139: 39–42.
20. Nakamura, Y, Tsuji, S, Tonogai, Y. Analysis of proanthocyanins in grape seed extracts, health foods and grape seed oils. *J Health Sci* 2003; 49: 45–54.
21. Sechrist J, Pachuski J, Sherma J. Quantification of lutein in dietary supplements by reversed-phase high-performance thin-layer chromatography with visible-mode densitometry. *Acta Chromatogr* 2002; 12: 151–158.
22. Breithaupt D E, Schlatterer J. Lutein and zeaxanthin in new dietary supplements – analysis and quantification. *Eur Food Res Technol* 2005; 220: 648–652.
23. Howes J B, Howes L G. Content of isoflavone-containing preparations. *Med J Aust* 2002 176: 135–136.
24. Penalvo J L, Heinonen S-M, Nurmi T *et al.* Plant lignans in soy-based health supplements. *J Agric Food Chem* 2004; 52: 4133–4138.
25. Chua R, Anderson K, Chen J, Hu M. Quality, labeling accuracy, and cost comparison of purified soy isoflavonoid products. *J Altern Comp Med* 2004; 10: 1053–1060.
26. Setchell K D R, Brown N M, Desai P *et al.* Bioavailability of pure isoflavones in healthy humans and analysis of commercial soy isoflavone supplements. *J Nutr* 2001; 131: 1362S–1375S.
27. Manning J, Roberts J C. Analysis of catechin content of commercial green tea products. *J Herb Pharmacother* 2003; 3: 19–32.
28. Persky A M, Hochhaus G, Brazeau G A. Validation of a simple liquid chromatography assay for creatine suitable for pharmacokinetic applications, determination of plasma protein binding and verification of percent labelled claim of various creatine products. *J Chromatogr B* 2003; 794: 157–165.
29. Dash A K, Sawhney A. A simple LC method with UV detection for the analysis of creatine and creatinine and its application to several creatine formulations. *J Pharm Biomed Anal* 2002; 29: 939–945.
30. Feifer A H, Fleshner N E, Klotz L. Analytical accuracy and reliability of commonly used nutritional supplements in prostate disease. *J Urol* 2002, 168: 150–154.
31. Cavazza A, Corradini C, Lauria A *et al.* Rapid analysis of essential and

branched-chain amino acids in nutraceutical products by micellar electrokinetic capillary chromatography. *J Agric Food Chem* 2000; 48: 3324–3329.

32. Anon. Emotional aspirin. *Consumer Reports* 2000; 60–62.

33. Drug Store News. www.drugstorenews.com (2000) (accessed 20 March 2000).

34. Parasrampuria J, Schwartz, K. Quality control of dehydroepiandrosterone dietary supplement products. *JAMA* 1998; 280: 1565.

35. Thompson R D, Carlson M. Liquid chromatrographic determination of dehydroepiandrosterone (DHEA) in dietary supplement products. *J AOAC Int* 2000; 83: 847–857.

36. Nurmi T, Mazur W, Heinonen S *et al.* Isoflavone content of the soy based supplements. *J Pharm Biomed Anal* 2002, 28: 1–11.

37. Yu L, Adams D, Watkins B A. Comparison of commercial supplements containing conjugated linoleic acids. *J Food Compost Anal* 2003; 16: 419–428.

38. Spence J D. Thornton T, Muir A D, Westcott N D. The effect of flax seed cultivars with differing content of alpha-linolenic acid and lignans on responses to mental stress. *J Am Coll Nutr* 2003; 22: 494–501.

39. Nesbitt P D, Thompson L U. Lignans in homemade and commercial products containing flaxseed. *Nutr Cancer* 1997; 29: 222–227.

40. Horie H, Mukai T, Kohata K. Simultaneous determination of qualitatively important components in green tea infusions using capillary electrophoresis. *J Chromatogr A* 1997; 758: 332–335.

41. Aucamp J P, Hara Y, Apostolides Z. Simultaneous analysis of tea catechins, caffeic, gallic acid, theanine and ascorbic acid by micellar electrokinetic capillary chromatography. *J Chromatogr A* 2000; 876: 235–242.

42. Le Gall G, Colquhoun I J, Defernez M. Metabolite profiling using H NMR spectroscopy for quality assessment of green tea, *Camellia sinensis* (L.). *J Agric Food Chem* 2004; 52: 692–700.

43. Khokhar S, Magnusdottir S G M. Total phenol, catechin, and caffeine contents of teas commonly consumed in the United Kingdom. *J Agric Food Chem* 2002; 50: 565–570.

44. Bonoli M, Colabufalo P, Pelillo M *et al.* Fast determination of catechins and xanthines in tea beverages by micellar electrokinetic chromatography. *J Agric Food Chem* 2003; 51: 1141–1147.

45. Henning S M, Fajardo-Lira C, Lee H W *et al.* Catechin content of 18 teas and a green tea extract supplement correlates with the antioxidant capacity. *Nutr Cancer* 2003; 45: 226–235.

46. Chen Z, Zhu Q Y, Tsang D, Huang Y. Degradation of green tea catechins in tea drinks. *J Agric Food Chem* 2001; 49: 477–482.

47. Nikfardjam M P, Schmitt K, Ruhl E H *et al.* Investigation of pure grape juices on their content of resveratrols. *Deutsche Lebensmittel-Rundschau* 2000; 96: 319–324.

48. Burns J, Yokota T, Ashihara H *et al.* Plant foods and herbal sources of resveratrol. *J Agric Food Chem* 2002; 50: 3337–3340.

49. Murphy P A, Song T, Buseman G *et al.* Isoflavones in retail and institutional soy foods. *J Agric Food Chem* 1999; 47: 2697–2704.

50. Murphy P A, Song T, Buseman G, Barua K. Isoflavones in soy-based infant formulas. *J Agric Food Chem* 1997; 45: 4635–4638.

51. Setchell K D R, Cole S J. Variations in isoflavone levels in soy foods and soy protein isolates and issues related to isoflavone databases and food labeling. *J Agric Food Chem* 2003; 51: 4146–4155.

52. Cabrera L, Rivero B, Magraner J *et al*. Stability studies of tablets containing 5 mg of policosanol. *Boll Chim Farm* 2003; 142: 277–284.

53. Harris R C, Almada A L, Harris D B *et al*. The creatine content of Creatine Serum and the change in the plasma concentration with ingestion of a single dose. *J Sport Sci* 2004; 22: 851–857.

54. Food Standards Agency. Survey of dioxins and dioxin-like PCBs in fish oil supplements. http://www.food.gov.uk/science/surveillance/fsis-2002/26diox (accessed 4 November 2005).

55. Williamson B L, Tomlinson A J, Mishra P K *et al*. Structural characterisation of contaminants found in commercial preparations of melatonin: similarities to case-related compounds from L-tryptophan associated with eosinophilia-myalgia syndrome. *Chem Res Toxicol* 1998; 11: 234–240.

56. Philen R M, Hill R H, Flanders W D *et al*. Tryptophan contaminants associated with eosinophilia-myalgia syndrome. *Am J Epidemiol* 1993; 138: 154–159.

57. Maughan R J, King D S, Lea T. Dietary supplements. *J Sports Sci* 2004; 22: 95–113.

58. Lachance P A. Nutraceutical/drug/anti-terrorism safety assurance through traceability. *Toxicol Lett* 2004; 150: 25–27.

59. Hahm H, Kujawa J, Augsburger L. Comparison of melatonin products against USP's nutritional supplements standards and other criteria. *J Am Pharm Assoc* 1999; 39: 27–31.

60. Cabrera L, Gonzalez V, Uribarri E *et al*. Study of the stability of tablets containing 10 mg of policosanol as active principle. *Boll Chim Farm* 2002; 141: 223–229.

61. Cooperman T, Obermeyer W, Webb D. *Guide to Buying Vitamins and Supplements. What's Really in the Bottle?* New York: ConsumerLab.com, 2003.

62. Anon. The glucosamine game. *Health Which* 2003; April: 6.

63. Lockwood GB. Nutraceutical supplements. In: *Encyclopedia of Pharmaceutical Technology*. New York: Marcel Dekker, 2005: 1–23.

24

Conclusions

Over the last 20 years there has been rapid growth in the availability and usage of nutraceuticals. This has been caused in part by the mass of information that has become available in the lay media and via the Internet sources, but also because of increased awareness of health issues among the general public. The perception that conventional medicines cannot successfully treat all diseases and that many modern pharmaceuticals are ineffective in certain disease states and have marked side-effects has led many people to look to the nutraceuticals for alternative therapies. Nutraceuticals are arguably the first complementary medicines whose use has been justified in biochemical terms, on the basis that because many illnesses are exacerbated or caused by simple deficiency states, it follows that disease states may be treated by high doses of essential nutrients. There is also clear evidence that supplementation with nutraceuticals may generally improve health, particularly in the prevention of diseases.

Future trends influencing consumers

Increasing awareness of health issues by the public, coupled with an ageing population increasingly affected by disease states associated with ageing, has seen a growth in the demand for nutraceuticals. Even before old age, many health-conscious consumers are using nutraceuticals, often in the form of 'lifestyle' self-improvement treatments. Although consumption of nutraceuticals is increasing, as is consumption of a wide range of complementary medicines, it is not strictly a holistic form of treatment because treatment does not involve diagnosis by a trained complementary practitioner. However, unlike the use of other complementary therapies, use of a number of nutraceuticals, particularly those with antioxidant activity, can be expected to have beneficial effects on the 'whole body', not just the symptoms of a particular disease state. Some nutraceuticals, such as the glycoaminoglycans (GAGs), have been claimed to be disease modifying, as they change the constitution of the cartilage by reducing degradation and stimulating biosynthesis of new material. Nutraceuticals allow consumers to take 'control' of their health by choosing medication with which they feel comfortable, without necessarily asking a physician.

Long-term self-medication with nutraceuticals has cost implications to consumers; if they qualify for health service or health insurance scheme reimbursement of conventional medicines, nutraceuticals may appear expensive by comparison. However, some nutraceuticals are now being supplied and subsidised by this route. An example of this is glucosamine in the UK, which has been made available on the National Health Service (NHS), meaning free supplies for elderly patients.

Consumers purchasing nutraceuticals are heavily targeted by manufacturers within the main social groups of users. Both advertising and wide-ranging media coverage of nutraceuticals is widely used to extol their benefits, and also to establish the products as a 'lifestyle choice'. In a move that will surely help consumers and lead to the appropriate use of safe products, GPs, pharmacists, nutritionists and nurses are all increasingly becoming aware of nutraceuticals via articles in their professional journals.

However, many indications discussed in this text are for serious disease states for which self-medication is inappropriate, whereas long-term use of nutraceuticals for disease prevention can be safe and beneficial. Examples where nutraceuticals may be used for serious diseases include flaxseed oil and carnitine for cardiovascular disease, and a wide range of antioxidants for the prevention of cancer. At present, consumers may try dietary supplements for many indications believing them to be safer than synthetic substances, but this presumption of safety may be erroneous, and most importantly, proper medical diagnosis is essential to enable prescribing of effective conventional medicines for serious diseases. Worryingly, it has recently been reported that an increasing number of diabetic patients are self-medicating with complementary medicines.[1]

Lastly, different chemical forms of nutraceuticals (e.g. in the case of glucosamine) and different formulations may be available on the open market compared with those used in scientific research and clinical trials, and consequently expected benefits may not be seen. Consumer-friendly terms must be used on or with formulated nutraceuticals to relay scientifically correct, proven information, and to instruct patients to consult a physician if there is any doubt of serious ailment.

The general public is increasingly bombarded with dietary health advice and slogans, such as:

- 'The French paradox'
- 'The Mediterranean diet'
- 'Five a day (fruits)'
- 'Consume oily fish'
- 'Consume 25 g of soy per day',

which inveitably leads to confusion. In addition, health product manu-facturers portray their products as being an easy way to satisfy these guidelines. What actually is the overall evidence for following these exhortations and other advice to take nutraceuticals?

This text has attempted to explain the evidence for these claims. By far the most detailed scientific and medical evidence for beneficial dietary supplementation is available for soy and teas. These have been the inspiration for thousands of publications on their health benefits to date, as evidenced by their extensive conclusions in the previous chapters. The great body of literature on these two is evidence of the scientific community's desire to find 'new' medicinal agents to alleviate or cure the increasingly common disease states afflicting an ageing population, particularly that of the developed world. Much of the epidemiological data for these two are firmly based on historical and modern use.

The majority of the nutraceuticals discussed in the preceding chapters have often been consumed in traditional diets without any knowledge of their benefits, but these also have often recently become the focus of epidemiological studies.

Naturally, there is often confusion to resolve when trying to evaluate the active component of a specific diet, for example in a Mediterranean diet, which contains many purported beneficial sub-stances, many of which are referred to in the previous chapters. Similarly, the benefits of wine may be explained either on the basis of its grape seed proanthocyanidin extract (GSPE) content or its resveratrol, or a substance yet to be identified and researched. Only now is detailed clinical evidence becoming available as to the effects of individual components.

Overall, the general public has a huge interest in complementary medicines, and wants straightforward answers. The preceding chapters will by now have answered most of the questions posed in the Intro-duction:

- Nutraceuticals have been defined and described
- Clinical evidence has been outlined to explain how well they work
- Medical advice should be requested from qualified practitioners
- Adverse effects and interactions with medicines have been outlined
- Quality has been discussed in detail
- Diet modification is possible with a number of nutraceuticals occurring in realistic levels in common foods, but it is extremely difficult to obtain therapeutic levels of a number of nutraceuticals from diet alone
- Detailed information has been laid out explaining the evidence for use of nutraceuticals in prevention and treatment of diseases.

Future trends facing manufacturers

Always aware of production costs and profits, manufacturers are being forced in two directions to become successful. On the one hand, they are purchasing more raw and formulated nutraceuticals from developing countries, particularly from East Asia, allowing them to sell at lower prices while increasing profit. This is due to lower production costs in these countries, and also because of less strict compliance with safety regulations pertaining to Western countries. On the other hand, they are investing capital in high-tech plant using novel biotechnology to make products of consistently higher purity.

In an obviously expanding industry, manufacturers are frequently bringing new products onto the market, associated with media hype and new claims that are not necessarily substantiated. Increasingly, a number of combination products and novel formulations are being marketed. Nutraceutical supplementation for the treatment and prevention of a range of long-term disease states is being encouraged, for example the use of soy and green tea products for cancer prevention, which other schemes of complementary medicine cannot offer because of the lack of research data.

Because new medicines are harder to find and more expensive and riskier to develop than ever before, many companies that have produced conventional pharmaceuticals in the past are now merging to survive or are turning to nutraceuticals. For example Du Pont, Abbott Laboratories and Warner Lambert. Novartis Consumer Health, the nutrition division of the Swiss drugs group Novartis, announced a joint venture with the Quaker Oats Company in February 2000, forming the Altus Food Company to sell functional foods in the USA. This venture was the first union between a drugs company and a food company. Novartis

Consumer Health has also launched the Aviva range of functional foods that are available in supermarkets and pharmacies. Mergers of this kind offer the companies involved a very large market and more alliances are likely, as joint ventures help to share knowledge, risk, flexibility, expertise and cost.

Some nutraceuticals are available as functional foods, which are foods that have been altered by their addition to increase health. One example is Columbus Healthier eggs, introduced in October 1998 by Dean Farms, Tring, Hertfordshire. These eggs are rich in n-3 fatty acids as a result of the hens being fed a diet rich in n-3 fats. All major British supermarkets now stock these eggs. Similarly, OmegaTech has launched DHA Gold eggs, rich in both n-3 fatty acids and docosahexaenoic acid (DHA). Another example was the introduction of Burgen bread in September 1997 by Allied Bakeries, the largest bread manufacturer in the UK. This bread is a wholegrain loaf with soya and flaxseed, which has been very successful commercially in Australia. The pack claims that the bread is 'high in natural plant oestrogens, believed to help menopausal symptoms', which clearly relates to the scientific research on soy and flaxseed in these therapeutic areas.

The agritech business is increasingly interested in producing new plant sources of nutraceutical ingredients. Monsanto has recently announced plans to develop genetically modified soy containing genes from fish, in order to produce a combination of soy isoflavones incorporating the n-3 fatty acids DHA and eicosapentaenoic acid (EPA).[2]

Scientific community, regulatory authorities and consumer organisations

The scientific community is increasingly interested in therapeutic applications of nutraceuticals, and levels of research are increasing. A survey of scientific publications in journals over the period 1993–2003 for four therapeutic applications of nutraceuticals, using MEDLINE via Cambridge Scientific Abstracts, shows a rise in the number of publications over the period (Figure 24.1). Particularly high levels of interest in soy for the prevention of cancer are shown.

At the same time government sponsorship of clinical trials has grown, such as the GAIT trial for GAGs, and increased research funding is available for nutraceutical research. Regulatory authorities are taking more control of the supply of nutraceuticals and regulating the health claims, and sponsoring writing of analytical monographs which are invaluable for their routine quality assurance. AOAC monographs have

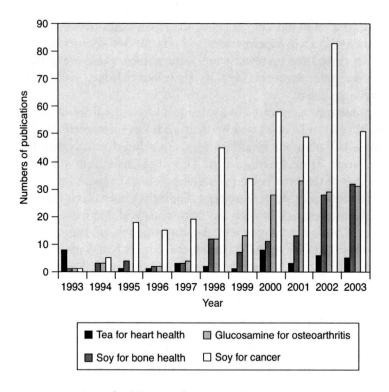

Figure 24.1 Numbers of publications for selected therapeutic applications of nutraceuticals.

now been published for glucosamine in both raw materials and supplement formulations, and monographs are expected soon for coenzyme Q10, *n*-3 polyunsaturated fatty acids and chondroitin sulfate.[3] Consumer organisations now routinely publish detailed analytical profiles of ranges of products, which enables consumers to choose the best quality. The body of evidence for a number of nutraceuticals is increasing rapidly, and the future for consumers improves with each new development.

Although data are now available to show that a number of nutraceuticals may help protect against a number of life-threatening diseases, there is still insufficient evidence to substantiate the use of certain nutraceuticals in a range of disease states for which they are being sold. Government support is required for increased research in these areas, and in the long term, reduced health costs would justify the money spent.

New horizons

Progress in treating diseases is being accelerated by the availability of genomic information, and pharmaceutical companies are using genotyping in their clinical trials to predict efficacy, drug safety and toxicity. This development in pharmacogenomics is being used to study a patient's response to medication, and the parallel science of 'nutrigenomics' has been developed to study the effect of nutraceuticals and dietary components on health. Nutrigenomics may allow the use of a particular individual's genetic information to predict specific personalised nutraceutical supplementation to prevent diseases or maintain health.

Overall

We are currently seeing unprecedented availability of nutraceuticals and a continuing range of new entities, new therapeutic applications, new formulations to improve compliance and increased awareness of healthcare professionals. Sensible use of scientifically and medically validated nutraceuticals will undoubtedly improve the health of sections of the population who take advantage of these developments.

There are a number of nutraceuticals with applications in a range of therapeutic areas. Some of them show comparable efficacy to conventionally prescribed pharmaceuticals. Many more nutraceuticals are also available, with an increasing range of therapeutic applications, adding to further consumption. Compared with both conventional pharmaceuticals and complementary medicines, nutraceuticals generally have lower incidences of adverse effects and drug interactions, but as global consumption rises, so does the incidence of side-effects and drug interactions. Overall however, the risk–benefit use of these products is not nearly as well documented as for conventional pharmaceuticals, and the absence of a wide range of documented adverse effects and drug interactions does not mean that these products are devoid of these properties. From details reported on drug interactions it would obviously be in the interests of patient safety if all use of dietary supplementation was made available to healthcare prescribers. Most of the disease states for which nutraceuticals are used are increasingly prevalent in ageing populations, which are increasingly affected by more than one disease, and we are likely to see more interactions and complications.[4]

With the introduction of government campaigns such as the 'Five-A-Day' programme, designed to increase public awareness of the need for a healthy lifestyle and diet, combined with ever-increasing knowledge of the potential health benefits attributable to certain dietary factors and the publication of new dietary recommendations, it is possible that such nutraceutical products will become commonplace adjuvants to many individuals' healthy lifestyles in the near future.

References

1. Marra J. The state of dietary supplements. *Nutraceuticals World* 2004; September: 50–57.
2. Associated Press, *New York Times*, 9 February 2006. Reviewed in 'Grapevine', *Nutraceuticals World* April 2006: 16.
3. Roman, M. The AOAC validation effort for dietary supplements. *Nutraceuticals World* 2005; November: 82–86.
4. Lockwood G B. Nutraceutical supplements. In: *Encyclopedia of Pharmaceutical Technology*. New York: Marcel Dekker, 2005: 1–23.

Index

Suffixes on page numbers:
'f' refers to figures
't' refers to tables